# HEALTH CARE SYSTEM AND HOSPITAL ADMINISTRATION

## 7

## MANAGEMENT TECHNIQUES AND GOOD GOVERNANCE

# HEALTH CARE SYSTEM AND HOSPITAL ADMINISTRATION

## 7

## MANAGEMENT TECHNIQUES AND GOOD GOVERNANCE


**DR. S.L. GOEL**

Professor of Public Administration (Retd.),
Panjab University, Chandigarh
Editor, Indian Journal of Public Administration, IIPA, New Delhi
Former Member, UGC, Former Member Distance Education Council
Former Member All India Board of Management, AICTE
Member, Executive Council, IIPA, New Delhi.
Former Vice-President, IIPA, New Delhi.
Emeritus Fellow, University Grants Commission
Former Director, State Bank of India (Local Board) Chandigarh
Former Director, National Horticulture Board, Ministry of Agriculture,
Government of India, New Delhi.



**DEEP & DEEP PUBLICATIONS PVT. LTD.**

F-159, Rajouri Garden, New Delhi-110027

HEALTH CARE SYSTEM AND HOSPITAL ADMINISTRATION
Vol. 7—Management Techniques and Good Governance

ISBN 978-81-8450-197-1 (Vol. 7)
ISBN 978-81-8450-198-8 (Set)



Typeset by S.S. COMPOSERS
3190, Mohindra Park, Shakur Basti, Delhi-110034.

Printed in India at MAYUR ENTERPRISES
WZ Plot No. 3, Gujjar Market, Tihar Village, New Delhi-110018.

Published by DEEP & DEEP PUBLICATIONS PVT. LTD.
F-159, Rajouri Garden, New Delhi-110027.
Phones: 25435369, 25440916
E-mail: ddpbooks@yahoo.co.in • ddpubs@gmail.com
*Showroom:*
2/13, Ansari Road, Daryaganj, New Delhi-110002 • Telefax: 23245122

# Contents

# Preface

11th Five Year Plan stresses on improving the governance. All our efforts to achieve rapid and inclusive development will only bear fruit if we can ensure good governance both in the implementation of public programmes and in governments interaction with the ordinary citizens. Corruption is now seen to be endemic in all spheres of life and this problem needs to be urgently redressed. Better design of projects, implementation mechanisms and procedures can reduce the scope for corruption. Much more needs to be done by both the Centre and the States to lessen the discretionary power of government, ensure greater transparency and accountability, and create awareness among citizens. The Right to Information Act empowers the people to demand improved governance, and as government we must be ready to respond to this demand.

Health Administration faces a great challenge in improving the health status of the population. Good Governance of health services can be a positive force in proving good health services to all without discrimination. Its services have to be so devised that they may be within the reach of all alike. Improvement in health policy formulations and implementation of health programmes arising therefrom are crucial to our development and progress. We have to be conscious of the need to make health administration more efficient and socially responsive. We have to accept the challenges of health problems and overcome them. Health administration that does not respond to the demands of rapidly changing social and economic conditions will one day cease to be effective. Indeed, it has not only to respond but to anticipate problems in order to be effective.

There is no doubt in my mind that the health administrators have the capacity to undertake such tasks. What is needed is determination and commitment. It can raise the level of consciousness to help develop health administrators who are sensitive to their environment, committed to socio-economic justice and trained to severe professionalism in administration.

There is a need to vitalise health management. World Health Report 2000 has also endorsed this. Unfortunately, health system can also misuse their power and squander their potential. Poorly structured, badly led, inefficiently organised and inadequately funded health systems can do more harm than good.

This report finds that many countries are falling far short of their potential, and most are making inadequate efforts in terms of responsiveness and fairness of financial contribution. There are serious shortcomings in the performance of one or more functions in virtually all countries. These failings result in very large number of preventable deaths and disabilities in each country; in unnecessary suffering, in injustice and denial of basic rights of individuals. The impact is most severe on the poor, who are driven deeper into poverty by lack of financial protection against ill-health. In trying to buy health from their own pockets, sometimes they only succeed inclining the pockets of others.

The ultimate responsibility for the overall performance of a country's health system lies with government, which in turn should involve all sectors of society in its stewardship. The careful and responsible management of the well-being of the population is the very essence of good government. For every country it means establishing the best and fairest health system possible with available resources. The health of the people is always a national priority government responsibility for it is continuous and permanent. Ministry of health must therefore take on a large part of the stewardship of health systems.

The World Health Report, 2000, Health Systems: Improving Performance by WHO, has also felt the need of good management system.

Governments should be the "stewards" of their national resources, maintaining and improving them for the benefit of their populations. In health, this means being ultimately responsible for the careful management of their citizens' well-being. Stewardship in health is the very essence of good government. For every country it means establishing the best and fairest health system possible. The health of the people must always be a national priority: government's responsibility for it is continuous and permanent. Ministry of health must take on a large part of the stewardship of health systems.

Even Ninth Five Year Plan has also recommended a sound administrative set-up:

(a) Creation of a functional, reliable health management information system and training and deployment of health manpower with requisite professional competence.
(b) Multi-professional education to promote team work.
(c) Skill upgradation of all categories of health personnel, as a part of structured continuing education.
(d) Improving operational efficiency through health services research.
(e) Increasing awareness of the community through health education.
(f) Increasing accountability and responsiveness of health needs of the people by increasing utilisation of the Panchayati Raj institutions in local planning and monitoring.
(g) Making use of available local and community resources so that operational efficiency and quality of services improve and the services are made more responsive to user's needs.

This state of hopelessness and frustration among the people is not because of the lack of professional knowledge or competence but due to poor administration of health services. Administration can provide the means whereby the most effective use can be made of the knowledge and skills of the personnel responsible for the health care delivery system. The benefits of modern science and technology can reach the people only if such services are properly planned and effectively implemented.

The design of an administrative system is a basic aid to the achievement of its primary objectives; if the design is unsound, the achievement of objectives is likely to fall short of expectations. This requires the capabilities to design and manage the health care administration.

The development of health and medical services has been promoted greatly by advances made in professional skills and technical proficiencies, but it seems apparent that the parallel advance has not been made in the art and science of health care administration.

The education and training of personnel responsible for the delivery of health care, in the art and science of Health Care Administration is of great significance as most of them devote 20 per cent to 80 percent of their time in various aspects of Health Care Administration. Besides, a large number of health personnel have the primary responsibility of administering a health complex, whether at the state headquarters or at district health centre complex or at primary health centre. Many of the intermediary functionaries of health care are responsible for supervision, coordination and control of health care. The key health administrators are exclusively responsible for policy-making, planning and designing administrative structures to provide the best health care to all.

At present, all these functionaries have been discharging these administrative responsibilities without proper education or training in administration with special reference to health care administration, obviously resulting in poor health care delivery systems. Dr. H. Mahler, former Director-General of WHO, rightly remarked at the Post-Graduate Institute of Medical Education and Research, Chandigarh: "It is a pity that a country like India with its rich intellectual background has still to grapple with basic health problems even many years after independence." This holds true of most of the countries in the developing world. Unless the training of the health and medical professionals includes a study of the principles, practice and philosophy of health care administration, they are ill-prepared for the jobs for which they are appointed.

Eleventh Five Year Plan, 2007-2012, Vol. II observes that the Drawbacks of the Public Health System are:

- Centralized planning instead of decentralized planning and using locally relevant strategies.
- Institutions based on population norms rather than habitations.
- Fragmented disease specific approach rather than comprehensive health care.

- Semi-used or dysfunctional health infrastructure
- Inadequate provision of human resources
- No prescribed standard of quality
- Inability of system to mobilite action in areas of safe water, sanitation, hygiene, .and nutrition (key determinants of health in the context of our country)— lack of convergence.
- Inability to mobilize AYUSH and RMPs and other locally available human resources

**Vertical Programmes**

*Technology-centric*

- See the disease as being caused by an agent (parasite/virus/ bacteria) and fail to see its social and ecological setting.
- Response is heavily dependent on technology.

*Fragmented*

- Only one or two of all the factors that go into the disease setting (and that too in isolation) are addressed.

*Administration*

- The entire planning and packaging is done centrally.
- Only local aspect is the application (under a chain of command).
- Limited role for community participation.

*The Result*

- An inappropriate package for local needs.
- Local people are indifferent sometimes even resistant.
- Even the administration cannot in perpetuity keep its attention on the programme alone.

**Need for this Book**

The question arises as to how we can develop the administrative skill and capability along with the professional competence among the personnel responsible for health care administration? This can be made possible by two methods. The first is to incorporate the teaching and research of health care administration in the syllabus of under-graduate and post-graduate medical education. The second method is to impart training to the personnel already engaged in health care administration, especially through executive development programmes. A few steps have been taken in this direction, such as the setting up of the National Institute of Health and Family Welfare for the training of personnel in health and family welfare administration; starting of diploma courses in health and hospital administration; starting a distance education programme in health and hospital management by NIHFW; arranging seminars on various aspects of hospital administration, etc.

The success of these methods depends upon the availability of well-prepared literature in health care administration based on the researches and case studies. The literature in this form is non-existent. Most of the available literature relating to the health care administration has tended to be historical or broadly descriptive. In a publication from Pittsburgh University, it has been affirmed that "In health administration, there are few theoreticians, few training centres, few books, and an absolute dearth of strict scientific investigations."

Whatever scanty literature is available on Health Care Administration is in the context of the developed world and hence totally unsuited to the different political, social, economic and cultural milieu of the developing world. Conventional health practices designed on the basis of Western models have proved inappropriate and beyond the capacity of the developing world. Why has Health Care Administration literature not been developed for such a long time? A contributory factor in this regard has been the dichotomy between Public Health and Medical Care specialists and social scientists. Both worked in their narrow grooves without benefiting each other. Fortunately, in recent years this dichotomy has been disappearing progressively. Even in the WHO, there has been a growing consciousness that the social scientists have an increasing role to play in regard to the formulation of curative, preventive, promotive and rehabilitative health policies and programmes, along with the medical scientists to solve the complex health care problems of a rapidly increasing population. A healthy trend is emerging wherein some health administrators are feeling interested in learning the social sciences relevant and useful to the understanding of their field. Some of the social scientists are feeling motivated to analyse the whole process of health care administration to help these experts in finding solutions to various problems outside their domain. Encouraged by such trends, the author has written earlier three books on Health Care Administration, three volumes on Hospital Administration followed by 4 volumes of Hospital Administration and a book on Family Planning Administration and Beyond.

The present Volume 7, i.e. "Management Techniques and Good Governance" has been divided into 19 chapters. Chapter 1 deals with nature, scope and role of Good Governance in the delivery of health to services people efficiently. Chapter 2 focuses on role of health in Socio-economic development as health is wealth. Chapters 3, 4, 5 examine the role of planning, decision-making and Supervision in delivery of health services. Chapters, 6, 7, 8 discuss communication, co-ordination, control, Headquarters, Field Relationship and Organisation analysis as instruments of promoting good health. Chapters 9, 10, 11 deals with Method Study and

Works Measurement, Management of Interpersonal relations and Motivation and Morale to enhance the organisational climate essential for good health services. Chapters 12, 13 and 14 examine Time Management, Human Resource Development and Organisational Development which are important for enhancing the Capability and Capacity of health personnel. Chapters 15, 16 and 17 deals with Management of the Employees Health, Management Techniques for Inculcating Aesthetic Sense among health and medical personnel as well as selfless services for building Health System on Truth, Beauty and Goodness. Chapters 18 and 19 deal with Techniques to Promote Human Excellence among health experts and Modernizing Health and Medical Care System.

All the chapters are supplemented with specially designed charts, tables, graphs and case studies. It is thus of utmost importance that the best brains in the country are attracted to the health and medical services. They should not only be motivated to enter the services but also remain there with full professionalism, motivation and devotion to duty. This necessitates a positive look at all the major parameters of their induction and retention. These are as follows:

(i) The personnel at the top level must understand that the most difficult thing in government, as Napoleon said, is not the selection of men but to take work from them. Good administrators know about this tact.

(ii) There is a need for delegation of work. The basis of Sardar Patel's success was that he delegated work, trusted the chosen men and that he rarely interfered with them. Nehru said that he did not quarrel with his tools, but he had a way of interfering with them.

(iii) Delay is often the deadliest aspect of administration. Napoleon owed his success to the maxim he prescribed for his men, to be speedy, to use dispatch and not to forget that the world was created in six days.

(iv) Politically motivated intrusions into the career civil service should be discouraged.

(v) Protect personnel from unjust adverse treatment.

(vi) Reward superior performance systematically.

(vii) Rationalize the process of sacking incompetent employees.

(viii) Create a basic understanding of modern management especially computer and information technology.

At the level of individual organisation, what is required is a mission orientation, which provides clear and understandable goals, fully owned by the senior management and accepted by the operational staff. The purpose of establishing a mission orientation is to:

- Clarify the goals of the organisation in the mind to the management.
- Clarify for staff the purpose of their jobs in meeting oraganizational goals.
- Make clear the policy of the government to ensure that it is interpreted accurately by staff.
- Create and sustain pride in belonging to the organisation.
- Provide targets to aim for and against which results can be assessed.

It is hoped that this book on "Health Care System and Hospital Administration: Management Techniques and Good Governance" would make a modest contribution to the knowledge and existing literature in this expanding field. Besides, this would help the academicians, national health officials, public health administrators, medical research workers and the policy makers and planners in the proper understanding of health care delivery system. I will consider my labour well rewarded if the findings of the study are translated to provide decent health care to the millions of people living in rural areas, urban slums and tribal areas. Comments and suggestions from the readers would always be welcome.

Chandigarh S.L. GOEL

1

CHAPTER

# Nature and Scope of Health Care Administration and Good Governance

> Health is a positive state of well-being in which harmonious developments of mental and physical capacities of individuals lead to the enjoyment of a rich and full life. It implies adjustment of individual to his total environment—Physical and Social.
>
> —*First Five Year Plan*

## A. MEANING AND SIGNIFICANCE OF HEALTH AND FACTORS INFLUENCING IT

### Significance of Health

In the new millennium, the people are realising and improving their health not only through government machinery but by their own efforts. It is being realised globally that health is one's own responsibility and depends to a substantial extent on the lifestyle of the people and not entirely only on health intervention by hospitals. Therefore, in the new millennium, we have to find out ways and means of promoting people's health through other methods as well.

Dr. Diroshi Nakajima, Director General, World Health Organisation in his message in the World Health Report, 1998, "Life in the 21st Century: A Vision For All" rightly says that "The progress and achievement of the past 50 years are solid foundations for a healthier and better world. It is already time to build on them. We can pass no greater gift to the next generation than a healthier future. That is our vision. Together, the people of the world can make a reality."

It is a recognised fact from the times immemorial that Good health is a prerequisite to human productivity and the development process. It is essential to economic and technological development. A healthy community is the infrastructure upon which to build an economically viable society. The progress of society greatly depends on the quality of its people. Unhealthy people can hardly be expected to make any valid contribution towards developmental programmes.

Health is man's greatest possession, for it lays a solid foundation for his happiness. Charaka, the renowned Ayurvedic physician is known to have said: "Health is vital for ethical, artistic, material and spiritual development of man." Buddha has said that of all the gains, the gains of health are the highest and the best. Health is not only basic to leading a happy life for an individual but it is also necessary for all productive activities in the society. Who would deny that a soldier who is not keeping good health cannot be expected to defend the frontiers of his country even when he is provided with the latest sophisticated weapons? Similarly, who would deny that an unhealthy farmer with the best possible technological know-how would not succeed in producing the best that can be expected of him? Obviously what is true of an unhealthy soldier or an unhealthy farmer is also true of other categories of workers. Thus, no industry can expect the optimum output if it does not employ healthy workers or does not make and provide adequate facilities for proper maintenance of their health.

Undoubtedly, professional efficiency, good health and development are interrelated. Yet, health cannot be bestowed upon people if they themselves do not make any effort to maintain a proper balance between their external and internal environments.

Y.S. Tajesekhara Reddy, Honourable Chief Minister of Andhra Pradesh in its Convocation Address on April 23, 2005 clarify that Human development and improving the quality of life of people are the ultimate goals of all activities of any government. Quality of life and development can be achieved only with healthy mind and body. Health is the vital ingredient of all developmental activities.

Whatever one may say, a disease-stricken society afflicted with diseases can hardly hope to extricate itself from the clutches of poverty and ignorance that keep it backward and underdeveloped in many areas of life. A nation can become truly healthy only when it succeeds in overcoming all these deficiencies stemming from cultural, social, economic and other causes. A nation that is ill-fed can hardly afford to exhibit efficiency in any field. In fact, an epidemic or endemic disease in any part of the world can pose a potential danger to all mankind and even a challenge to modern science. The Planning Commission has stressed the vital importance of public health in the enrichment of community life. It has been stated:

> "Health is fundamental to the national progress in any sphere. In terms of resources for economic development, nothing can be considered of higher importance than the health of the people which is a measure of their energy and capacity as well as of the potential man-hours for productive work in relation to the total number of

persons maintained by the nation. For the efficiency of industry and of agriculture, the health of the worker is an essential consideration."

In his address to 31st Session of WHO Regional Committee for South-East Asia held at Ulan Botor, Mongolia (22-28 Aug., 1978), Dr. Nyam Osor, Minister of Public Health, Mongolia read a passage from a poem by Dashdorjiin Natragdorj, which glorifies "Health." It is being reproduced below.

"Happiness, happiness, happiness
It may be of different origin on this earth
But the happiness of being healthy
Is the real happiness."[1]

Thus, there can be no two opinions that health is basic to national progress and in terms of resources for economic development nothing could be of greater significance than the health of the people. To quote Herophilas, C., 300 B.C.

"When health is absent
Wisdom cannot reveal itself
Art cannot manifest, Strength cannot fight,
Wealth becomes useless
And Intelligence cannot be applied."[2]

As such, good health must be a primary objective of national development programmes. It is a precursor to improving the quality of life for a major portion of mankind.

**Meaning of Health**

Health is viewed differently by different people all over the world. The World Health Organisation defined health as "a state of complete physical, mental, and social well-being and not merely an absence of disease or infirmity." Rehabilitation health has also become an integral part of health services making coverage of health broad-based depicts the important activities under each head—preventive, promotive, curative and rehabilitative. (See Chart 1.1)

"Health is a positive state of well-being in which harmonious development of mental and physical capacities of the individuals lead to the enjoyment of a rich and full life. It implies adjustment of the individuals to his total environment—physical and social."

Some people even define it as a condition under which an individual is able to mobilise all his resources—intellectual, emotional and physical for optimum living. Thus, health is not static; on the contrary, it fluctuates on a scale which ranges between optimum health as defined by WHO to

CHART 1.1

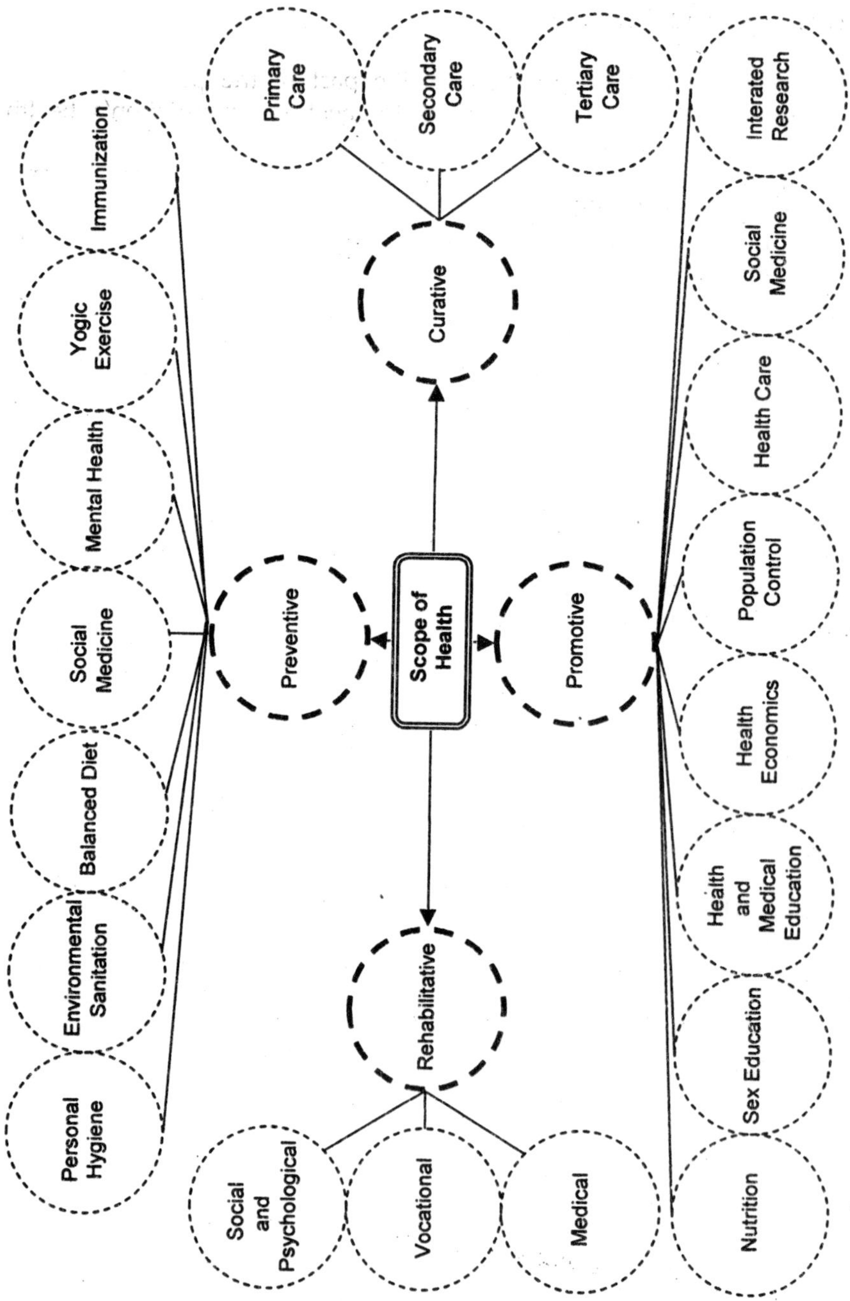
Scope of Health
Preventive
Curative
Promotive
Rehabilitative
Immunization
Yogic Exercise
Mental Health
Social Medicine
Balanced Diet
Environmental Sanitation
Personal Hygiene
Primary Care
Secondary Care
Tertiary Care
Interated Research
Social Medicine
Health Care
Population Control
Health Economics
Health and Medical Education
Sex Education
Nutrition
Social and Psychological
Vocational
Medical

complete lack of health. Dr. E. Berthet, Secretary-General of the International Union for Health Education, Paris, defines health as follows:

> "We no longer ought to define health only in terms of sickness but rather in relation to the harmonious development of every individual's personality. After all, it represents a balanced measure of a person's total potential—whether biological, psychological and social; and to the notion of individual health we should add the concepts of family and community health."[3]

Health is not only curative but also includes preventive, promotive and rehabilitative services. Under each head, there are a large number of areas. The need is to devote health efforts on all aspects and not concentrate only on curative services.

Sangita Reddy, ED, Appollo Hospitals Group clearly mention in *The Economic Times,* dated 13 Nov., 2007 that every health care system around the world is constantly working to meet with three objectives. Equitable access, high quality and low cost. For care providers, these are often competing objectives, with the tradeoffs among these goals usually ridden with economic, social and political implications.

The inherent challenge in reconciling the three objectives is common to every health care system, and not unique to any particular country. For instance, many countries have learnt that higher spending does not correlate with higher quality or better outcomes, as is usually perceived by consumers. In fact, the first of the measures that we need to adopt to reduce health care costs focuses on reducing higher spends.

Dr. Diroshi Nikajima, Former Director General of WHO (*World Health,* Nov.-Dec. 1994) rightly say that Improving the health of nations is therefore dependent on reducing inequities both between countries and between the rich and poor within a country.

The basic elements of our strategy for action need be:

- Ensuring that the poorest and most vulnerable groups of the population have access to primary health care. This means redirecting often scarce money as well as personnel to the front line of the health care system at community and district levels. It also means increasing their access to information about health.
- Protecting the poorest from risks to health which are beyond their control; protection from environmental hazards; protection from crime and violence; access to adequate food, shelter, water and sanitation; and, above all, the ability to earn an income. These are the basic minimum needs for health and development.
- Building strong commitment to health among top political leaders in all countries. This includes assuming responsibility, at the highest level, for monitoring the reduction of health inequities.

S.C. Seal, in his presidential address, defined health as "flexible state of body and mind which may be described in terms of a range within which a person may sway from the condition wherein he is at the peak of enjoyment of physical, mental and emotional experiences, having regard to environment, age, sex and other biological characteristics due to the operation of internal or external stimuli and can regain that position without outside aid."[4]

Health has found an important place in the constitutions of all states and the UN agencies. Of the 30 Articles of the Universal Declaration of Human Rights, Art. 25 is particularly concerned with the right to health. Everyone has the right to a standard of living adequate for the health and well-being of himself and of his family, including food, clothing, housing and medical care and necessary services and the right to security in the event of unemployment, sickness, disability, widowhood, old age or other lack of the livelihood, in circumstances beyond his control. Motherhood and childhood are entitled to special care and assistance. All children whether born in or out of wedlock shall enjoy the same social protection.

The preamble to the WHO Constitution also states that the enjoyment of the highest attainable standard of health is a fundamental right of every human being and that governments are responsible for the health of their people and can fulfil that responsibility by taking appropriate health and social welfare measures.

**Factors Influencing Health**

A variety of factors influence human development both favourably and unfavourably. Some of these factors are: environmental—natural or manmade; physical, chemical, biological and social; economic, cultural factors: education, genetic factors; pre-natal health development factors and nutritional factors. Thus, the promotion of health cannot be achieved by measures that derive from any single health discipline, nor can health measures be considered independently of the broader educational, social, economic and administrative factors that are crucial to human development. That is why, Inter-Sectoral coordination is essential. Obviously, the relationship between socio-economic development and progress of health is of extreme importance. In fact, every aspect of economy has a health component which has an important bearing on the overall socio-economic development. Thus, as stated in a WHO paper on public health: "The health component and other components of the total system necessarily interact. Health not only affects the remainder of the socio-economic complex but also, affected by it, sometimes unfavourably."[5] We shall discuss this in detail in a separate chapter on "Inter-Sectoral Coordination."

Because of this intimate relationship, it has been mentioned in the First Five Year Plan, "If this subject is regarded in the proper light as one which is concerned with everything affecting the health of the community it must be admitted to be the biggest and the most important problem of India."[6]

Socio-economic development consists of various components related to the productive shares of activities. Health programmes cannot be related unilaterally to either the economic or the social spheres as they influence both and are influenced by both. There, obviously, is a need for a unified and integrated approach to public health, i.e., to combine services for nutrition improvement, communicable disease-control, better maternal and child-health and family-welfare. Thus, conventional linear planning and the execution of separate programmes cannot meet the needs of human development. As stated by T. Adeoye Lambo in his article, 'Total Health' in *World Health*:

> "It is now apparent that a more balanced consideration of the biological, social and cultural aspects of health is needed. Life is a process and not a substance, a living system based upon the primacy of continuity and inter-relatedness throughout the universe. . . . If man and his family are to remain in empathy with the emerging necessities in the developing milieu, an adequate design of inter-disciplinary tools will have to be made to assist in this task of providing a total health package."[7]

In general, the factors influencing health could be classified into three broad categories: hereditary, environmental and personal. Similarly, the various conditions which play a vital role in determining one's health status can be put under four major areas, viz., mental health, social health, spiritual health and physical health.

## B. PRINCIPLES, MEANING AND OBJECTIVES OF HEALTH ADMINISTRATION

### Principles for Health Care Administrators

The Health Care administrators need to be aware of certain basic principles for the formulation of health policies. Some of these principles are stated below:

(a) Health opportunities need not be related to the purchasing power of the people.

(b) While planning Public Health Programmes for the benefit of the whole community, care should be taken to see that medical facilities are accessible to the poor people inhabiting the rural areas, urban slums and tribal areas.

(c) Investment on preventive as well as curative health programmes and activities should be considered as beneficial. However, the priority may be given to the preventive health care, i.e., changing lifestyles of the people as we know that prevention is better than cure.

(d) Doctors should be trained to act as social physicians as well to promote healthy and happier life.
(e) Health should not be considered in isolation from other socio-economic factors.
(f) Health consciousness should be fostered through health education and by providing opportunities for the participation of the individuals in the health programme.
(g) Sound Health Administrative structures may be designed for the implementation of the health policy.
(h) All the systems of medicine must be encouraged to provide decent health to the people in a coordinated fashion.
(i) Utilize community resources optimally and encourage local participation to promote self-help programmes at the village level.
(j) Ensure that basic health services are available, accessible and acceptable to the people.

**Meaning of Health Administration—Good Governanace**

We have already defined the term 'Health'. Let us define the term 'Administration'. Administration is at the centre of all human affairs. Its principal aspects are formulation of policy and its implementation for the attainment in an optimum manner of stated ends in the shape of services or products. Administration is an activity which demands correct analysis and accurate orientation. According to Simon. "In its broadest sense, administration can be defined as the activities of groups cooperating to accomplish common goals."[8] In the words of Marx:

> "Administration is determined action taken in the pursuit of a conscious purpose. It is the systematic ordering of affairs and the calculated use of resources aimed at making those things happen which one wants to happen—and forestalling everything to the contrary."[9]

In simple words, administration may be defined as the management of affairs with the use of well thought-out principles and practices and rationalised techniques to achieve certain objectives. Pfiffner and Presthus define administration as "the organisation and direction of human and material resources to achieve desired ends."[10]

Administration consists of a structure or an organisation of various institutions essential for its functioning; the processes, procedures and interaction of various constituents; and the techniques and skills of human relations. It is the management of human affairs concerned with the needs of carrying out specific objectives. Administration is involved in all fields of human endeavour where there is a planned effort. It is a force which lays down the objectives—which an organisation and its management are to strive for and the broad policies under which to operate.

Administration provides the means whereby the most effective use can be made of the knowledge and skills of those giving the service. It is a way of conceptual thinking for attaining pre-determined goals of group efforts. Now administration is judged by Good Governance:

Good Governance is an essential ingredient for health development of the country. The Government of India and State Governments come out with new ideas and approaches but these do not succeed when put to action because of lack of good governance. Good Governance is of paramount importance in these times of far reaching changes. In this backdrop of major changes, we need to re-orient ourselves to deliver ways and means to promote good governance. No government of course can hope to survive without a strong and effective good governance nor can an health system exist without the support of those it was established to serve.

S.G. Barve feels that Good Governance is more an art than a science and there can be very few esoteric principles about it. It is a question of performance rather than theory or action. There are no sensational short-cuts to good governance. There are no spectacular situation. What is wanted is a long and patient siege. Another outstanding deficiency is failure to locate definite responsibility at different points and levels of the administrative hierarchy. This location of responsibility has to be finally carried down to the level of the individual functionary.

The issue of good governance has, in recent times, emerged at the forefront of the agenda for sustainable human development. It is imperative that this process while being sustainable in terms of resources over generations and across space, recognizes the legitimate claim of each person in a society to be an active and a productive participant. Empowering people for meaningful participation in this development process is one of the key interventions of the government of India in its attempt to usher in sustainable development.

Good governance implies utmost concern for people's welfare wherein the government and its bureaucracy follow policies and discharge their duties with a deep sense of commitment; respecting the rule of law in a manner which is transparent, ensuring human rights and dignity, probity and public accountability.

In the new millennium, the greatest challenge before the largest democracy of the world, is to steer the overall growth in the country. In the lines of fairness, equality, equity, justice and sustainability especially when the role of the Government itself is being redefined, Good Governance is of paramount significance in these times of far reaching changes and ushering in an era of globalization, liberalization and privatization.

The fact that India is the second most populous country that survives on just 2.4% of world's landmass, creates its own population-resources tension. Combined with the colonial legacy of systems that sub-served the exploitative objectives of the then colonial administration; has made the task of change much more difficult. Thus, despite the creation of an enabling framework for sustainable development, India continues to face enormous challenges in search of options for development that are environmentally sound and suitable to its specific social conditions through good governance.

Combating poverty and its eventual eradication which is vital for health has been the central theme of all that major policies and programmes of the Government of India since Independence. In the decades of the 90's, the focused intervention of the government of various social development sectors bore fruit. At the beginning of the 90's an estimated 320 million people, or 36% of the total population, were below the poverty line, however, by the end of the decade, India succeeded in bringing down the number of people living below the poverty line by 18.75% to 260 million. In absolute numbers, a huge 60 million people were brought above the poverty line in 10 year's time.

Despite the impressive statistics, the nation is aware that the absolute number of people still living below the poverty line is huge. The proportions of poor people in rural and urban areas are 27% and 23.62% respectively.

Notwithstanding the significant progress in the areas of poverty eradication, improvement of literacy rates and health standards, etc. and the emergence of an enabling framework for sustainable development, Indian continues to face enormous challenges in achieving sustainable development. There still remains a disparity between India and the rest of the world on various social development indicators. India has taken it as a challenge to reduce the poverty ratio, ensure attendance of children in schools, reduce gender gaps in literacy and wage rates by 50%, reduce population growth, attain at least 75%, literacy reduce infant mortality to 45 per 1000 live births, reduce maternal mortality rate to 2 per 1000 live births, increase forest cover to 25%, provide sustained access to drinking water in rural areas and to clean up major stretches of polluted rivers.

Jayshree Sengupta in an article, "Growth is not For All: Rural India being kept in a different Basket" in *The Tribune,* dated 29.11.06 feels that after all, how can any city have the growth of slums and skyscraper side by side as in Mumbai, without problems? Unless the government increases and prioritizes its expenditure on infrastructure—building more roads and irrigation systems—rural India will not be participating in the high growth process.

Unless state governments see to it that health care is improved substantially and education is not only accessible to all but is of good quality, there can never be a stable back up to a buoyant and rising India. There is little time for waiting for public-private partnership in achieving the goals in infrastructure, education, health, housing and drinking water availability.

The Government in India, both at the Centre and the states, share the concern for ensuing responsive, accountable, transparent, decentralized and people-friendly health administration at all levels. There is, however, considerable frustration and dissatisfaction amongst the people, especially the weaker sections of society, about the apathy, irresponsiveness and lack of accountability of health experts and workers even as the expenditure on staff continues to increase. There is increasing anxiety about growing instances of corruption and criminalisation in public life and administration. The people, particularly the vulnerable groups, are also greatly concerned about the deterioration in the performance of agencies concerned with health and social welfare.

All these problems are symptoms of bad governance otherwise in 60 years of independence, we could have achieved a good health care system and welfare of all categories of people. What is needed is constant practice of good governance? Anyone deviating from good governance practices need be dealt strictly.

Hargopal in his article, "Good Governance: Human Rights Perspective" rightly stresses that, "A day-long Conference of Chief Secretaries held on 2-11-2004 under the Chairmanship of Cabinet Secretary focusing on good governance, administrative reforms and related issues had agreed to have a Model Code of Governance which would enshrine the fundamental principles and benchmarks of good governance and would look at governance from the point of view of the citizens and outline the framework for good governance, based on identifiable benchmarks for comparison and evaluation, which can be a States to follow." Accordingly, a Model Code of Governance, which is in the form of a road-map for the administration was finalized and sent to all Chief Secretaries of States/UTs on 14-4-2005. The main components of the Model Code cover action points under the heads. (i) Improving Service Delivery, (ii) Development of Programmes for Weaker Sections and Backward Areas, (iii) Technology and System Improvement, (iv) Financial Management and Budget Sanctity, (v) Accountability and Transparency, (vi) Public Service Morale and Anti-Corruption Measures, and (vii) Incentivising Reforms.

The Prime Minister had announced during the National Conference of District Collectors in May 2005, the institution of awards for excellence in Public Administration. Accordingly, the Department of Administration Reforms and Public Grievances has instituted Award Scheme titled, Prime Minsiter's Award for excellence in Public Administration during the financial year 2005-06 for the recognition of the meritorious and outstanding contribution made by Civil Servants in the following areas:

- Implementation of innovative schemes/projects; Bringing about perceptible systemic changes and building up institutions.
- Making public delivery systems efficient and corruption-free; Showing innovation and adaptation to meet the stake-holder's requirements.
- Extraordinarily performance in emergent situations like floods, earthquakes, etc.; and
- Setting high standards of services and continued improvement, showing high leadership qualities and improving employees motivation, etc.

Indian administration is certainly the core of all human affairs. India is certainly on the cross-roads of her national destiny, facing a serious challenge to our politics and administration, i.e. chronic delays, lack of sympathy and humane approach, time consuming meetings, corrupt practices, lack of work culture, criminalization of politics, insensitive and callous, etc. All these are the obstacles in the path of good governance which can be removed by personnel in government both political and administrative to reassure good governance.

We are now experimenting on human welfare, human development, in our country. We had never done it before on the colossal scale that we are doing today. We had the necessary philosophy and ideas; but the implementation was arrested in later centuries. Therefore, the stress today should be on practical implementation, faster and still faster, and watching a new India, healthy and strong, rising on the horizon. This should be the great watchword of all administration in the Centre and the States, down to the Zilla Parishad and Gram Panchayat institutions. in our country.

Now let us define the term 'Health Administration'. It is a branch of Public Administration which deals with matters relating to the promotion of health, preventive services, medical care, rehabilitation, the delivery of health services, the development of health manpower and the medical education and training, The purpose of Public Health Administration is to provide total health services to the people with economy and efficiency. Health Administration must use the knowledge of health economics to achieve economy. Three French teachers of Health Economics (Professor P. Bonamour, F. Guyot and D. Jolly) defined Health Economics as: "that branch of knowledge which seeks to optimize medical action, that is, to study ways of spreading the available resources so as to ensure the best possible state of health for the population, within the limited means."[11]

Efficiency in health administration can be achieved through proper policy formulation and its implementation. Health administration is the force which can help the health system in the formation of sound health policy and its implementation. One of he best definitions of Health Administration is given by C.E.A. Winslow who defined it as 'The science and art of preventing diseases'; "prolonging life, promoting health efficiency through organized community effort for the sanitation of the environment, the control of communicable diseases, the education of the individual in personal hygiene, the organisation of medical and nursing services for the early diagnosis and preventive treatment of disease, the development of social machinery to ensure to every citizen a standard of living adequate for the maintenance of health, so organizing these benefits as to enable every citizen to realize his birth right of health and longevity."[12] Thus, Public Health Administration is the application of administrative processes and methods which are used in carrying out the objectives of health in an organized community. The term community refers to the entire population of functionally defined geographics area that has developed common interests, activities and interrelations.

According to Beaton:

> "Public Health is the planning, carrying-out and evaluation of health measures and systems services that both maintain and improve the health of a population group and prevent and control diseases within that population group."[13]

There has been an increase in the variety, number and complexity of functions that have to be performed by the health administration, because of scientific and technological advancement. The health administration has not been modernized correspondingly to make use of the new technology. A serious imbalance exists between aspirations and performances. There is a widespread belief prevalent among the experts in the field of Health Administration that there is an urgent need for better management of health services if higher standards of health and health care are to be achieved.

The following are typical of the symptoms that demonstrate the need for better management:

(a) Overlapping, conflicting and competing organisations within the health 'system'. Where the system is composed of unrelated parts, it is not possible to manage a coherent health programme because no administrative structure can execute it.

(b) Widely scattered funding mechanism with little control over costs. Many health services have little idea of the true cost of some of their facilities or services.

(c) Decisions on the mixture of facilities and services without reference to population needs and with no information about those who do not use the services. Medical management thus tends to be based on currently met demand, not a need.[14]

Good management provides the surplus investment which nourishes the processes of industrialization and modernization of society. Good administration furnishes the infrastructure of services which secure the order, stability and security which are the prerequisites of economic and social development. Carefully recruited and periodically trained or retrained personnel are needed for both spheres of operation. We would, therefore, like to conclude with Charles Beard, who wrote, at the end of his long career:

> "There is no subject more important than this subject of Public Administration. The future of civilised government, and even, I think of civilisation itself, rests upon our ability to develop a science, philosophy and practice of administration competent to discharge the public functions of a civilized society."[15]

There is no doubt that medicine has accumulated a long list of triumphs as regards the care containment, or amelioration of established somatic diseases. Yet, it knows almost nothing of social aspects of disease and its treatment. In the past not much attention has been paid by the medical and other scientists to such causes of social disease as parental inadequacy, overcrowding, poverty, malnutrition, inadequate occupational and educational opportunities, the non-therapeutic uses of leisures, the misuse of mass media or the suppression of underprivileged section of the community. Medicine today with all its success or failures and the kind of demand it faces, is increasingly becoming a part of larger societal concern. The health administrators have to become aware of the tact that the obligatory relationship of social, mental and somatic disease requires looking fresh, at medicine's expanding role. They have to think in terms of planning and execution of comprehensive medical care programmes, including preservation of health and prevention as well as cure of disease. Already, continuity of home care has become a new slogan in the medical circle, particularly in the developing countries. While all the aims appear laudable, they are rarely achieved except for the cure of disease part. Obviously, as the successes of medical science pile up, the sub-division of medical labour increases with its attendant technical incompetence, discontinuity of care and high cost. These considerations coupled with the present defensive isolation of the medical world in the bastion of acute curative, specialized and technical medicine, the hospitals prevent the giving of comprehensive care and the development of the true 'health centre' as a focal point for community health care. All this must be studied as the most crucial area of health administration.[15a]

In the developing countries in particular, the emphasis has hanged from the physical environment 'to preventive medicine'. A great deal of attention is now being paid to man's relationship with is total complex social environment. The occurrence and spread of disease is being looked at in relation to numerous interacting factors in man's physical, biological, socio-economic and cultural environment. Thus, the discipline of health administration is faced with many new challenges and nothing much can be achieved by it without looking at health problems from a holistic point of view.

One of the basic principles of public health administration relevant both to developed and developing countries should be that scarce resources, including that of medical manpower, should not be utilized only for the purpose of creating high power clinical establishments to treat rare diseases rather than using them for the successful functioning of public health services to combat common health problems, particularly of vulnerable groups, like pregnant women, educating mothers and young children. Similarly, medical education can be reoriented and medical services reorganised with the involvement and cooperation of medical and social scientists.

**Objectives of Public Health Administration**

Good governance would promote welfare state in its true connotation wherein people would be looked after by Government as part and parcel of government machinery. B.K. Ghokhale writes, "The welfare state is one which is wedded to the principle of promoting the general happiness and welfare of the people. It regards itself more as an agency of social services than as an instrument of power. It drawn up all types of plans according to its resources, the genius of the people and the ability and integrity of the administrators."

There are numerous objectives of public health administration. The following deserve special attention:

(a) Increasing the average length of human life.
(b) Decreasing the mortality rate, particularly infant mortality rate, due to those diseases which can be easily prevented or remedied.
(c) Decreasing the morbidity rate.
(d) Increasing the physical, mental and social well-being of the individual.
(e) Increasing the pace of adjustment of individual to his environment.
(f) Providing total health care to enrich quality of life.

The important activities in the domain of health which need the attention of health administration have been well-enumerated in the 'Charter of Health' adopted by the Regional Committee for South-East Asia. The objectives of the Charter include:

(a) The provision of primary health care services to the rural population and under-served groups in urban areas, aiming at full coverage.
(b) The development of health manpower which will maintain its sensitivity and relevance to the health service delivery system.
(c) The provision of safe water to rural and urban communities and improvement of the facilities for waste-water disposal and basic sanitation.
(d) The reduction of mortality and morbidity among infants, children and mothers; and the regulation of fertility so as to achieve a balance between population growth and economic development.
(e) The implementation of effective measures for the surveillance, prevention and control of the major communicable diseases, with prevention and control of malaria being given the highest priority and due importance being given to an integrated multi-immunization programme.
(f) The promotion and formulation of national and regional food

and nutrition policies and the development of common programme jointly with the other economic and social sectors concerned. The Health Charter should serve as a spring board to renewed activities, for the health and happiness of humanity. The same idea has been beautifully expressed in the Vedic benediction:

May all humanity be happy
May all be without disease
May all witness auspicious sights
May none have to undergo suffering

"In practice, it is difficult to achieve the ideals of public health as mentioned in the Constitution of World Health Organisation. Even the most advanced countries have not been able to meet this ideal.

So, the Health Administrators in the developing countries must focus their attention on achieving a level health which they can afford. They must proceed gradually in the pursuit of this ideal. 'Health Administration', whether in developed or developing countries, are faced with a number of managerial problems ranging from the provision of the most basic health and sanitary measures to the best use of finite resources in elaborate medical care system. All countries, however, have one basic problem in common—how can one best improve the health status of the population? This problem has become more pressing owing to changes in the needs and expectations of communities to developments in health and other technologies, and to the urgent need to link health improvement with socio-economic development."[16]

The purpose of public health administration is to enrich the quality of life leading to ethical, artistic, material and spiritual development of man.

If the ideal of health administration is to provide better medical care to the people then we shall have to see that in a given situation we make the best possible use of our resources in terms of personnel and finance to achieve optimum results. For instance, in a developing country like India, the health administrator should normally be concerned with the following:

(a) that the patients are treated as close to their homes as possible in the smallest, cheapest and simply equipped unit such as a sub-centre which is capable of looking after them adequately;
(b) that the medical services should be organised and administered in such a way that the quality of medical care improves gradually;
(c) that medical care services should be organised from the bottom-up and not from the top-down;
(d) that the services planned should meet the needs of the people;
(e) that all members of the health and medical personnel function as a well-knit team; and

(f) that new categories of health personnel such as multi-purpose health workers and community health workers should be given suitable training to provide simple medical care and preventive services to large sections of the community.

In any developmental and welfare administration, that is the only right attitude. The administration takes money from the people as taxes, only to restore it back in hundred-fold and in thousand-fold measure to the people as welfare measures. How is the administration able to perform this miracle? Because the men who handle that money have that yoga-bala, energy of yoga, within them; they have imaginative sympathy; they have efficiency; they have dedication; they are always conscious that they are basically citizens of free India, who are called upon to perform of tremendous national function and mission. That attitude achieves a revolutionary miracle within them; they become dynamic persons instead of remaining static individuals. In such an environment, good governance can flourish.[17]

In the case of virtual epidemic of behavioural disorders, modern health care must place a new emphasis on solving the human side of medicine. As stated by Maureen A. Backy, "The crucial link between the person providing health care and the persons receiving it, is often very weak indeed. Modern medicine tends to emphasize technical solution and, overlook the value of close personal contact and relationship.[18]

## C. NATURE AND SCOPE OF HEALTH ADMINISTRATION

### Health Administration as a Science and an Art

Health administration is becoming complex day-by-day. Man is acquiring undreamt of powers, for scientific progress makes him everyday more capable of shaping the world and his destiny. He has the potentiality to bring about socio-economic revolution for the harmonious and healthy development of the people. The world has the resources and know-how to achieve a significant improvement in wealth care. But improved health will not percolate to the majority of the people as a natural consequence of economic growth. It requires an efficient administrative and managerial system to translate the benefits of science and technology to the people. Unfortunately, developing countries have failed to produce the expected system. The weakness, ineptitude and general inefficiency of their governmental systems are massive obstacles not only in their development but even in their survival.[19] These deficiencies prevent the vast flood of money, talent and material from achieving their objective. It is accepted that inability to manage efficiently or utilise effectively the available and potential resources is the common ill of all the less-developed countries. It follows that successful development demands a sound programme for managerial improvement.[20] Thus, the administrative inadequacies in a national government have a retarding influence on socio-economic development. Charles F. Nicklas, Public Administration Advisor to the Philippines Government, remarked:

> "The success of management improvement efforts and indeed the quality of public administration depends to a very great and undeniable extent upon the concepts, philosophies, interests and characteristics of key officials at the top echelons of the government hierarchy. Without the proper attitude and impetus at these levels, the cause of improved management and operation in government faced constant frustration. . . . It is, therefore, essential in the interest of progress that the individuals be endowed with the desire to see that the public service is administered in the most efficient, effective and economic manner possible and possess the knowledge and breadth of understanding necessary to fulfil that desire.[21]

Public health administration is an area of activity which calls for specialised knowledge and techniques which can help the people to achieve the health care. Until and unless, we understand all the implications of such an administration, we may not be able to reap the potential benefits of health organisations. This is a definite art which can be learnt and practiced to produce pre-designed output. Health administration is an art as it can help to direct and guide the efforts of those involved in such an enterprise towards some specific ends or objectives efficiently. There is a great need to make this art perfect and professional. A professionally efficient and competent administration is able to serve the people better. Besides, the health personnel must be dedicated to their profession.

Dr. H. Mahler is very critical about the inability of health workers in contemporary society to influence those social and environmental factors which truly determine public health. He states:

> "There persist widespread negative attitudes among health professionals towards the health care of the poorest strata in the rural and urban populations in the developing countries. Most of these attitudes imply-with a repetitiveness of an old gramophone record caught in a narrow, arrogant, condescending and different groove—that these poor people are too apathetic, too superstitious, too illiterate to benefit from the health care potentially available to them. . . . Health professionals and those who train them should be much more radical in accepting a social responsibility for the health needs of the people in these poor rural and urban communities so that they can act as agents for change.[22]

Thus, we can say that there is a need to train health administrators and workers in the new art of Public Health Administration so that they can take the benefits of the modern science to the common man and maintain the spirit of Geneva Declaration.[23]

"Now being admitted to the profession of Medicine, I solemnly pledge to concentrate my life to the service of humanity. I will give respect and gratitude to my deserving teachers. I will practice medicine with conscience and dignity. The health and life of my patients will be my first consideration. I will hold in confidence all that my patient confides in me. I will maintain the honour and noble traditions of the medical profession. My colleagues will be my brothers. I will not permit considerations of race, religion, nationality; party politics or social standing to intervene between my duty and my patient. I will maintain the utmost respect of human life. Even under threat I will not use my knowledge contrary to the laws of humanity. These promises I make freely and upon my honour." The same feeling has been expressed in the Tokyo Declaration. To quote the preamble to the Declaration of Tokyo: "It is the privilege of the medical doctor to practice medicine in the service of humanity, to preserve and restore bodily and mental health without distinction as to persons, to comfort and to ease the sufferings of his or her patients."[24]

Prof. J.S. Neki has rightly said in this connection that "to help, to heal, to reconstruct, to comfort—and all along the line to act with compassion all these bear testimony to the moral consciousness of the doctor. Whatever the new strains imposed upon medical ethics, this structure will survive and continue to guide doctors in their professional conduct. . . . Legal and juridical obligations they have, of necessity, to fulfil. But these are not genuine ethics. Genuine ethics has to be ingrained into character and does not have to depend upon external controls."[25]

Now the question arises whether public health administration is a science or not. It is definitely not a science like the physical sciences as it cannot claim certainty. It is a science similar to other Social Sciences like Economics, Sociology, etc. We are applying scientific methods in health administration for careful planning, analysis and the design of the procedures. We can make the instruments of Health Care Administration more perfect through careful practice and research and thus reach definite universal principles. We should be clear here that the universal principles in human organisations would differ to a great extent depending upon the ecological differences, prevalent in different areas. We can say that 'scientific societies', and the exchange of knowledge and hypotheses natural scientists have advanced the exactness of knowledge in the domain of natural science, so we may expect administrative societies, and the exchanges among administrators to advance the exactness of knowledge in the domain of administration.

Thus public health administration is both a science and an art. In order to advance—the cause of this budding discipline for the present and the future academic scholars and practitioners, we may concentrate on its principles, philosophy and practice. The developing world is faced with the problems of limited resources, infinite needs and competing demands in the domain of health. In order to provide the health services (preventive, promotive, curative and rehabilitative) to the total population—sick and the healthy, the developing world would have to provide an effective system of health administration. If these components are combined fruitfully, it is sure that the health administration can deliver the desired goods and services to its constituents.

**Scope of Health Care Administration**

In order to translate the aims and objectives of the public health organisations, the scope of health administration is expanding. Besides curative, preventive, promotive aspects, Health Administration studies social medicine which is concerned with the study of man as a total individual for the understanding of health and disease. The British Medical Association considers this concept from the angle:

> "That the health of the people depends primarily upon the social and environmental conditions under which they live and work, upon security against fear and want, upon nutritional standards, upon educational facilities and upon the facilities for exercise and leisure."

Social medicine includes social anatomy, social psychology, social pathology and social therapy. There is also a new term, i.e., Medical Geography-linking medicine with geography. Medical Geography views disease as maladjustment to the environment to which numerous factors contribute; disease, therefore, becomes an anthropological phenomenon with geographical distribution. Thus, to understand the implications of health, it is necessary to have knowledge of the ecology of man. Such understanding would throw a flood of light on problems of diagnosis and treatment.

We can see the expanding and diversified field of medical science from the Table 1.1 depicting the various stages of the development from 1850-2000. To quote W.L. Barton:

> "If this era is to have success there must be a move from the concept of health as being the total responsibility of a professionalized service to a new emphasis on self-reliant health care. . . . The emerging science of the new era calls for a clear definition of objective, purpose and function, so as to identify the required competence, distinctive skills and body of knowledge in terms that can be clearly understood by the people and the politicians as well as by the professional leadership involved. It demands daring leadership, not afraid to step forward from the basic professions from which they came; to face the challenges and difficulties of education in the new fields and to direct with courage; through competence in public health, the team of equals."[26]

Health administration is concerned with 'what' and 'how' of the health. 'What' is the subject matter; covering preventive, promotive, curative and rehabilitative services. It also covers professional training of the health and medical personnel and the role of the International Health Administration and its impact on the national health administration. It is very difficult to classify the subject matter of health administration in watertight compartments. We have to focus on an integrated philosophy of health, medical care is defined by the WHO as:

> "A programme of services that should make available to the individual, and thereby to the community, all facilities of medical and allied sciences necessary to promote and maintain health of mind and body. This programme should take into account the physical, social and family environment, with a view to the prevention of disease, the restoration of health and the alleviation of disability. The extent of these services will vary according to local conditions."[27]

We have to view health administration from a broader viewpoint. It encompasses many other factors, which influence health care administration. The broadening scope of health care administration can be seen from the Table given on the next page. (Table 1.1) The various activities which can come under each sub-head can be seen from the Table 1.1.

As regards 'how', it is the technique of management, i.e., the principles of management which can make the health administration successful and fruitful. These principles have been classified by different management experts into a number of functions. Clough[28] gives only two-making decisions and providing leadership. R.C. Davis[29] gives three — planning, organising and controlling. Newman, Summer and Warren[30] list four—organising, planning, leading and controlling. Terry[31] notes planning, organising, actuating and controlling.

Koontz and O'Donnell[32] list five functions: planning, organising, staffing, direction and control. Hicks[33] covers six functions: creating, planning, organising, motivating, communicating and controlling. Dales[34] goes one step further, i.e. seven functions-planning, organising, staffing, direction, control, innovation and representation. Many experts on Administrative Management feel that management is a basic operative force in all complex; purposive organisations. It is the function of executive leadership anywhere. It means that management skills are transferable. But there are writers who argue that there are fundamental differences between managing one organisation and the other. Earnest Dale, for instance, says that the universality of management principles is contradicted by observed examples of the difficulties faced by managers who work in widely different type of organisation from the one in which they were successful. As such, we should be careful in applying the general principles of management to health organisations within the peculiar environment surrounding them.

We must understand the difference between administration and management, though, we have used the term interchangeably. Orday Tead has made a distinction between these two terms in the following words: Administration is the process and agency which is responsible for the determination of the aims for which an organisation and its management are to strive, which establishes the broad policies under which they are to operate and which gives general oversight to the continuing effectiveness of the total operation in reaching the objectives sought. And he goes on to say that "management is the process and agency which directs and guides the operations of an organisation in the realising of established aims."[35]

To quote Mcfarland: "In government agencies administration is preferred over management, although in recent years the term management has become widely used in government agencies. Another possible distinction refers to the levels of organisation. In business, the term administration refers to the activities of the higher levels in the managerial ranks. Still another distinction related to organisational level is that administration refers to the determination of major aims and policies, while management to the carrying out of the operations designed to accomplish the aims and effectuate the policies. Here, again, the distinction is not only widely followed but it exists."[36]

Peter F. Drucker has rightly observed: "Our society has become, within an incredibly short fifty years, a society of institutions. It has become a pluralist society in which every major social task has been entrusted to large organisations from producing economic goods and services to health care, from social security and welfare to education; from the search for new knowledge to the protection of the natural environments."

Now let us discuss some of the definitions of management which can be understood and applied by Health Administrators and managers. Management may be defined as the art of securing maximum result with a minimum of effort so as to secure maximum prosperity and happiness for both employer and employee and gives the public the best possible service.[37]

Peter F. Drucker has rightly pointed out that, "Management is the crucial factor in economic and social development. It was obvious that the economists' traditional view of development as a function of savings and capital investment do not produce management and economic development. On the contrary, management produces economic and social development, and with it savings and capital investment. It becomes apparent that the developing countries are not underdeveloped, they are under managed."[38] Massie says that: "Management is defined as the process by which a cooperative group directs action towards common goals."[39] Terry has rightly said that, "management is a distinct process consisting of planning, organising, actuating, and controlling, performed to determine and accomplish the objectives by the use of people and resources."[40]

According to A. Dasgupta, "Management is the creation and control of technological and human environment of an organisation in which human skill and capacities of individuals and groups find full scope for their effective use in order to accomplish the objectives for which an enterprise has been set-up. It is involved in the relationship of the individual, group, the organisation and the environment."[41]

To Stanely Vance, "Management is simply the process of decision-making and control over the action of human beings for the express purpose of attaining predetermined goals."[42]

According to Lundy, "Management is principally the task of planning, coordinating, motivating and controlling the efforts of others towards a specific objective."[43] The health sector has wide and varied relationships with other sectors of the social system. Individual and community health depend on a multiplicity of factors, such as nutrition and other basic biological requirements, personal and psychological security, culturally supported behavioural patterns, Legislation, Education, opportunity for participation of the community in planning and implementation, protection against exposure to pathogens; and accessibility of treatment to reduce the impact of disease. Indeed, it is hard to think of a community activity that has no relationship to health. This view makes health the result of occurrences in many sectors of the social system; it implies that what occurs in those sectors may support, negate or offset the preventive and therapeutic interventions of the health sector. These considerations have enlarged the objectives of health administration from the mere provision of health services to the improvement of community health by all available means.

The health administration studies all aspects for the delivery of health care services (Chart 1.2). In this context, health administration studies the role of public, private and voluntary efforts in meeting health challenges. Health administration also studies the structure and functioning of international health administration, government administration at all levels, private administration and voluntary administration, which help the people in improving their health status. A recent development in health administration has been the encouragement to the traditional medical systems to help the needy people. According to Dr. P.N.V. Kurup, Former Adviser to the Government of India for indigenous system of medicine:

> "In our anxiety to make an effective comprehensive health service available as soon as possible to the maximum number of people, the available material, financial and manpower resources that are rooted in traditional medical practices should not be overlooked. Against this background the traditional systems of medicine can play a vital role as an additional or alternative approach in a country's Health Delivery Programme."[44]

China has used this system with definite results. Thus, health administration studies the role of all the systems of medicine which help in the improvement of the health status of the people. However, in order to make a really good contribution, it has to adopt a multi-disciplinary approach. In the West, the health administrators are increasingly relying on the application of behavioural administrative sciences—anthropology,

CHART 1.2

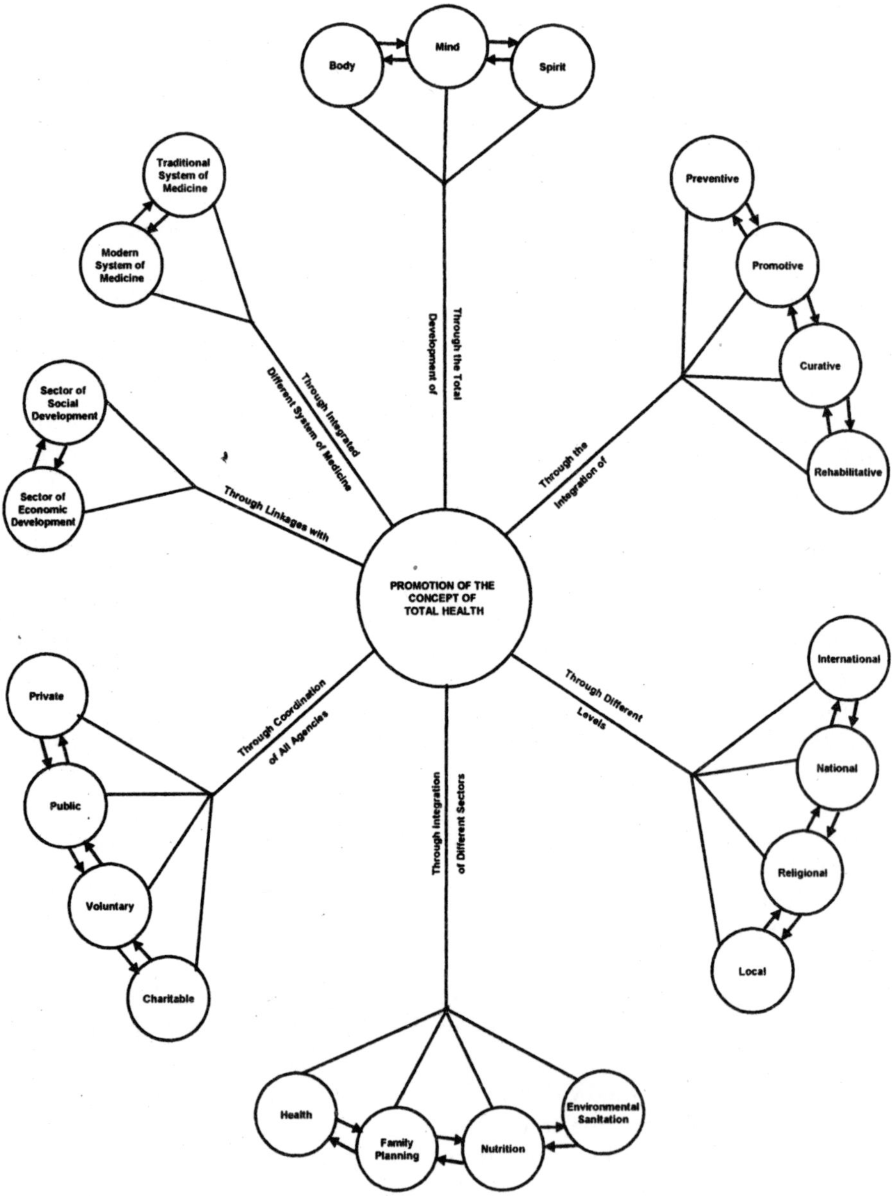


sociology, social psychology and public administration, in the identification and solution of administrative problems in the area of health. Thus, this needs to be achieved with a much greater pace in a developing country like India. It cannot be delayed in view of the kind of problems we face today. In the present context, the health administrator has to acquire a broader outlook and a strong will and determination to grapple with the existing mind-boggling health problems.

### Research and Monitoring in Health Administration

There is a need for conducting systematic research on many aspects of health care administration. By using operational research methods and techniques, one can assess the extent to which scientific knowledge is utilised for bringing about improvement in the health level of the bulk of the people at the lowest cost. Research in health administration is concerned with administrative, economic and organisational aspects of the delivery of health and medical services.

Success of health care administration depends not only on research investigations in the medical field, but also on the researches in other allied fields and particularly on the application of the procedures and practices as evolved in these fields. It may be stressed that operational research has special relevance to health administration in India because of inadequacy of organising health services and also due to several shortcomings of policy-making. However, nothing much can be achieved without providing the necessary training to personnel engaged in public health programmes and activities. The Central and the state ministries of health and family welfare have to play a special role in this regard. There is a definite need for studying the patterns of utilization of health services, both in the rural and urban areas. By identifying factors affecting delivery of health care services, they can possibly plan to overcome them. The Union Government has already done a good job in this direction by establishing a National Institute of Health and Family Welfare Administration, which is actively engaged in various types of research relating to health and hospital administration. Some universities are also offering an independent course on health administration. The universities must be encouraged to take up research projects in health and hospital administration, as the dichotomy between the social scientists and medical personnel is fast fading.

### Monitoring and Surveillance in Health Administration

Unplanned development in the area of health has led to many unforeseen problems, which are directly or indirectly related to certain deficiencies in the planning processes. Thus, there is a great need to develop specific guidelines for monitoring the public health programmes and activities so as to yield maximum benefits to the largest number of people. The governments, both at the Centre and the State levels, need to be made aware of malfunctioning of health organisations in time, so that remedial measures could be adopted. In all communities where a central organisation exists, there are some devices to keep Government informed about the health of the people they govern. There is a need to examine these devices so that these could be further modified to yield the desired results. By applying modified devices one could provide a sensitive indication of trends in health and development to the health planners for taking appropriate decisions regarding adoption of remedial measures.

Health surveillance is the comparison and interpretation of data generated through monitoring or from any other sources to determine the impact of health measures on the health status of populations. "Surveillance means the epidemiological study of a disease as a dynamic process involving the ecology of the infectious agent, the host, the reservoirs, the vectors, and the environment as well as the complex mechanisms concerned in the spread of infection and the extent to which the spread occurs."[45]

## D. INDICATORS: MEASURING IMPACT OF HEALTHCARE ADMINISTRATION

Health is generally referred to as a measurable quantity, but the concept is elusive and words cannot define it with precision. A WHO study indicated that among the problems of measurement of levels of living, that of the measurement of health levels occupies central position. Health, a very broad concept, lends itself poorly to objective measurement; direct measurement of health status is often impossible and, in practice, indicators concern status that deviate from health but can be measured-indicators of the health status of individuals or groups; indicators of environmental conditions that may have an effect on health status; and the indicators of the activities of health services The distinction between health and 'sickness' is not always well-defined. Most people would agree that it is desirable to prevent illness and premature death. However, the prevalent indices are:

### Death Rate

All over the world, death rates have been coming down and the average age at death has been moving up during the fifty-year' period between (1950-2000). It has been estimated that for the world as a whole, life expectancy at birth has increased from 40 to 72 years—the developed countries averaging an increase from 56 to 82 years and the developing countries from 32 to 62 years.

### Infant Mortality Rate

It means the number of infants who die under one year of age out of every 1,000 who are born alive. During the last fifty years it has come down substantially.

### Incidence and Prevalence of Disease

In most countries of the world, a system operates that enables both the local and the central health administration to know fairly and quickly about variations in the occurrence of the notifiable infectious diseases and about the outbreak of epidemics. The system has come in for heavy criticism because reporting is often patchy, incomplete and unreliable. But with all these limitations, these statistics, looked at over the years, do provide an enormously useful record of the long-term gradual decline of many infectious diseases, as well as of sudden epidemics, their rise and fall, and their passage from one community to another or from one country to another.[46]

**Admission Rate of Patients to the Hospitals in the Area**

Hospitalisation statistics are essential for administering a hospital service and for planning and evaluating the services. They cannot provide a full and undistorted picture of the health or ill-health, of the population served. However, with experience, health statisticians and health administrators learn to interpret the statistics and can often determine what is going on in the community.

**Surveys and Special Enquiries**

Such health surveys or morbidity surveys can be of various kinds. They may involve medical examinations or special disease finding (surveys) tests or they may be performed through household visits and enquiries. National sickness surveys have been carried out in many countries including Canada, Denmark, Japan. India, UK, USA, for the past 20 years. However, although continuous health surveys have great value within a country, something less elaborate is needed for comparing levels of health in different places and for recognizing important changes over the course of time. It would be good if we could devise a simple but general health index, that would summarise the state of health of a population in one single figure that would be easy to monitor and interpret—something like the GNP in the economic field. But so far this has not been possible as health is not a readily quantifiable entity or attribute.

**Proportional Mortality Ratio**

It is defined as the number of deaths at the ages of 50 and over as the percentage of total deaths. If all persons survive up to 50 years of age, then the index would be 100, if no one reaches this age, the index would be zero.

**Expectation of Life**

The expectation of life at birth is generally considered to be the single important indicator of the health status of a population.[47] It will be seen from the above mentioned indicators that there is no comprehensive measure of a nation's health.[48]

**Limitations of Health Administration**

Health is concerned with qualitative improvement and it is not subject to exact measurement. Any health organisation can be successful if the following facts, peculiar to health management, are taken into consideration:

(a) The nature of the object being managed;
(b) Public attitudes to that object;

(c) The difficulty of placing a value on 'health';
(d) The multiplicity of aims and objectives and of the criteria applied to them;
(e) The long interval between decision and outcome and the associated uncertainty surrounding decision-making;
(f) Orientation to 'service' rather than 'production';
(g) The involvement of several professions in the management process;
(h) Political intervention;
(i) The scope for public involvement; and
(j) The need to coordinate many different agencies, officials, private and voluntary.

All these factors must be taken into consideration while administering the health development. Health administrators should be sensitive to all these limitations and plan and administer health services most conducive to the satisfaction of the population. It is really difficult to have a single model to solve the health problems in a country or area. A single model has not been devised for the solution of health problems. However, we can design any workable model, suitable for a given area.

The ideal index which combines the effects of a number of components measured independently, is yet to be developed, although it can be stated that such an index should satisfy the following requirements:[49]

(a) *Availability*: It should be possible to obtain the data required without special and complex investigations.
(b) *Completeness of coverage*: The index should be derived from data covering the population of an entire country or that part of it to which the index is supposed to refer.
(c) *Quality*: The national data should not vary with time and place in such a way as to have any substantial effect on the index.
(d) *Universality*: The index should, as far as possible, be the expression of a group of factors that determine and affect the level of health.
(e) *Calculation*: The index should be calculated in as simple a manner as possible and the calculation should not be costly in terms of the resources required.
(f) *Acceptance*: The index should be widely accepted and used and no doubts should exist in respect of the methods employed for developing the index or for interpreting it,
(g) *Specificity*: The index should reflect changes only in those phenomena of which it is the expression.
(h) *Reproduction*: When the index is used by different specialists under different conditions at different times, the results should be identical.

(i) Sensitiveness: The index should be sensitive to changes in the phenomena concerned. Allowance should be made for the effect of inflation of these index.

(j) Validity: The index should be a true expression of the factors of which it is supposed to be a measure. Some form of independent external evidence of this should be provided.

Moreover, health cannot be measured in isolation. It is a part of much broader spectrum of inter-related and interdependent conditions, and no picture of health status can be complete without also taking into account the socio-economic and environmental circumstances like income, education, housing, environment, clothing, food, climate. pollution and still other factors that influence levels of health and disease at least as much as the activities of the health services themselves.

**Health Care Administration in the New Millennium**

In the new millennium, we have to keep the inherent and potential dangers of affluence and industrialisation leading to excessive use of alcohol, smoking, sex and drugs, which directly or indirectly affect health of the people causing misery and devastation. John Bland in his editorial. "The Price of Progress" cautions the developing countries not to venture such lopsided development. To quote him:[50]

One of the paradoxes of the modern age is that. just when the world is making a concerted lunge towards industrialization and advanced technology, which are Universally viewed as desirable, this same "progress" appears to confront mankind with a growing number of acute public health problems.

The more roads and cars we build, the more people die prematurely in traffic accidents. The greater the earnings, the greater are the spending on alcoholic drink and tobacco. As medicaments and chemical products proliferate so the risks increase of accidental poisoning particularly of children. Opportunities for better and further education have never seemed brighter, yet the sinister cult of narcotic drugs is still gaining ground among young people. And the race for ever more source of industrial energy brings in its train increasing hazards to the ecology and to human health from fumes, pollutants, oil slicks at sea and radioactive leaks from nuclear power plants.

Is this "price of progress" an inescapable consequence? Perhaps it is not. Those countries that are regarded as industrialized are trying hard to mitigate the drawbacks and dangers, and they are alerted to potential new dangers that might threaten man and nature. Now the writing is on the wall for the fast-developing Third World countries; many of them are already taking wise steps to avoid making the old mistakes. Forewarned is forearmed.

What is required in new millennium to promote positive health? Policy-makers and planners of health should devise ways and means to popularise simple lifestyle conducive to health. This has been stressed in Vedas and ancient scriptures from India. Mauritius Non-Communicable Diseases Study Group in their article "Lifestyle Hazards" rightly stresses the dangers of modern lifestyle, and the methods to change simple lifestyle conducive to health. To quote them:

In the space of a few decades, there have been remarkable reductions in morbidity and mortality due to infectious and parasitic diseases in most developing countries in all regions of the world. However, other threats to health in the form of the so-called "Western degenerative" or "lifestyle" diseases are emerging at rates that far outstrip what would be expected from the fact that people are living longer.

In many developing nations, already beset with economic, social and other health problems, the rates of heart disease, diabetes and hypertension are as high as or even higher than in major developed nations. These chronic diseases impose a destructive drain on communities through their association with sickness and premature death.

Primary preventive activities will focus on behavioural and structural changes related to smoking, health nutrition, and levels of physical activity in the community. Secondary prevention targets include improved case detection, expanded health education services, and an upgrading of follow-up and rehabilitation facilities.[51]

Dr. Jean Paul Jardel is also an advocate of healthy lifestyle. To quote him,[52]

> "Health for all by the year 2000" is the social objective which the Member States of WHO set for themselves in 1977. It will only be attained if major health problems and their deeply underlying causes are resolutely tackled by appropriate strategies. Health for all does not mean merely providing more and better services to care for patients, alleviate suffering and prevent disablement and premature death. It also implies preventing the occurrence of disease and encouraging healthy lifestyles in an environment conducive to health. Charles Boelen in his article, "Just Imagine" analyses the causes of critical health situation in developing countries. He however believes that we must harness our human capital to provide decent health services to the people. In 21st century, we have to produce health manpower to generate dynamic change in the society to make people healthier. To quote him.[53]

Plenty of reports attribute the critical health situation of poor countries to political instability, inadequate infrastructure, incompetent management, absence or migration of managers, chaos, natural disasters, even general indifference or pessimism, or a combination of these factors. Such reports are certainly revealing, but they are too gloomy and do not offer enough hope. Let us look more positively at the real potential for development that those countries have.

The one natural resource that all of them have in abundance is the human resource. Unlike gold or diamonds or oil or copper, there is no need to dig for human beings, because there are such great numbers of them easily available and ready for work. But this raw material has not yet been sufficiently refined to make it a formidable potential for health development.

Personnel trained for Health in new millennium should be innovative, imaginative and creative. Innovation will convert inspiration into solutions and ideas into products that will be world class . . . there is a definition of an innovator. It says that innovator is one, who does not know that it cannot be done. We will require leaders who will instill this spirit in everyone.[54]

More than half a century ago, Albert Einstein had suggested that we would require a new manner of thinking if mankind is to survive. We cannot have plans of economic development where the human is a bystander. In the new human centred development the balance of five Es', namely, ecology, environment, economics, equity and ethics will have to be achieved. Mere economic development with disregard to equity and ethics will take us nowhere; just as economic development disregarding ecology and environment will be fatal. May be we should look at the issue of equity again. We often talk about equity—which is based on subsidy. But this is not sustainable.

The world 'equity' must be substituted with 'dignity'. This can come only through the process of self-employment, which alone can bring self-empowerment. The new engineers and technologists can contribute to making this happen.[55] Health in new millennium need be viewed in a holistic concept—combination of biological, social and cultural aspects. Modern medicine studies man in detail, but man is an indivisible whole of such enormous complexity that, at the present state of our knowledge and with our present crude techniques, it is impossible to grasp the whole truth about him. There is a tendency to separate a part of the truth from the web and present it for the whole. This is the unsatisfactory state in which the social and biomedical sciences now find themselves, and what is true of the natural and medical sciences is equally true of the whole body of knowledge from which has not yet been possible to deduce any consistent laws of life. (See Chart 1.3)

In short, Good Governance would mean:

(a) Making administration responsive;
(b) Making administration citizen-friendly;
(c) Making administration transparent; and
(d) Making administration ethical;[56]

**Making Public Services Excellent**

It is now apparent that a more balanced consideration of the biological, social and cultural aspects of health is needed. Life is a process and not a substance—a living system based upon the primacy of continuity

CHART 1.3

**Good Governance in New and Emerging Areas**

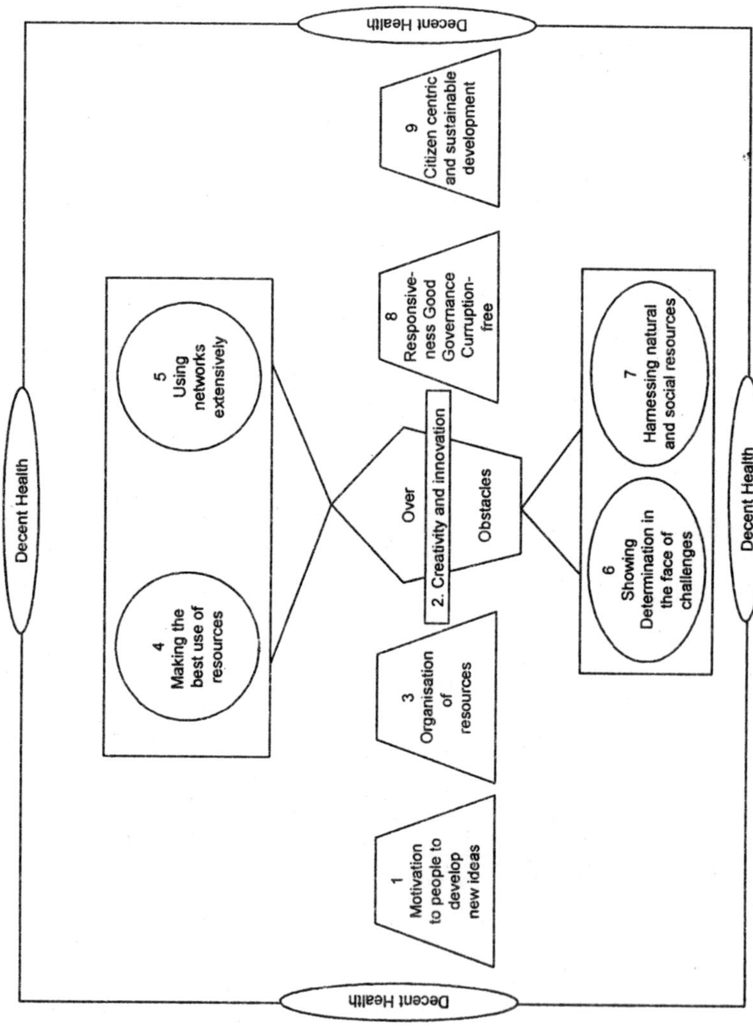

and interrelatedness throughout the universe. The history of human culture is not an evolution but a continuous development, which is not broken at each generation as organic evaluations.

### Essentials of Health Administration

Health administration, to be effective and efficient, needs to have the following ingredients which are also the ingredients of good governance.

*1. Administrative Innovations (See Chart 1.4)*

Reorganisation of administrative structures and procedures are essential to wee out impediments through innovation. Administrative innovation is the *sine qua non* for health administration through good governance. The organisational reforms in India have thus tended to exist mainly in form rather than in real substance—leaving little impact on the efficiency of the system. We cannot have effective administration without a close fit between policy objectives. What has been lacking in India's administrative reforms in the past four decades is the congruence between strategy, structure and substance leading to lead governance.

*2. People's participation*

It is essential to make use of the potential energy of the people through their involvement for better health. T.K. Moulik opines that 'participation in development process implies stimulating individuals to take initiative and mobilizing people to work for overall societal development." To quote ILO, "Participation involves collectively organized and continued efforts by the people themselves in setting goals, pooling resources together and taking actions which aim at improving their living conditions." This is also essential for good governance.

*3. Definite Policies, Programmes and Projects.*

Formulations of health goals and policies precisely reflecting the needs of the people in essential through good governance.

*4. Monitoring*

There is a need of monitoring and evaluation to locate problems and inject improvements for consistent health development.

*5. Use of Modern Management Techniques*

Using modern management techniques for optimizing personnel, financial and material resources for health promotion is essential.

*6. Achievement Orientation*

The emphasis should be on achievement and not mere paper planning.

CHART 1.4

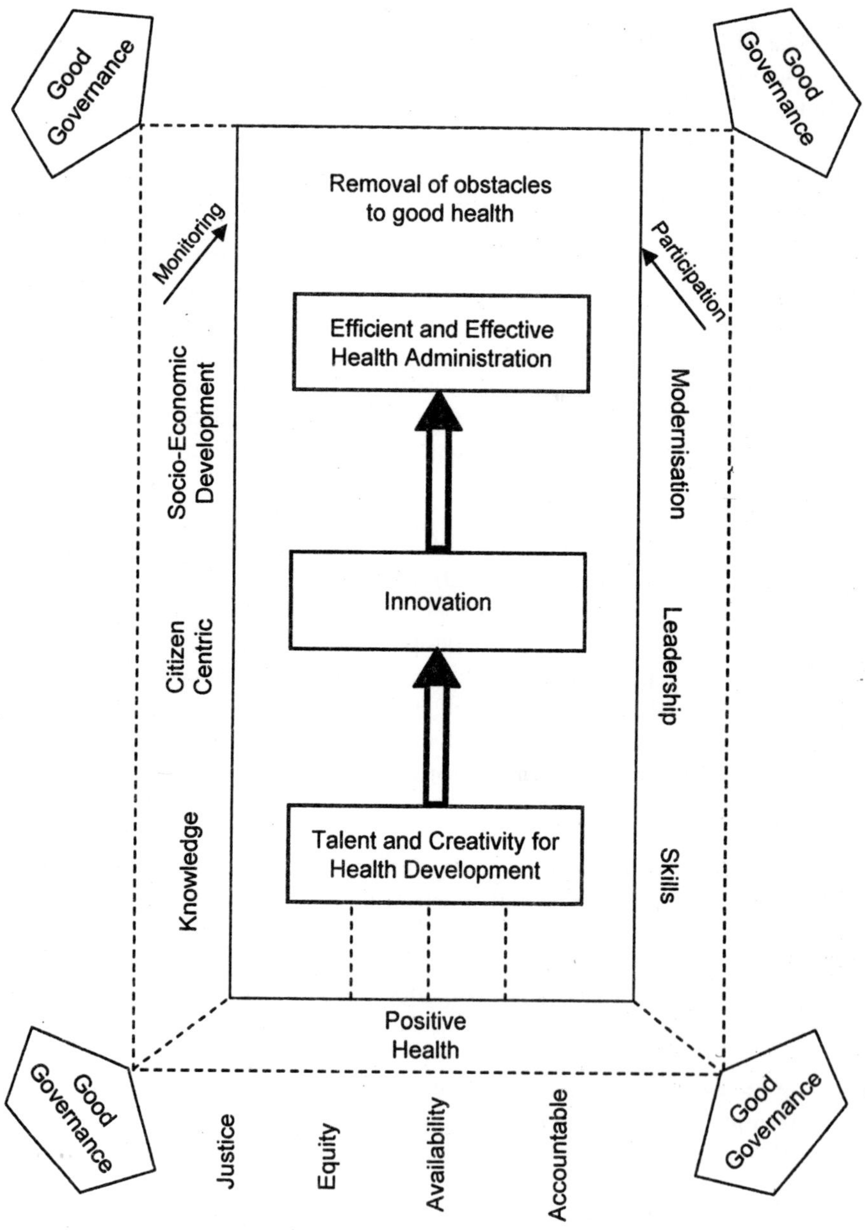
Good Governance
Good Governance
Removal of obstacles to good health
Monitoring
Participation
Efficient and Effective Health Administration
Socio-Economic Development
Modernisation
Innovation
Citizen Centric
Leadership
Talent and Creativity for Health Development
Knowledge
Skills
Positive Health
Good Governance
Good Governance
Justice
Equity
Availability
Accountable

*7. Commitment and Dedication*

These are essential to health development. Commitment and dedication too can provide extra power to development and are an insurance against possible fallouts.

Health administration could not achieve much in developing countries. Since development administration is engaged in all the essential services like health, education, social welfare, etc. which concern every individual, therefore good governance is of great significance in providing best services in these areas to the people. Inspite of the existence of infrastructure, technical know-how, we have not been able to provide decent development-oriented services because of poor governance.

The three most vital players in the arena are the Elected Ruling Government, the Appointed Administrative Machinery and the Demanding Public. While the ultimate responsibility and answerability/accountability rests with the first component, the actual job of delivering results rests on the administrative machinery. It is, in the ultimate analysis a joint team effort of the three but any weak link can jeopardize the outcomes and efforts of any other causing bad governance.

## Notes and References


1. WHO, SEARO, S.E. AJRC 31, p. 59.
2. Govt. of India, First Five Year Plan, p. 488.
3. WHO, *World Health*, May 1979, p. 23.
4. S.C. Seal. (1961), Presidential Address, 50th Science Congress, Delhi.
5. WHO, Public Health Papers, No. 49, 1973, p. 9.
6. Govt. of India, First Five Year Plan, p. 511.
7. WHO, *World Health*, December 1975, p. 3.
8. H. Simon, et. at, Public Administration, p. 3.
9. Marx (ed.), Elements of Public Administration, p. 3.
10. Pfiffner and Presthus, Public Administration, New York, p. 3.
11. WHO, *World Health*, May 1979, p. 14.
12. J.J. Hanlon, (1964), Principles of Public Health Administration, C.V. Mosby.
13. G.H. Beaton, (1974), Canad J. Public Health Paper, p. 463.
14. WHO, Public Health Papers, 55, Geneva; 1974, p. 8.
15. Dimock and Dimock, Public Administration, p. 2.

15a. Threat V., Guranattee, Challenges and Responses: Health in South-East Asia Region, Tata McGraw Hill. New Delhi, 1977, pp. 44-46.

16. WHO, Technical Report Series (596), Application of System Analysis to Health Management, Geneva, 1976, pp. 5-6.
17. Swami Ranjananathananda, "Democratic Administration in the light of Practical Vedanta, Madras, Sri Ramakrishna Mission, 2003, pp. 123-24.
18. WHO, *World Health*, December 1975, p. 6.
19. David S. Brown, "Improving the Administrative Capability of the Aid Receiving Countries," *Public Administration Review*, June 1964, p. 64.
20. J.I., Iboka, "Developing the Administration in a Developing Country," *International Review of Administrative Science*, Vol. XXXVLII, No. 2, 1972, p. 293.
21. Charles F. Nicklas, in the book "Approaches to Development Politics Administration and Change," Edited by Montegomery and Sifiin, New York, 1966, p 188.

22. Text of Address by Dr. H. Mahler, Director General. WHO, to Thirtieth Session of WHO: Regional Committee for South-East Asia, 2-8 August, 1977, Bangkok, Thailand, Published in South-East Asia, Region Office: Final Report and Minutes of the Meeting of the Thirtieth Session, New Delhi, September 1977, pp. 69-70
23. Geneva Declaration.
24. "I Swear by Apollo" by Christians Viedma, *World Health*, The Magazine of the WHO, July 1979, p. 28.
25. J.S. Neki, Medical Ethics, "A Viewpoint from the Developing World," *World Health*, July 1979.
26. W.L. Barton, "Alma-Ata: Signpost to a New Health Era", *World Health*, July 1979, p. 14.
27. WHO, Technical Report Series, No. 176.
28. Donald J. Clough, "Concepts in Management Science", Prentice-Hall, Englewood Cliffs, NJ., 1963, p. 2.
29. Ralph C. Davis, Industrial Organisation and Management, Harper, New York, 1956, p. 54.
30. Summer Newman, Warren, The Process of Management, Prentice-Hall, Englewood, Englewood Cliffs, N.Y. 1967, p. 10.
31. George R. Terry, Principles of Management (Homewood, III, Irwin, 1965), p. 52.
32. Koontz and O'Donnell, Management—A Book of Readings, McGraw Hill Book Co., London, 1968, p. 1.
33. Herbert G. Hicks, The Management of Organisations, McGraw Hill, New York, 1967, p. 156.
34. Earnest Dale, Management Theory and Practice, McGraw Hill, New York. 1967, p. 57.
35. Tead Orday, The Art of Administration, McGraw Hill Book Company, Inc, New York, 1951, p. 101.
36. Mcfarland Dalton. Management: Principles and Practice, IVth Ed., 1970, p. 7.
37. John F. Mee. Management Thought in a Dynamic Economy, New York, 3.
38. Peter F. Drucker, *op. cit.*, pp. 13-14.
39. Massie Joseph, Essentials of Management, New Delhi, 1973.
40. George R. Terry, 'Principles of Management', Homewood, Illinois, 6, 1968, p. 4.
41. A. Dasgupta, Indian Business: A Management, Delhi, 1969, p. 60.
42. Vauce Stanley, Industrial Administration, New York, 1959.
43. James L. Lundy, Effective Industrial Management, New Delhi, 1968, p. 1, (Ed).
44. WHO, *World Health*, Nov. 1977, p. 15.
45. WHO, *WHO Chronicle*, 20, 315 (1966).
46. WHO, Technical Report Series, No. 137, p. 25.
47. WHO, *World Health*, Nov. 1974.
48. WHO, Public Health Papers, Geneva, 1974, p. 17.
49. WHO, Technical Reports Series, 472, p. 20.
50. John Bland, "The Price of Programme", in *World Health*, June 1979, p. 23.
51. Mauritius Non-Communicable Diseases Study Group, "Lifestyle Hazards" in *World Health*, June 1989, pp. 18-19.
52. Jean Paul Jardel, "Knowledge's in Strength" in *World Health*, June 1989. p. 3.
53. Carles Boelen, "Just Imagine" in *World Health*, March, 1990, pp. 23-24.
54. Dr. R.A. Mashekat, "A Five Point New Millennium Indian Agenda", in *University News*, Vol. 37, No. 38, Sept. 20, 1999, pp. 19-22 (Convocation Address at the 30th Convocation of IIT, New Delhi).
55. *Ibid.*, p. 17.
56. T. Adeoye Lambo, "Total Health" in *World Health*, December, 1975, p. 3.

**2**
**CHAPTER**

# *Health and Socio-economic Development*

## MEANING AND GOALS OF DEVELOPMENT (see Chart 2.1)

The word 'development' is so often used in our daily life that we hardly care to think of its real meaning. The meaning of the term 'develop' is to unfold itself or to grow into a fuller or mature condition. And 'ment' stands for instrument of action, an act or process. So, in simple words development is to discover or unfold any hidden field. Development can be defined as a process of directed change towards some objectives which are accepted as desirable goals. Development implies progressive improvements in the living conditions and quality of life enjoyed by society and shared by its members. It is a continuing process that takes place in all societies.

As stated in Dag Harnmarskjold Report, entitled What Now, Another Development Dialogue, 1975: 1/2, the goal of development is to ensure:

> "Development of every man and woman, and not just the growth of things, which are merely means 'for development geared to the satisfaction of needs beginning with the basic needs of the poor. . . 'and for' development to ensure the humanisation of man by the satisfaction of his needs for expression, creativity, conviviality, and for deciding his own destiny."

Development is a process of growth in the direction of modernity, especially towards nation-building and socio-economic progress. It has been stressed that "development is the rational process of organising and carrying out prudently conceived and staffed programmes or projects as one would organize and carry out military or engineering operations." Development has been defined in the same report, What Now Published by the Dag Hammarskjold Foundation, Uppasala, Sweden. It states:

CHART 2.1

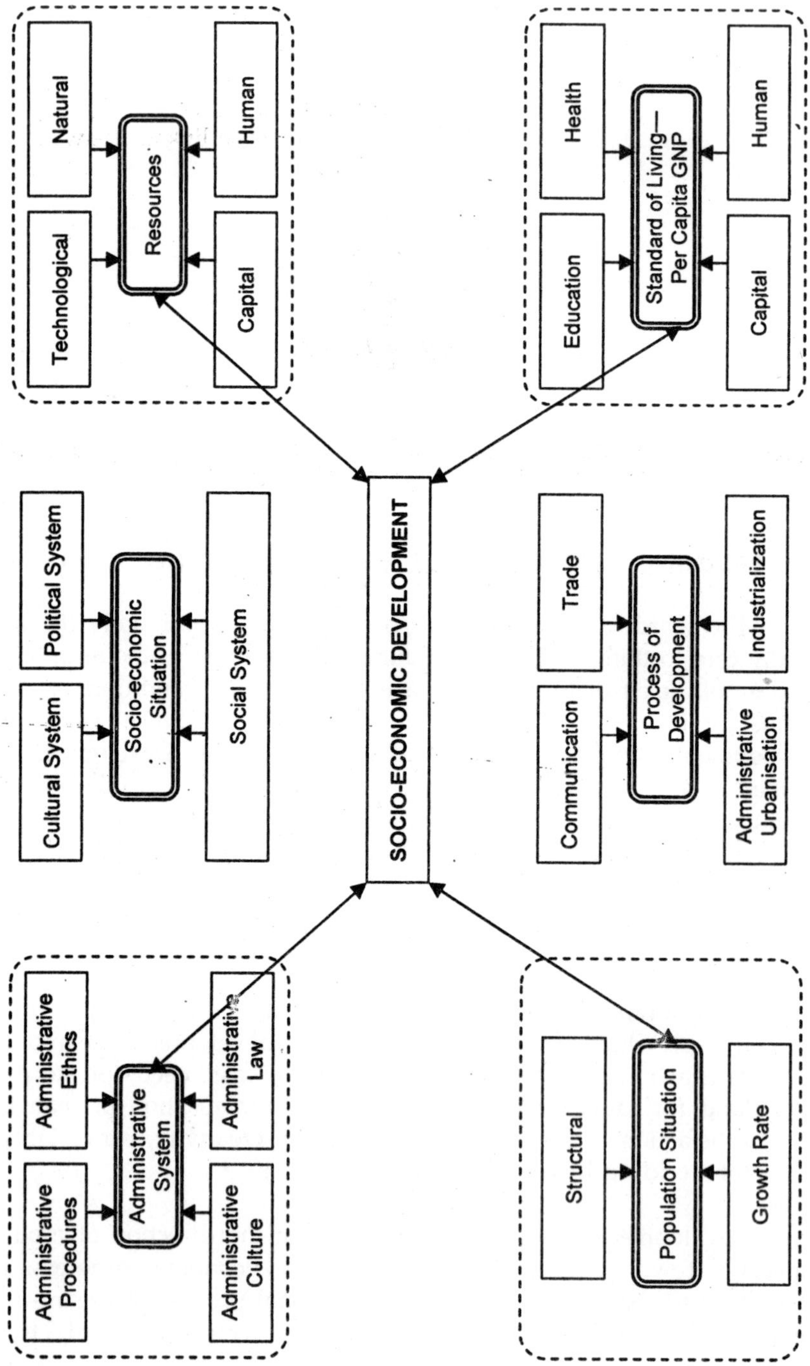
Technological
Natural
Resources
Capital
Human
Cultural System
Political System
Socio-economic Situation
Social System
Administrative Procedures
Administrative Ethics
Administrative System
Administrative Culture
Administrative Law
SOCIO-ECONOMIC DEVELOPMENT
Education
Health
Standard of Living—Per Capita GNP
Capital
Human
Communication
Trade
Process of Development
Administrative Urbanisation
Industrialization
Structural
Population Situation
Growth Rate

> "Development is a whole; it is an integral, value loaded, cultural process; it encompasses the natural environment, social relations, education, production, consumption and well-being. Development is endogenous; it brings from the heart of each society, which relies first on its own strength and resources and defines in sovereignty the vision of its future, cooperating with societies sharing its problems and aspirations."[1]

We must be clear that the development is indeed a dynamic concept. Development implies growth plus social change. Nevertheless, development has often been conceived of primarily in economic terms, since sustained economic changes are necessary for the achievement of many social goals. This is not wholly correct. According to Dr. Candua, former Director-General of the WHO:

> "Among the objectives of the development are health and productivity. They are reciprocal and complementary. Without health, productivity can hardly flourish. On the other hand, productivity may increase means and opportunities for better health."[2]

Only a man who is healthy, enjoys working and is rewarded by a high degree of productivity. The hierarchy of goals of development may be shown in the form of a pyramid wherein at the base are basic minimum needs followed by economic and social necessities for bare subsistence. The fulfilment of these needs leads to a higher set of socio-political needs and ultimately to the goal of the full flowering of human personality or 'total development' and the release of the creative energies of every individual.[3]

| | |
|---|---|
| (4) Cultural | (4) full development of human potential and creativity, |
| (3) Socio-political | (3) equity of distributive justice, social equality, redistribution of assets, democracy, |
| (2) Economic-social | (2) higher growth with greater equity, mass consciousness, and |
| (1) Basic minimum needs | (1) eradication of abject poverty and unemployment—access to minimum income and public services through employment with people participation. |

According to Mr. K.S. Dadzie, United Nations Director-General for Development and International Economic Cooperation,

> "The final aim of development must be the constant increase of the well-being of the entire population on the basis of its full participation in the process of development and a fair distribution of benefits therefrom."

Thus, the main aim of development should be to enrich the quality of life. Dr. T. Adeoya Lambo, Deputy Director-General, WHO, in his article "Towards Justice in Health" in *World Health* (July, 1979) has rightly said:

> "What is happening around us shakes our complacency, challenges our faith in human progress and imbues us with an intense feeling of shame, doubt and guilt. In a world where the gigantic scientific and phenomenal technological achievements command our admiration and almost fetish acceptance, we are witnessing an intolerable degradation of man. Our pride in belonging to a generation that for the first time since the genesis of man has set foot on another planet cannot, however, disguise the awful truth that it may be easier to travel to the moon than to erase from the surface of the earth, the image of inevitable poverty, human exploitation, injustice and the degradation of human welfare."

Our first concern is to redefine the whole purpose of development. Any process of growth that does not lead to human fulfilment or, even worse, that inhibits it is a travesty of the idea of development.

## ASPECTS OF DEVELOPMENT

In fact, there the two aspects of development-economic and social, which cannot be isolated one from the other. P.C. Sikligar in his article, "Social Development: A Profile" in IJPA, April-June, 1998, rightly stresses the complimentary role of economic and social development. To quote him:

> "The term social development was separated from economic development in 1950s by the United Nations in their report on the World Social Situation, giving an impression that the human factors, like cultural dimension, value, social security, social justice, social welfare, social service, social policy, social work, political orientation, environmental issues, etc. were neglected since time immemorial in the framework of economic development. Earlier, social development was perceived as economic growth. Later on global economists also realised the importance of human factors which were neglected to economic development. Keeping in mind the human orientations, they accepted that the entire economic development could not become social development but it could only be a part of social development. In later stages, sociologists considered inclusion of needs of social values in the process of development. They emphasised that social development is more than economic development and the necessity to ensure development in all fields related to society's dimensions. In other words, it could be said that economic development could be helpful in the process of social development in a vital manner."

## PERSPECTIVES OF ECONOMIC DEVELOPMENT: NEED OF SOCIAL DEVELOPMENT THRUST

Economic development—a high growth rate of the national product is a means to an end, i.e., it cannot in itself be the ultimate objective—the final goal of a dynamic society. Economic growth is never more than the method of obtaining the means through which a nation plans to achieve some form of social progress or social change. Developing nations have become increasingly conscious of the social aspects of economic planning. It is now generally realized that economic growth should be a means towards the eradication of hunger, illiteracy, disease, and reduction of existing social and economic inequalities. The consequences of growth without development are too painful to be ignored.[4] The correlation between economic growth and social development has tended to be low in the Asian, African and Latin American countries. In a recent study[5] this relationship has been critically examined. For this purpose, the authors devised a method of measuring development which combines social, economic and political factors. They, then studied the relationship between this measure and the per capita GNP—a usually accepted economic growth index among 74 developing countries. They found that per capita GNP is responsible only for about half of the variation in the indicators of meaningful development, bearing out the conclusion that economic growth has often failed to be really reflected in socio-economic development. The late Max Milikan had said:

> "There is a growing recognition that economic growth alone will not automatically bring with it all the virtues of modernization."[6]

In other words, there is a realisation that development is a social as well as an economic process. Because of this intimate relationship, it is very difficult to isolate social development from the economic context.

> "If this inter-relationship is not taken into account material advances may be accompanied by loss of social cohesion, insecurity, delinquency, mental stress and other social ills. In fact, the trend is now for economic planning to give way to the socio-economic planning that involves planning for the social goals, with economic development as means rather than an end."[7]

Many writers have defined economic development in a broader sense. Myrdal has defined it as nothing less than the "upward movement of the entire social system,[8] or it may be interpreted as the attainment of ideals of modernisation "such as rise in productivity, industrialization, social and economic equalisation, development of modern knowledge, improved institution and attitudes, and a rationally coordinated system of policy measures that may on the one hand remove the host of undesirable conditions in the social system that have perpetuated a state of under development while on the other hand promote better nourishment, better health, better education, better living conditions, etc."[9] After over a quarter of a century's experience and experiments with economic growth models based on western models, we find that this model stands as the 'God that failed'.

Nobel Laureate, Jan Tinbergen has rightly said:

> "The poor countries should reject the aim of initiating western patterns of life. Development is not linear process, and the aim of development is not to 'catch up' economically, socially, politically or culturally. Many aspects of western life have become wasteful and senseless and do not contribute to people's real happiness. For poor nations to attempt to imitate the rich may only mean that they trade one set of problems for another and in doing so discard or destroy much that is valuable in terms of their human resources and values."[10]

Thus began in the early seventies a search for another development (social development). To quote Mr. Mahbub Al Haq:

> "We are taught to take care of our GNP, since this would take care of poverty. Let us reverse this and take care first of poverty itself since GNP can take care of itself, for it is only a convenient summation, and not a motivation for human effort."[11]

## PERSPECTIVES OF SOCIAL DEVELOPMENT (see Chart 2.2)

Social development is a broad concept encompassing improvement in the social status of the people enriching human capital. Social development lays stress on provision of health services—education, housing, cultural amenities, protection of children, a change in the status of women, regulation of labour and improved status for workers and reduction of disease, poverty and other social illness.

According to T.K.N. Unnithan,[12]

> "Social development may be seen as a process of ushering in a new order of existence. The quality of life and the quality of social relations which exist would indicate the level of the order of existence."

ECAFE meeting of the Working Party on Social Development held at Bangkok redefines the social development as:

> "The greater capacity of the social system, social structure, institutions and policy to utilize resources to generate favourable

CHART 2.2

**Health as Management Tool for Development**

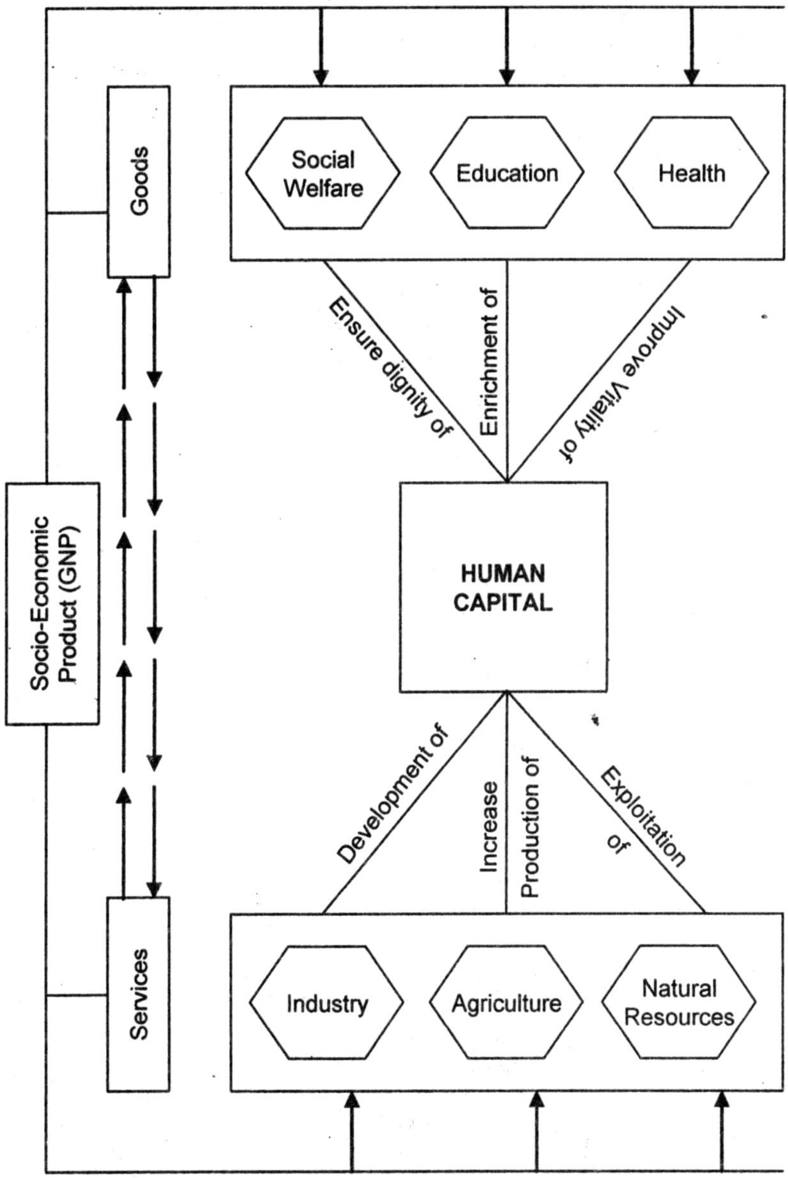

changes in levels of living interpreted in the broad sense as related to accepted social values, and a better distribution of income, wealth and opportunities."[13]

This is a comprehensive definition given by ECAFE (now ESCAP) in terms of the capacity of the social system to bring about favourable changes in the levels of living. The name of ECAFE has been changed to ESCAP to indicate the change in thrust to social development.

Social development is more concerned with the investment in human beings. A unit of investment in education, health, social welfare, etc., is, in the ultimate analysis, as productive as a unit of investment in agriculture, industry or trade. Research undertaken at the United Nations Research Institute for Social Development (UNRISD) in Geneva has indicated that developing countries, which have relatively high scores on social indicators, also tend to have high growth rates. Therefore, we must take a comprehensive view of development. Such a view of the development process would enable the planners to estimate realistically the social and economic changes and to accelerate those already taking place. Planning for 'people' must replace merely planning for aggregate production growth. According to Dr. Salima Omer, Associate Professor, University of Nebraska, USA, social development is a:

> "process that aims at the total development of people . . . social development is inter-sectoral, inter-regional and inter-disciplinary and visualises institutional and structural reforms to provide greater social justice."[14]

It has been realised increasingly over the years that social development is necessary not only to provide opportunities to individuals for self-development but also as a vital contribution to economic development. The distinction between social and economic development is no longer tenable. Economic development is necessary to achieve most social goals and social development which is in turn is necessary to achieve most economic goals. The purpose of development is to permit people to lead economically productive and socially satisfying lives.

The emphasis of the strategy of UN Second Development Decade (1971-80) as well is on growth with social justice, removal of poverty and substantial rise in the level of employment. This strategy is fully based on the idea of total development, i.e. combining the social and economic development. To quote the strategy:

> "As the ultimate purpose of development is to provide increasing opportunities to all people for a better life, it is essential to bring about a more equitable distribution of income and wealth for promoting both social justice and efficiency of production, to raise substantially the level of employments, to achieve greater degree of

income, security, to expand improved facilities for education, health, nutrition, housing and social welfare, and to safeguard the environment. Thus, qualitative and structural changes in the society must go hand in hand with rapid economic growth, and existing disparities—regional, sectoral and social should be substantially reduced."[15]

Dr. Mahler has very succinctly remarked in this connection:

"Economic growth, without being specifically attuned to human needs and human realizations, is not worth very much. Once more you hear everywhere people speaking about nuclear energy, oil energy, solar energy, wind energy and everybody seems to be overlooking the fact that without human energy, there would be no kind of progress either socially or economically."[16]

Recently, four Asian scholars viewed development in terms of fundamental humanistic values rather than in narrow techno-economic terms. They mentioned five core principles, which stand inseparably together—

(1) Man as the end of development—which is therefore, to be judged by what it does to him.
(2) Delineation of man, in the sense that he feels at home with the process of development in which he becomes the subject as well as the object.
(3) Development of collective personality of man in which he finds his richest experience.
(4) Participation as the true form of democracy.
(5) Self-reliance as the expression of man's faith in his own abilities.[17]

The three most vital players in the arena are the Elected Ruling Government, the appointment Administrative Machinery and the Demanding Public. While the ultimate responsibility and answerability/ accountability rests with the first component, the actual job of delivering results rests on the administrative machinery. It is, in the ultimate analysis a joint team effort of the three but any weak link can jeopardize the outcomes and efforts of any other causing bad governance.

It may be useful to conclude with the remarks that the process of development is holistic in nature, encompassing political, social, economic and cultural aspects.

## HEALTHCARE ADMINISTRATION AS A COMPONENT OF SOCIO-ECONOMIC DEVELOPMENT

In this work, we shall deal with one of the social services, i.e., health services. The health component and other components of the socio-economic system necessarily interact. Health not only affects the remainder of the socio-economic complex, but is also affected by it, sometimes favourably, sometimes unfavourably. K.S. Dodzie, United Nations Director-General for Development and International Economic Cooperation in his article, "The UN Answers the Challenge" in *World Health* (November, 1979) has rightly said: "The promotion and protection of the health of the people is essential to sustained economic and social development and contributes to a better quality of life and to world peace." The major areas in which health affects socio-economic development include problems arising out of the rate of population growth, rapid industrialisation and urbanisation, mental stress and social instability, environmental pollution and the growing disparity of living standards within and among nations. It needs to be reiterated here that social development not only continuously interacts with economic development but that the various aspects of social development keep on interacting with one another. 'A sound mind in a sound body' is an old proverb. Thus, changes in one sector of social activity produce changes in the other. We must see that these chain reactions are conducive to the attainment of overall objective of social development. Myrdal has summed up the position very succinctly as:

> "Standards of both health and education depend, in turn, on the whole social milieu, especially the prevailing attitudes and institutions."

In an overall and integrated concept of social and economic development of a country, health cannot be considered exclusively as an end itself. One must take into account also its role as one of the social sectors in overall development and try to establish measurable relationships between health and the microscopic variables, such as consumption, productivity and labour on which it depends or with which it is involved most directly. In other words, it is necessary to determine the investment in health required for development or the rate of development. The benefits accruing from health programmes are less difficult to measure. It is rarely, if ever, possible to identify all the consequences of a health programme, especially the long-term consequences. A health care is primarily a social service. Health programmes are mostly established because they contribute to the satisfaction of primary human needs, irrespective of economic considerations except in so far as they can be afforded and constitute an asset for the future. For this and other reasons, the cost and other data required to evaluate the contribution made by health programmes to development are rarely completely available, even when it would be feasible to obtain them.

To plan for health, that is, to meet the basic needs of the community and, at the same time, to satisfy the requirements of the overall pace for development is a complex process. It will be possible to achieve it fully when the economic benefits obtained with a specific health measure can be expressed in quantitative terms and when it is possible to measure precisely the degree of benefit to health from activities which are carried on outside this direct operational sphere. While health planners have always assumed that there is a good correlation between health and socio-economic development, doubts have been expressed by the general planners regarding such a correlation. Research is still in its infancy in this area. H. Leibenstein has rightly said that data on general relationship indicated that health and education were the most evident among the large 'residual' of factors that proved statistically more important than the usual economic indicators in explaining economic development.[18]

Prof. D. Banerji stresses the role of health as a contributor to economic growth and the need to integrate health activities into general economic activities so that the former do not interfere with the latter or *vice-versa*. Dr. E.J. Thierry in his article, "Laying the Foundations", succinctly remarked that:

> "Health is man's most precious possession; it influences all his activities; it shapes the destinies of people. Without it, there can be no solid foundation for man's happiness. Nevertheless, all too often, social planners, forget this simple truth and leave health out of account: Integration of health schemes in overall development plans are of paramount importance."[19]

The tasks assigned to health economists in cooperation with planners include the development of instruments for measuring social phenomenon; the identification of the fields of health where the maximum results can be obtained with the available resources and the provision of and in improving the management of health services (e.g., in hospital establishment).[20]

Though progress has been made in the analysis and estimation of cost and benefits in public programmes, but cost-benefit analysis in public health area has lagged behind. The economics of health is a newer term than medical economics: it encompasses the medical care industry, extends into such fields as the analysis of the economic costs of diseases and the benefits of control programmes, return from investment in education and training, etc. Many have tried to evaluate man or, in other words, to put a price upon his economic worth. One of the earliest attempts was that of Sir William Petty (1623-87) who originated many ideas later used by the political economists. Adam Smith used in his Wealth of Nations and other works; Dublin Lotka and Spiegelman have attempted to translate the figures of life expectancy into terms of financial values to the community. It was observed that the period of infancy and early childhood represent a drain upon family and community resources. This investment made towards a productive age is therefore a loss to the community, not only in the investment made but also of future earnings of the individual. But, loss due to sickness, on the other hand, is limited to the duration of illness when the individual remains unproductive or underproductive from ill-health. Let us now mention the possible direct and positive effects of health on socio-economic development.

1. Many uninhabitable areas can be made fit for settlement and thus it can help in the exploitation of idle resources of that area, e.g., in Haryana, an area of Pehowa Block was made fit through the Malaria Eradication Programme. The area was infested with malarial parasites and was unfit for human settlement. Various studies have indicated the useful consequences of disease eradication programmes on agricultural development and ultimately economic growth.
2. It can help in the lowering of absenteeism rate resulting from poor health caused by diseases. Here, we must be cautious about its limitations in the developing countries where there is widespread unemployment or underemployment and where a sick person is readily replaceable without affecting the socio-economic conditions in these countries.[21]
3. Good health can promote good labour morale and productivity; i.e., a healthy worker can work full-time and has a greater productivity potential. According to Benjamin, in these countries "where health conditions are worst and relatively simple, their low cost health programmes can produce dramatic lessening of the ability and disability of the labour force."[22]
4. Good health affects intelligence, improper nutrition and lack of mother-care can cause mental retardation and other mental problems. A study carried out by Correa and Cummins in "Contribution of Nutrition to Economic Growth covering 18 Countries for the period 1950-62, reveals that in 9 countries of Latin America, there was an increase in the national product, whereas the contribution was zero in the economically developed countries. The poorer the country, the greater the role of improved nutrition in its development.[23]
5. Good health is a basic right and produces civic consciousness. We should not look at health only as a means of economic development. What is more important is to view economic growth as contributing to the betterment of the health of the people, as it must be recognised that health is a basic human right, Thanis Kraivixien, the Prime Minister of Thailand, rightly said in his inaugural address to the 30th WHO Regional Committee for South-East Asia, held at Bangkok, Thailand (28 August, 1977);

"Any society should consider that a high quality of life, and the happiness of the people, which can only be obtained through a sufficient level of health, is not only a basic prerequisite to development but should be the basic objective of any development effort."[24]

6. Better health is generally associated with better capability and leadership. In a study by ILO on qualitative difference in the labour force, health was found to be the factor most clearly related to difference in economic growth.[25] According to Myrdal: The required personal qualities are certainly multiple and probably have a synergistic action. However, there can be no doubt that health plays an essential part."[26]
7. Better health induces positive attitudes conducive to economic growth and modernisation. The individuals become better citizens as they hope for future betterment and work hard to make the future more pleasant and enjoyable. Improved health may induce in the people to increase productivity and motivation to reduce family size.[27] The people with good health are generally enthusiastic and try to achieve higher and higher goals in life.

Let us now review some studies which have analysed the loss resulting from poor health or diseases. Sirton made an assessment of the financial loss due to malaria to the individual and the family alone at not less than Rs. 11,000 lakhs annually. In this conservative estimate of the annual financial loss to the country due to malaria; Sinton arrived at the figures of Rs. 1,000 crores. He stated:

> "It constitutes one of the most important causes of economic misfortune engendering poverty, diminishing the quantity and quality of food supply, lowering the physical and intellectual standards of the nation and hampering increased prosperity and economic progress in every way."[28]

Tuberculosis is a widespread and contagious disease. A study was carried out by Dr. A.S. Sen and Dr. R.N. Basu, Consultant and Senior Research Officer, Planning Commission, Government of India, to measure the cost of tuberculosis in India.[29] They found that the total losses from mortality, morbidity and the direct cost[30] of the disease amounted to Rs. 420.4 crores, Rs. 288.58 crores and Rs. 29.68 crores respectively. The production loss due to mortality and morbidity from tuberculosis has been very large. As compared to these losses, the amount of direct expenditure which is being incurred on the control programme is very small. The annual direct cost for a population of about six million works out at Rs. 0.49 per person per annum. Hence, the eradication of tuberculosis is not only a social welfare activity but an ultimate economic gain.

Because of this inter-relationship, economic development cannot be isolated from the social context, health programmes cannot be related unilaterally to either the economic or the social spheres, as they influence both and are influenced by both. Thus, there is a need to promote, encourage and support research on the standardization of nomenclature, systems of health statistics, indices of health and socio-economic development, evaluation methods, and health economics theory and practice. The World Health Assembly Technical Discussion on the contribution of Health Programmes to socio-economic development (1972) arrived at the following general agreement:

> "It was recognised as a basic principle that health programmes are rarely ever justified solely on economic grounds, but rather as the means of, maintaining and improving health, which is perhaps the most important single factor in improving the quality of human life. It was accepted without question that health is an objective in its own right and represents one of the most important manifestations of social progress."[31]

Thus, there is a clear indication of the need for knitting together social and economic components of development plans to attain intended objectives of development of the people, within a time schedule and resource schedule.

All the countries of Asia, Africa and Latin America should apply development planning to accelerate socio-economic development, guided by social justice.[32] Development planning relates to a teleologically-determined manipulation of policy measures and instruments devised so as to stimulate the authors of the socio-economic scene to act in the most conducive to the achievement of the national socio-economic development objectives and goals.[33] Thahane defines it as a "process of organizing national economic and social effort for the promotion or achievement of clearly defined national development goals."

The process of Development Planning can help us to get the benefits of modernisation which depends upon the "Systematic, sustained and purposeful application of human energies to the rational control of man's physical and social environment for various human purposes."[34]

The people inhabiting the developing world expect their governments to pull them out of the morass of distressing under development. This would be possible only provided the efforts of the Governments are comprehensive, selective, coordinated and sustained. Besides, timely action, backed by a strong will and determination at all decision-making and operational levels, can change the complexion of our socio-economic scene.

In the 21st century, development is going to pose a great challenge, because health of the people, which is a major component of development faces many challenges. We suggest here some ideas, which can promote health of the community and ultimately promote socio-economic development.

On the basis of our discussion and analysis, the following suggestions are given to revitalize the health care delivery system to meet the challenges and fulfil the basic health needs of the people.

(i) Will and determination on the part of the political elite, to accept innovative measures to meet the population's health needs and priorities.
(ii) Identification and implementation of a clear and comprehensive National Health Policy.
(iii) Decentralised planning, involving the participation of the target communities.
(iv) Mobilisation of existing and untapped resources—community, government (local and national), bilateral, multilateral and non-governmental—to provide adequate health care for all.
(v) Establishment of appropriate administrative structures with necessary competence and capability and devolution of authority and responsibility for the implementation and development of the programme in a team spirit and a well-designed information system to help in planning, implementation and evaluation.
(vi) Manpower development for national health needs.
(vii) Strengthening existing rural establishment and graded extension of national administrative structures to provide adequate and accessible referral, supervisory, logistical and other supporting services to ensure the judicious use of health services.
(viii) More allocation of financial resources based on the principles of equitable distribution and maximum utility.
(ix) Encouraging integration and coordination.
(x) Reorientation of Medical Education to suit the needs of the community.
(xi) Designing health technology to suit the environment and making the best use of existing technology of traditional system of medicine.
(xii) Improving research and development capacity to solve health problems.
(xiii) Devising measures to promote the use of simple, standardised equipment and drugs, placing reliance on available local resources whenever possible to foster self-reliance.
(xiv) The preventive health measures are crucial for sustained improvement and must be intensified to attain:
   (a) Total coverage of the entire urban and rural population in the country with assured potable drinking water supply and sewerage;
   (b) The disposal of urban wastes should also be given a high priority to ensure clean environment;
   (c) For improving the environmental sanitation and hygiene,

high priority must be given to town and country planning, provision of better working and living conditions, removal of congestion through the increased tempo of housing construction, slum clearance and prevention of water and air pollution;

(d) The nutritional status of the population must be raised and total prevention of food adulteration and drugs control should be achieved through rigorous controls; and

(e) Health education should be an integral part of all health programmes.

It is hoped that the implementation of these suggestions would ensure wider and more evenly distributed health care based on social justice, greater involvement and satisfaction of the beneficiaries and more efficient and more economical health services in new millennium.

O.P. Diwivedi[35] in his article, "Development Administration: an Over View" suggests challenges of sustainable development in the new millennium.

The challenge before the leaders and administrators of developing nations is then, how to achieve sustainable development and yet provide basic human needs (the provision of food, appropriate habitat, health and education), as well as social justice, removal of poverty and self-reliance with very limited resources.

They will have to be more self-reliant in the 21st Century, as they cannot expect the same level of development and as the attention of the West turns more towards helping Eastern Europe. So they must consider being self-reliant and using their own resources among and between themselves much more than they have done so far. For this they will require a cadre of professionally trained and dedicated administrators, as well as moral and just politicians who can stand against the forces of corrupt politics and unscrupulous commercial and business interests. Specially, development administrators have an obligation to serve the public in a manner which strengthens the integrity and process of governance. Such is the challenge and duty for the leaders and administrators of developing nations in the 21st Century.

Good Governance can provide all the inputs based on knowledge, creativity, innovation and motivation. People's participation, for development/productivity/efficiency and fulfil the dreams of millions of people enshrined in the constitution, budgetary, documents, five years plan and often repeated promises of the executives. Good Governance can transform a developing country like India into a developed world where India can be counted among the few top countries of the world. It is expected that the executive machinery of the government of any political party should attend seriously politically intractable problems, avoid tendency to retain power by depriving citizens of basic human rights or manipulating ethnic conflict. The party should attend to all the problems affecting socio-economic development and for promoting the process of good governance leading to development modernization, dynamism. This will make resurgent of modern India contemplated by the leadership who got us Independence. The need of the hour is to develop dynamism, development, democracy through good governance based on innovation, creativity, talent, skill, etc. in order to usher an era where there is no poverty, no exploitation, no fear, as well as all follow the ethical values. The need of good Governance is of great significance in the new and emerging areas which have to take their roots.[35]

## Notes and References


1. Milton J. Esman, .'The Politics of Development Administration," in Montgomery and Stimn, (eds.); Approaches to Development of Politics, Administration and Change, New York, McGraw Hill, 1965, p. 9.
2. Message from Dr. M.G. Candua, Director-General of the WHO, in the *World Health,* March 1969, p. 5.
3. R.C. Malhotra, 'An Alternative Strategy for Self-sustained Development with focus on Participation by the Poor at the Local Lever, paper presented to Consultative Meeting on Alternate Strategy for Development with Focus on Local-level Planning Development (from Oct. 4 to Nov. 1978)—UN Asian and Pacific Development Institute, Bangkok, April 1979, p. 5.
4. Salvatore Schiavo—Campo and Hans W. Sorger, Perspective of Economic Development (Houghton, Mifflin Co., Boston, 1970.)
5. Irma Adelman and Cyntila T. Morris, Society, Politics and Economic Development, John Hoptrus Press, 1967.
6. Max Milikan, "A Strategy for Development", Centre for Social and Economic Information, Executive Briefing Paper I, New York, 1970.
7. WHO, Public Health Paper, "Inter-relationship between Health Programmes and Socio-economic Development", 49, Geneva, 1973, p. 32.
8. Gunnar Myrdal, Asian Drama, New York, 1968, p. 1869.
9. C.E. Black, The Dynamics of Modernization, New York, 1966, pp. 55-60.
10. Jan, Tinbergen, Reshaping the International Order: a Report to the Club of Rome, New York, E.P. Dutton and Co. Inc., 1976, Chapter 5, pp. 61-64.
11. Aly, Haq., Mahbub, The Poverty Curtain, p. 48.
12. T.K.N. Unnithan, "Development Processes in an Underdeveloped Country (India)" in Carle C. Zimmerman and Richard E. Dumors (eds.); Sociology of Underdevelopment, Jaipur, Rawat, 1976 (Asian ed.), p. 402.
13. ECAFE, Seminar on Meeting of the Working Party on Social Development, (Bangkok, 8-15, December 1970).
14. UN, Asian and Pacific Development Institute, Proceedings of a Consultative Meeting, Bangkok, April 1979, p. II.
15. UN General Assembly Resolution, 24th October, 1973, para 83.
16. Text of Address of Dr. H. Mahler, Director General, WHO—WHO Regional Committee for South-East Asia, Thirteenth Session, Bangkok, Thailand, 28 Aug., 1977, Published in Final Report and Minutes of the Meeting of the Thirteenth Session, WHO, New Delhi, Sept. 1977, p. 64.
17. Haque, Wahidul, Niranjan Mehta, Anjsur Rahman and Poona Wignaraja, "Towards A Theory of Rural Development,", Development Dialogue, 1977; Dag Hammarskjold Foundation, Uppasala, Sweden in B.P. Desai; Planning in India (1951-78), Vikas Publishing House, Ghaziabad (UP), 1979, p. 158.

18. H. Leibenstein, Theories Non-traditional Inputs and Interpretation of Economic History in P. Deprez (eds.) Population and Economic History Association, Winnipeg University of Manifolia, 1968.

19. Dr. F.J. Thierry, "Laying the Foundation" in *World Health*, March 1969, p.13.

20. D.C. Banerji, (1967), "Health Economics in Developing Countries", *Indian Medical Journal*, Ass. 49, pp. 417-21.

21. WHO, Public Health Papers, No. 64, p. 20.

22. B. Benjamin, Social and Economic Factors Affecting Mortality in Confluence, Surveys of Research in the Social Services, Vol. V. (Hague Mauton Co.), 1965.

23. H. Correa and G. Cummins (1970): "Contribution of Nutrition to Economic Growth," *American Journal Clin. Nutr*, 23, 560-63 in World Health Papers, 49, p. 47.

24. WHO, SEARO: SEA/RC. 30, p. 64.

25. Galenson and G. Pyatt, The Quality of Labour and Economic Development in Certain Countries, Geneva, ILO, 1964.

26. G. Myrdal, Asian Drama—An Inquiry into the Poverty of Nations, New York, Pantheon, 1968.

27. M. Perlman, "On Health, Population Change, and Economic Developments", in M. Perlman and other (eds.), Spatial, Regional and Population Economics, Essays in Honour of Edgar M. Hoover (New York and Breach, 1972), pp. 293-310.

28. J.A. Sinon, "What Malaria Costs in India Nationally, Socially and Economically", condensed and reprinted in *Health Bulletin* in 1958, No. 26, Government of India Press, p. 125.

29. A.S. Sen and B.N. Basu, Economics of Health—The Cost of Tuberculosis Planning Commission, Government of India, Health Division, 1968, pp. 1-35.

30. Direct Cost means expenditure on hospitals, clinics, drugs, research, training, BCG vaccination, etc.

31. WHO: World Health Assembly, 1972, A/25, Technical Discussion, 66, p. 6.

32. UN: Proceedings of the Inter-regional Seminar on Organisation and Administration of Development Planning Agencies, Vol. I, p. 113 (Sales No. E.74 II, H. 2).

33. T.T. Thahane, Planning for Development, in John Barratt and others, (eds.), Accelerated Development in Southern Africa, London, Macmillan, 1974, p. 451.

34. Quoted in Marrico B. Jansen, ed., Changing Japanese Attitude Towards Modernisation, Princeton, 1965, pp. 23-24.

35. O.P. Diwivedi, "Development Administration: An Overview" in *UPA*, July-Sept. 1997, pp. 321-22.

3

CHAPTER

# Planning for Health Care

Health Planning is in essence an organised, conscious and continual exercise to select the best available alternatives which can meet the health needs of the people.

To plan is to produce a scheme for future action, to bring about specified results, at specified cost, in a specified period of time. It is a deliberate attempt to influence, exploit, bring about and control the nature, direction, extent, speed and effects of change. It may even attempt deliberately to create change. It is a carefully controlled and co-ordinated Quality. "

—*Cyril, L. Hudson*

## MEANING AND DEFINITIONS

Planning of community health services means the careful analysis, intelligent interpretation and orderly development of these services, in accordance with modern knowledge. Techniques and experience, to meet the health needs of a nation within its resources.[1] A health plan, is a predetermined course of action that is firmly based on the nature and extent of health problems, from which are devised priority goals.[2] Health planning is an aid to political and administrative authorities to decide how health services can be modernized and improved to provide effective and decent health care to the community. Health planning is not an Independent exercise, it is an integral part of the overall socio-economic development. National Health Planning has been defined as the orderly process of defining community health problems, identifying unmet needs and surveying the resources to meet them. Establishing priority goals that are realistic and feasible and projecting administrative action to accomplish the purpose of the proposed programme.[3] Planning is essentially a process of making choice between available alternatives at all levels of decision-

CHART 3.1

**Health Planning**

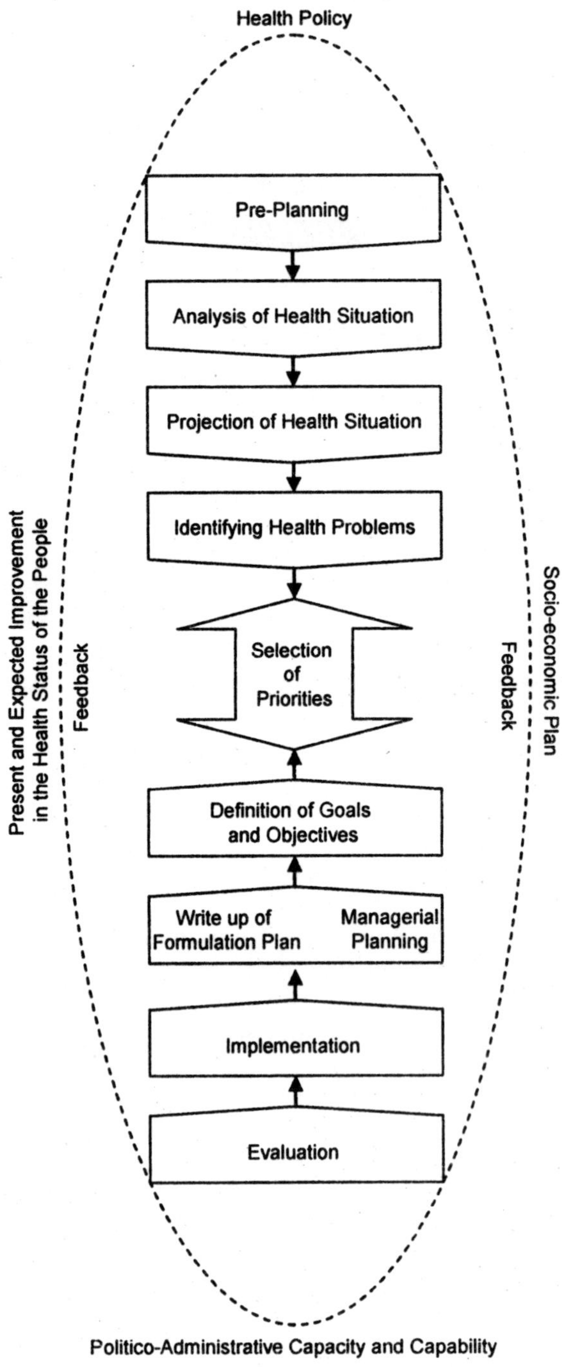

making. Planning is the exercise of intelligence to deal with facts and solutions as they are and find a way to solve problems. Planning is, in essence, an organised, conscious and continual attempt to select the best available alternatives to achieve specific goals. As expressed by Ackoff (1970, p. 1)

> "Planning is one of the most complex and difficult intellectual activities in which man can engage. Not to do it well is not a sin, but to settle it for doing it less than well is."

According to Dr. Montoya:

> "Health Planning is the phase of the total process which leads from the policy statements to the concrete identification of the populations whose needs and demands will be served; the indication of the types of activities that will be performed for those populations, with their general attributes, and the specification of the type of instruments that will be required to carry out the activities.[4]

A plan is a pre-determined course of action that is firmly based on the nature and extent of socio-economic problems, from which are devised priority goals. Planning involves choosing from among alternatives the proper course of action and calls for decision-making which is an intellectual process. Planning is not a guess work, it is conscious determination and projecting a course of action for the future and is based on objectives, facts and considered forecasts.

Planning then is just a rational approach to the future. According to Henri Fayol: "The plan of action is, at one and the same time, the result envisaged, line of action to be followed, the stage to go through, and methods to use. It is a kind of future picture wherein proximate events are outlined with some distinctness whilst remote events appear progressively less distinct."

Planning substitutes order to chaos and introduces rationality into decision-making process, it reduces random and haphazard activity. Planning makes personnel conscious of the objectives of the enterprise and thus encourages their involvement and participation. Planning promotes internal coordination and thus helps in making possible the integrated and coordinated effort, facilitates control as the top executives can compare the performance with the standard of targets laid down by the process of planning. Planning generates economy and efficiency. Terry has rightly stated that "Planning is the foundation of most successful action of an enterprise.

## DEVELOPMENT OF HEALTH PLANS

Development planning has assumed a role of far reaching importance in accelerating Socio-economic development in the developing as well as in the underdeveloped countries. It is through development plans that steady progress and modernization can be attained. These plans symbolize the national aspirations and as a whole place increasing responsibility on the governments for translating these aspirations into programmes of operation. Development Planning is an essential means for achieving a high rate of economic growth and for progressively modernizing the economy of a developing country.

Whatever mythology we may adopt, it can be successful only if it suits the prevailing environment in the developing countries. Simply transferring to the Third World the sophisticated techniques that are appropriate to the developed world will not meet the requirements, instead what is needed are simple methods that are easily adaptable. This would require that "talent for perspective among the personnel responsible for the plan formulation and implementations, and his work more effectively, an executive must develop a 'talent for perspective about himself'.

Planning is a rational process which involves a number of steps. We discuss here the important steps which may be kept in mind while planning health services at any level, i.e. Union, State or Local. Whatever be the methodology of planning, these basic steps are essential. However, the details of these steps may vary from country to country.

### I. Pre-Planning

Effective health planning would depend upon the interest of the government as manifested by clear policies framed by the political authorities and the health legislation enacted by the legislature. Besides, there should be an infrastructure to plan for health care. Administrative capability and skill in planning is the most important attribute of the health planning. The twenty-first session of the Regional Committee of South-East Asia held a technical discussion on National Health Planning in 1968. They mainly concentrated their deliberations on the pre-planning stage. The main recommendations of the technical discussion were:

"(a) Even though there are health planning units at present in some countries of the Region, it is necessary to strengthen these units as well as the relationship that exists between them and the National Planning Units.

(b) It is necessary to develop urgently realistic health plans as a part of development plans. This apart from other advantages, makes it possible for funds for health aspects of development projects to be obtained from the resources of such projects.

(c) In the pre-planning stage, the government should establish health planning units and health administrators should be adequately represented on the national planning bodies.

(d) Heads of planning units should be given a formal course of training."[5]

## 2. Analysis of Health Situation

The first step at this stage involves:

### *Assessment of the Present Health Situation*

This relates to a time from which the planning is to be done. It is nothing but setting up of a base line to help the planners to make projections for the planning period and to help in the evaluation of plans. Generally speaking, the following data would be required to analyse the present health situation:

(a) Characteristics of population—population (age, sex) cause of death statistics, morbidity data, environmental data responsible for the problems of environmental threats to health, cultural background.
(b) Data on health facilities such as hospitals, clinics, etc.—public, private and voluntary, their geographical distribution and utilisation by the community.
(c) Data on available resources, e.g., personnel, material and finance.
(d) Data on training institutions for health personnel.
(e) Data on nature and functions of health organisations.

The data collected would serve as the base for planning. Health statistics provide the key to a competent sound and efficient planning. It has been stated officially that health planning and effective operation of health services are only possible on the basis of reliable statistics.[6]

Dr. Chandrasekhar, Ex-minister of Health and Family Planning (India), emphasised the importance of this subject and said:

> "All over the region, greater efforts were needed to have better. Further, more adequate and more reliable, vital and health statistics. Health statistics were extremely poor not only in India but undoubtedly in the Region as a whole."

We can improve upon this data as suggested by the technical discussion on Health Statistics Requirements for National Health Planning by experts of the WHO Regional Committee:

"(1) The data collected should be relevant for planning purposes and sufficiently reliable for a realistic planning of health programmes and their subsequent evaluation.
(2) Closer coordination and collaboration between health statisticians, health planners, health administrators and decision-makers should be established for proper collection and utilization of health statistical data.[7]

(3) In view of the inadequate development of health statistical services and scarce statistical resources, production of superfluous data which are not required or utilised should be avoided.
(4) Training of health statistical personnel—at the professional, intermediate and lower levels—should be continued and strengthened.
(5) Data-processing facilities should be developed and strengthened.
(6) The most desirable form of organisation of health statistical services at the national level would be an adequately staffed single unit, preferably one of the same rank as other technical divisions of the Ministry of Health or of the Directorate of Health Services. Such a unit should coordinate all the health statistical activities in the country.
(7) An endeavour should be made to extend the coverage of cause-of-death statistics, but, where it is not possible to have the cause of death certified by a physician, it was felt that the reporting by auxiliary and lay personnel could be accepted."[8]

The second step under analysis is projection of the health situation over the plan period. This can be done on the basis of assumptions which can predict as to what is likely to happen at the end of plan period.

**3. Identifying Health Problems**

On the basis of the projected data, we can enumerate the health problems which need to be tackled by the plans. Current problems faced by the Health Care System, as analysed by Ninth Plan include:

1. Persistent gaps in manpower and infrastructure especially at the primary health care level.
2. Sub-optimal functioning of the infrastructure; poor referral services.
3. Plethora of hospitals not having appropriate manpower, diagnostic and therapeutic services and drugs in Government voluntary and private sector.
4. Massive interstate/interdistrict differences in performance as assessed by health and demographic indices; availability and utilisation of services are poorest in the most needy states districts.
5. Sub-optimal intersectoral coordination.
6. Increasing dual disease burden of communicable and non-communicable diseases because of ongoing demographic, lifestyle and environmental transitions.
7. Technological advances which widen the spectrum of possible interventions.

8. Increasing awareness and expectations of the population regarding health care services.
9. Escalating costs of health care, ever widening gaps between what is possible and what the individual or the country can afford.[9]

**4. Selection of Priorities**

Resources in the developing countries are limited. Myrdal has forthrighly said, "The now widely used term 'Developing countries' is one of these diplomatic euphuism the really important aspect of their situation and the meaning that seeks expression is not that they are developing, but they are under-developed, that they need to develop, and that they ought to develop, and in some cases are planning to develop."[10]

J. Brijant has also pointed out that, "The rates of economic growth for many of the less-developed countries provide a sombre picture for their future. They indicate that now and in the foreseeable future resources will be desperately limited. Indeed these limitations are relentless determinants of design of health services."[11]

Thus, available resources are insufficient to meet the needs of the people. Therefore, there is a need to select the pressing and urgent problems. There are a number of factors (Economical, Technical, Financial, Social, Political, Administrative, Ethical,, etc.) which must be taken into consideration while laying down the priorities. This can be decided with the help of techniques like cost-benefit analysis, cost-effectiveness. Priorities have to be determined at different levels. The first level is determination of priorities among various sectors of the economy. This would depend to a large extent, upon the political philosophy of the government.

**5. Definition of Goals and Objectives**

Goal is the direction in which the plan is to proceed and the term is used more in the case of long-term planning. Goals formulated are generally broad. A goal is usually described in terms of:

(a) what is to be attained;
(b) the extent to which it is to be attained;
(c) the population involved;
(d) the geographic areas in which the proposed programme will operate; and
(e) the length of time required for achieving these goals.[12]

The objective is a precise statement of the ends intended to be achieved. We must build the hierarchy of objectives, i.e. ultimate, intermediate and immediate. Immediate objectives are further divided into effort objectives and performance objectives (targets).

**6. Write-up of formulated Plan**

After deciding the priorities, goals and objectives, the next major step is to prepare a write-up of the plan. This may contain a schedule (time sequence for the plan to be implemented) and procedures (a set of rules for implementing the plan) and other details so that evaluation becomes easy and meaningful.

Before we embark upon the planning of health services, we must keep in mind the finances allocated for health. The finances allocated from 1st to 8th Plan vary from 3.3 to 1.75 per cent for health and .01 to 1.50 per cent for family planning which is quite inadequate.

**7. Strategy**

Strategy should be defined. Ninth Plan has laid down the following approach to be followed in Ninth Plan:

(i) An absolute and total commitment to improve access to, and enhance the quality of primary health care in urban and rural areas by providing an optimally functioning primary health care system as a pan of the Basic Minimum Services;

(ii) To improve the efficiency of existing health care infrastructure at primary, secondary and tertiary care settings through appropriate institutional strengthening, improvement of referral linkages and operationalisation of Health Management Information System (HMIS);

(iii) To promote the development of human resources for health, adequate in quantity and appropriate in quality so that access to essential health care services is available to all so that there is improvement in the health status of community, periodically organise programmes for continuing education in health sciences, update knowledge and upgrade skills of all workers and promote cohesive team work.

(iv) To improve the effectiveness of existing programs for control of communicable diseases to achieve horizontal integration of ongoing vertical programmes at the district and below district level; to strengthen the disease surveillance with the focus on rapid recognition, reporting and response at district level; to promote production and distribution of appropriate vaccines of assured quality at affordable cost; to improve water quality and environmental sanitation; to improve hospital infection, control and waste management;

(v) To develop and implement integrated non-communicable disease prevention and control program within the existing health care Infrastructure;

(vi) To undertake screening for common nutritional deficiencies especially in vulnerable group and initiate appropriate remedial measures; to evolve and effectively implement programmes for improving nutritional status, including micro-nutrient status of the population;

(vii) To strengthen programmes for prevention, detection and management of health consequences of the continuing deterioration of the ecosystems; to improve linkage between data from ongoing environmental monitoring and that on health status of the population residing in the area including health impact assessment as a part of environmental assessment in developmental projects;

(viii) To improve the safety of the work environment and workers' health in organised and unorganised industrial and agricultural sectors especially among vulnerable groups of the population.

(ix) To develop capabilities at all levels for emergency and disaster prevention and management; to implement appropriate management systems for emergency, disaster, accident and trauma care at all levels of health care;

(x) To ensure effective implementation of the provisions for food and drug safety; strengthen the food and drug administration both at the Centre and in the States;

(xi) To increase the involvement of ISM&H practitioners in meeting the health care needs of the population;

(xii) To enhance research capability with a view to strengthening basic, clinical and health systems research aimed at improving the quality and outreach of services at various levels of health care;

(xiii) To increase the involvement of voluntary, private organisations and self-help groups in the provision of health care and ensure inter-sectoral coordination in implementation of health programmes and health-related activities; and

(xiv) To enable the Panchayati Raj Institutions (PRI) in planning and monitoring of health programmes at the local level so that there is greater responsiveness to health needs of the people and greater accountability; to promote inter-sectoral coordination and utilise local and community resources for health care.[13]

**8. Implementation**

Plan implementation is an integral part of the planning process. It requires responsibility for translating the objectives of health plan into action. However, looking from the broader point of view, plan Implementation requires co-operation, co-ordination and commitment at all levels of the implementing machinery starting with the Ministries of Health at the Union and State levels through to the various non-secretariat organisations in the field at the district, block or village level. It is at the implementation level that the difficulties creep in resulting in lower output. Implementation must be watched properly and timely action should be taken to improve administrative, technical, financial or personnel inadequacies.

Planning and implementation are intimately connected. To quote Mr. Goetz: "Plans alone cannot make an enterprise successful. Action is required; the enterpise must operate. Plans can, however, focus action on purposes. They can forecast which actions will tend towards the ultimate objective, which tend away, which will likely offset one another, and which are merely irrelevant. Managerial Planning seeks to achieve a consistent and coordinated structure of operations focused on desired ends. Without plans, action must become merely random activity, producing nothing but chaos."[14]

Experience with the Five Year Plans has demonstrated that from the very start of the planning process, implementation is generally slow, even half-hearted, and there is a wide gap between the results achieved and the planned targets. Many of the schemes have consequently to be carried over to the next plan. It is a happy sign that the Government of India is keen to lay greater stress on implementation and that the highest priority is being given in the Plans to "Perationalize the Plan."

**9. Monitoring or Managerial Planning**

In developing countries, there is a large gap between planning and implementation. Monitoring can help in improving the situation through advance fixing of targets to be achieved in a short period of time. We can compare the achievement targets with the targets planned. If there is a gap between the two, we can locate the reasons and take remedial action. Monitoring helps to verify whether the performance is according to the time schedule.

**10. Evaluation**

Evaluation is a built-in device to measure the effectiveness of health planning. "Evaluation measures the degree to which objectives and targets are fulfiled and the quality of the result obtained. It measures the productivity of available resources in achieving clearly defined objectives. It measures how much output or cost effectiveness is achieved. It makes possible the re-allocation of priorities and of resources on the basis of changing health.[15] Dr. J.E. Asvall, Deputy Director, Bureau of Hospitals, Director General of Health Services, Oslo, Norway in his article, "Evaluation of Public Programme" mentions the problems of evaluation of health programmes. He says that inadequate evaluation is a serious weakness in health services. A key factor to the improvement of the whole health care system, evaluation has not so far been developed in the country to such a level that it fulfils the requirements of planning and management.[16] The ultimate test of evaluation should be perceptible change in the health status of the people and improvement of the quality of life. In a Foreword to the Fifth Five Year Plan, 1974-79, Prime Minister, Mrs. Indira Gandhi writes:

> "A plan is ultimately neither a mere catalogue of schemes nor a sophisticated exercise in numbers. It is a charter of the progress of a

people who refuse to be overwhelmed by the magnitude and vast variety of their problems and difficulties but are courageously struggling to map out a programme of action which will step by step and year by year help to overcome them.[17]

The following are some practical observations that may help in developing a realistic and readily implementable plan:

(i) If the plan is to be readily appreciated, it may have to be framed in terms of concepts and information in vogue among the development planners in general.
(ii) A plan should be acceptable not only to the planning authorities but to the people at large. Public acceptance, which is an essential prerequisite of public cooperation, may be won by means of a programme of plan publicity and wide public discussion of the plan. It is only through informing, motivating, encouraging and involving the people that we can best hope to improve their living condition.
(iii) A related point is that a buffer reserve of resources might be maintained to cope with sudden situations created by acts of nature.
(iv) There should be an effective mechanism to review the progress or regress and to ensure immediate re-adjustments to achieve pre-desinged output. There a need to divide the planning into programme of operation, such as annual development plans, investment plans, area plans in order to have the degree of clarity and ensure specific actions.
(v) There is a need to develop realistic targets to avoid frustration resulting from "Target Achievement Gap." Mr. H. Venkat Asubbiah, in his article, "Target Achievement Gap", in *The Tribune* (June 3, 1981) has rightly said that "the government's short-term policies and public pronouncements are increasingly tailbored to suit political exigencies of the moment. This inevitably further widens the gap between plan targets and actual achievements. More seriously, this also distorts national objectives."

## CONSTRAINTS ON HEALTH PLANNING

There are a large number of factors which stand in the way of effective health planning. We should try to overcome or minimize these constraints. These are as follows:

(a) Lack of adequate health information system for planning and monitoring and ultimately for evaluation.
(b) Natural resistance to change.

(c) The relatively low priority often accorded to health by political decision-maker and the public.
(d) The frequency of governmental, political, and administrative changes, with concurrent changes in commitments to support the plan.
(e) The imperfect state of the art of planning, i.e. absence of trained health administrator and planners, and particularly the lack of precise tools to measure need, demand, cost and benefit.
(f) The 'long time' lag between planning and implementation, particularly as regards the supply of additional health manpower and the enactment of necessary legislation.
(g) The traditional division of health professionals into compartments and the resultant lack of adequate inter-professional communication.
(h) The inflexibility of educational system.
(i) Inefficient administrative practices that limit the flexibility of the budgets, promote fragmented programmes, and result in inappropriate personnel system.
(j) Inadequate coordination of planning between the various ministries and departments concerned with socio-economic development.

## FORMULATION OF HEALTH PLAN IN INDIA

### Planning Machinery at Various Levels

Let us now discuss in brief the planning machinery responsible for the formulation of health plan in India. India has perhaps the largest tradition of planning in any non-socialist country. The nearest parallel to it in Western Europe is the French System of planning. The main difference, however, is that India has a federal structure of Government and achievement of socialist pattern of society is her avowed objective. The Planning Commission was established in March 1950, the Commission was required:

(a) to make an assessment of material, capital and human resources as well as formulate development plans for the most effective utilisation of these resources for improvement of social, human and economic conditions in the country;
(b) to indicate the obstacles in the way of planned economic and social development in the country and suggest ways and means to the government to deal with them;
(c) to suggest any change or addition to the administrative system for effective implementation of development plans proposed by it and approved by the government; and
(d) to carry out appraisals, from time to time, of the progress achieved in implementation of the development plans by the

administrative agencies or departments concerned and to suggest ways and means for improving the scale and quality of this implementation.

The Commission comprises a number of members at its head as well as a body of experts, administrators and housekeeping personnel which constitute its secretariat. So far as the members are concerned, some of them are whole-time while a few are part-time. For the preparation of Ninth Plan, for instance, there were 7 members, out of which 5 were whole-time experts including Vice-Chairman while 4 were ex-officio, i.e., Prime Minister, the Finance Minister, the External Affairs Minister and the Planning Minister. There is, however no fixed strength and thus the exact number of members may vary from time to time, depending upon several factors.

The Secretariat of the Commission includes three wings:

(i) General Divisions,
(ii) Subject Divisions. and
(iii) House-keeping Divisions.

There are at present 10 general divisions which concern themselves with the studies relating to the Plan as a whole. The branches are:

(a) Perspective Planning,
(b) Statistics and Surveys,
(c) Economic Research,
(d) Socio-Economic Research,
(e) Plan Coordination,
(f) Programme Administration,
(g) Multi-level Planning,
(h) Project and Information,
(i) Scientific Research, and
(j) Plan Information and Publicity.

There is also a Programme Evaluation Organisation which scientifically evaluates the results achieved in terms of the objectives and targets of various Sector plans, State plans, programme and projects which together comprise the National Development Plan.

Then there are 14 Subject Divisions:

(a) Agriculture,
(b) Land Reforms.
(c) Irrigation,
(d) Power,
(e) Transport,
(f) Communication,
(g) Education,

(h) Employee are Manpower,
(i) Health and Family Welfare,
(j) Housing and Urban development,
(k) Industry and Minerals,
(l) Village and Small Scale Industries,
(m) Social Planning, and
(n) Social Welfare.

These divisions maintain intimate relationship with their counterparts in the Central Ministries and State government departments. They collect, process and analyse relevant information and data as well as sponsor research for use by the Commission in the formulation of sector plans and programmes.

The House-keeping Divisions deals with records, Accounting and Routine Administration. The Subject Divisions carry out most of the Planning exercises. Each Division utilises working or expert groups on which the concerned Ministry is represented. At the Central level, a Health Planning Section was created in the Employment and Social Services Division of the Planning Commission in October 1951. In April 1956, it was made a separate and independent division. As a 'Subject Division' it helps the Planning Commission in the formulation of the health programmes and projects to be incorporated in the five-year and annual plans. It assists in evaluating performance, it carries out studies of special interest to health planning, e.g. manpower requirements of health programmes. The division works in close cooperation with the Ministry of Health and Family Welfare so that there may be an intimate relation between planners and those who carry out policies. Each division utilises working or expert group for preparation of the plan in their respective fields. The directions given to working groups are of a general nature in the beginning but become much more specific as the preparation of a five-year plan proceeds towards completion. The planning unit in the Ministry of Health and Family Welfare has the following functions:

(a) Compilation of national five-year health plan and supporting material;
(b) development of strategy for getting plans accepted and financed;
(c) preparation of the central, annual health plan and discussions with the Planning Commission and the Ministry of Finance;
(d) discussion and coordination with States on matters relating to planning developments and the financing and implementation of plans; and
(e) submission of progress reports on planning schemes to the Planning Commission.

Thus, the health plan prepared by the division in collaboration with the Ministry of Health and Family Welfare is reviewed by the members of the Planning Commission and is integrated with the total plan. Most of the health work is carried out at the State level. Health services are primarily the responsibility of the State. State Planning Boards have been set-up in many parts of India. These boards are to prepare the draft state plans by bringing about consultations between the experts, ministers, and other decision-makers as well as by seeking the views and demands of the district administration and other organisations. Except in a few States, the State planning boards have, however, yet to establish their role in a meaningful manner. They lack adequate expertise and creativity. Their position as the 'thinking tank' of the Government on social and economic problems has yet to be demonstrated and proved. *The Tribune* Editorial has rightly stated that:

> "In most States, the Planning Boards, like several 'autonomous' Corporations, have been made sanctuaries for disgruntled, defeated or troublesome politicians who tend to treat Plan funds as discretionary grants. Sinecures were deemed necessary to ensure the political support of such politicians in the struggle for ministerial survival amidst recurring toppling drives.

Inevitably, such political accommodation has led to the minimum involvement of economic experts who alone should comprise State Planning Boards. It is time the pollution of planning through politics was ended.[18]

The programme advisers are responsible for coordination and cooperation between the Union Minister of Health and Family Welfare, the Planning Boards at the State level, the Planning Bureau of the State Departments of Health, especially as regards the allocation of resources and the determination of priorities during the five-year plan.

The various groups concerned have strong preferences and influences. The programme advisors have to reconcile these conflicting interests without much friction. The Planning Commission submits the plan to the National Development Council. The Council comprises the Prime Minister as the Chairman and the Chief Ministers of States as Members while the Members of Planning Commission are its *ex-officio* members. Several Ministers of the Central Government may also be invited by the Chairman to attend the meetings as non-members, in order to put forward their viewpoints on matters within their respective ministerial jurisdiction. The Council may set-up a Committee for various subjects or fields of planning. The main functions of the Council may be summarised as:

(a) To formulate and prescribe guidelines for the preparation of the National Plan as well as to suggest ways and means for mobilisation of resources for the Plan.
(b) To discuss and scrutinizes the draft National Plan as prepared by the Planning Commission.
(c) To examine policy question arising in regard to the Plan.

(d) To review relevant questions relating to the implementation of the Plan.

The decision of the National Development Council along with the draft National Plan are sent to the Cabinets and Legislatures of all the governments in the country for discussion. These high powered organs of the Government have thus the final voice in regard to the nature and scope of plan as well as for the strategy and resources for its implementation.

How can we plan for attaining an acceptable level of health for all in 21st Century? The Government must make an unequivocal political commitment including required legislations and introduce the health reforms (as suggested by the expert agencies) that are essential if the delivery of health care to all by the legendary of new century is to become a reality.

The health administrators lack the art of health planning. This results in giving low priority to the programmes directly or indirectly affecting health services. In the past, the health administrator has rarely made a contribution in the planning process to the totality of the plan. He has been advocating only for expenditure on health services without realising that the programmes of education, agriculture, community development,, etc., also contribute indirectly to the health of the people. To quote Myrdal:

> "From the Planning point of view the effect of any particular policy measure in the health field depends on all the policy measures and is, by itself, indeterminate. This means that it is impossible to impute to any single measure or set of measures a definite return in terms of improved health conditions. A generalised model, in aggregate financial terms, visualizing a sum of inputs of preventive and curative measures giving rise to an output of improved health conditions, cannot be of any help in planning."[19]

Thus, there is a need of training health administrators in the art of planning. The WHO has been encouraging the training of health administrators in institutes of health administration. Strangely enough, it was found that most of the health experts trained in the art of planning were not engaged in planning activity resulting in the wastage of the resources of the sponsoring organisation and the training institutions. It is suggested that the young people from the health departments may be selected, trained and made responsible for planning. In the developing world, the senior positions are occupied by elder people who do not want to be trained. Thus, there is a need to create a special cadre for health planners, besides imparting general training for health planning to all. The training institutions should not be satisfied with their passive role of training health experts in the art of health planning but should see that the knowledge provided during training is being made use of effectively and the situation is improving. The health administrators lack the techniques of management and personal qualities which are essential for successful health planning. Planning is a complicated and complex process and health administrators have to convince all concerned for developing meaningful health planning. There are still a number of problems requiring solutions with regard to coordination, communication and inter-relationships between the many individuals and organisations involved. The head of the health planning team and the health project officer will have to develop considerable skill in the political, administrative and technical areas. The health administrators will have to work hard in preparing health plans acceptable to policy-makers.

Health planning methods need modifications to suit the social, political and economic environment prevailing in the country. We have already discussed in brief the different methods being used in different countries. The understanding of health planning process and methodology in different countries throughout the world will equip the health administrators with a broader horizon of health planning. There is still plenty of room for information to develop new patterns and variety of approaches. The health administrators should not adopt blindly any approach which has been successful in some countries.

They must find out the methods most suitable to the macro-environment prevailing in their own countries. The health planning should be based on the needs of the population. A population base, in contrast to an institutional disease, or diagnostic base, is absolutely necessary for objective planning and evaluation. The health planning should encourage people's participation. People should form an integral part of planning process. V. Subramaniam writes:

> "A people's plan cannot be a people's plan unless it has an inbuilt flexibility so that adjustment and mid-term corrections are possible in the light of several factors and circumstances which come to the fore during the implementation of the programrne."[20]

## CONCLUSION

During the Ninth Plan, efforts were further intensified to improve the health status of the population by optimising coverage and quality of care by identifying and rectifying the critical gaps in infrastructure manpower, equipment, essential diagnostic reagents and drugs. Efforts were directed to improve functional efficiency of the health care system through:

(a) Creation of a functional reliable health management information system and training and deployment of health manpower with requisite professional competence.
(b) Multi-professional education to promote team work.
(c) Skill upgradation of all categories of health personnel, as a part of structured continuing education.

(d) Improving operational efficiency through health services research.
(e) Increasing awareness of the community through health education.
(f) Increasing accountability and responsiveness to health needs of the people by increasing utilisation of the Panchayati Raj institutions in local planning and monitoring.
(g) Making use of available local and community resources so that operational efficiency and quality of services improve and the services are made more responsive to users needs.[21]

The success of socio-economic development in a developing country like ours depends upon the degree to which plan strategy has been carried out. The essence of development involves the setting up of a planning machinery with a view to utilizing the resources in an economical and efficient manner, so as to promote the well-being of the people and to increase the Gross National Product. The process of development planning can help us to get the benefits of modernization which depends upon "Systematic, sustained and purposeful application of human energies to the rational control of man's physical and social environment for various human purposes.[22]

It is clear that poor planning may upset the programme results. However, we may keep in mind that excessive planning can divert valuable managerial resources from the present utilization. Rigid enforcement of the detailed plans can kill the programmes by stifling initiative deviation from detailed task specifications should be allowed if high level targets are nevertheless achieved. Therefore, there is a need that the planning itself must be clearly anticipated in advance so as to ensure that it will make a positive contribution to the programme.

## Notes and References

1. WHO, Technical Reports Series, 215, 4, (1961).
2. WHO, Public Health Paper, 46, p. 9.
3. WHO, Public Health Paper, 44, p 15.
4. Dr Montoya, "Programme Technology In the Context of Health Planning", Unpublished.
5. Gunarantee, *op. cit.*, p 10.
6. WHO, *WHO Chronicle*, 1966, No. 20, pp. 301-9.
7. WHO, SEARO, 20th Session of the WHO Regional Committee for South-East Asia, New Delhi, October, 1970, p. 101.
8. WHO, SEARO, SEA, RC 24/16 Rev I, 1 October. 1971. p. 38, Annex. 4.
9. Ninth Five Year Plan, *op cit.*, p. 139.
10. G.Myrdal (1968), Asian Drama, an Inquiry into the Poverty of Nations, New York, Pantheon, Vol 3, p. 1841.
11. J. Brijant, 1969, Health and the Developing World, Ithaca and London, Council University Press, p 26.

12. WHO, Public Health Paper, 41, p. 31.
13. Ninth Five Year Plan. *op. cit.*, pp. 140-41.
14. Billy E. Goetz, Management Planning and Control, New York, McGraw Hill, 1949, p. 63.
15. WHO, 1967, Technical Reports Series No. 350.
16. WHO, *WHO Chronicle*, Vol. 27, No. I, pp. 3-5.
17. Govt. of India, Planning Commission, Fifth Five Year Plan, 1974-79, New Delhi, p. vii.
18. *The Tribune*, Chandigarh, 1st August, 1979.
19. G. Myrdal (1968), Asian Drama, an Inquiry into the Poverty of Nations, New York, *Pantheon*, Vol. 3, p. 1618.
20. Subnamaniam, V, "The Citizen and Planning" in the *Indian Journal of Public Administration* (New Delhi), Vol. XXI, 3, July-Sept, 1975, p. 57.
21. Ninth Five Year Plan, *op. cit.*, p. 139.
22. Quoted in Marrico, B. Jansen, ed., Changing Japanese Attitude towards Modernization, Princeton, 1965, pp. 23-24.

4

CHAPTER

# Decision-making

"The decision-making process involves problems to be solved, a number of conflicting objective to be reconciled, a number of possible alternative courses of action from which the 'bests' has to be chosen and some way of measuring the value or pay off of alternative courses of action."

—*Donald J. Clough*

## DECISION-MAKING

Good decision-making in a health system is essential for decent, health care to the people. Decision-making is done at all levels but it requires more rationality at state level health department, District health system and PHC as many decisions are taken at these levels to facilitate health services. It is very essential for health functionaries to understand the process of decision-making to take rational and realistic decisions to ensure good health services at a minimum cost. Let us understand the meaning of decision-making.

Webster's dictionary defines decision-making as "the art of determining in one's own mind upon an opinion or course of action." Shull and his associates define the decision-making process as ".... a conscious and human process, involving both individual and social phenomena, based upon factual and value premises, which includes a choice of one behavioural activity from among one or more alternatives with the intention of moving toward some desired state of affairs."[1]

According to Ishwar Dayal, "Decision is the commitment of the decision-maker to act, thereby committing the personnel, material and financial resources of the organisation towards the action objectives.[2]

Emory and Niland view a decision as only one step in an intellectual process of differentiating among relevant alternatives. It is . . . . ."the point of selection and·commitment . . . The decision-maker chooses the preferred purpose the most reasonable task statement, or the best course of action."[3] According to Hodge and Johnson, "Decision-making is to solve any obstacle (problem) that stands between decision-maker and the accomplishment of the organisation." According to Donald J. Clough: "The decision-making process involves a problems to be solved, a number of conflicting objective to be reconciled, a number of possible alternative courses of action from which the 'best' has to be chosen and some way of measuring the value or payoff of alternative courses of action."[4] According to Kreitner: "Decision-making is a process of identifying and choosing alternative course of action in a manner appropriate to the demand of the situation. The act of choosing, implies that alternative courses of action must be weighed and weeded out." According to Manley H. Jones: "Broadly, decision-making involves making organisation committed to adoption of a specific course of action and use of resources in a particular manner."

New health problems demand new solutions and top health functionaries who can come out from the routine are highly prized. This requires creativity in the sphere of decision-making. Newman has indicated the distinct stages the knowledge of which can help the health professionals at top level in this process:[5]

1. *Saturation*: to be familiar with the problem.
2. *Deliberation*: to consider alternate solutions and to rearrange them.
3. *Incubation*: to let the subconscious mind work on the problem.
4. *Illustration*: to get the new ideas and sensing that it may work.
5. *Accommodation*: to work out the new ideas so that it is a practical solution to the problem.[6]

Hicks gives the following types of creativity in sound decision-making:

1. *Innovation*: creativity to think totally new ideas.
2. *Synthesis*: creativity to absorb, combine and use ideas from different sources.
3. *Extension*: creativity to use old or new ideas.
4. *Duplication*: creativity to use others' successful ideas.

According to W. Brooke Groves, "Decision-making is the selection from two or more reasonable possibilities of a course that will, at the time and under circumstances, provide the most suitable solution of the problem at hand."[7]

## ESSENTIALS OF DECISION-MAKING

### Capabilities to take Worthwhile Decisions

The techniques of decision-making are important but more important is the skill and commitment on the part of the top health executives to take scientific decisions as these decisions would affect the lives of the millions of people. To be successful in developing decision-making skills, decision-makers must go beyond a willingness to accommodate to change; they must want to create change and to control the situation surrounding them because they have identified worthwhile things to do and they want to do these things. Men can't develop decision-making skills unless they are action-oriented and want to do worthwhile things.[8]

Louis A. Allen in his book, "Management and Organisation", has rightly said that a person is born with the talent for personal leadership but must learn management leadership. There is a need to equip the top executives in the art and science of decision-making rather than dealing merely with the operative management. Ralph Currier Davis in his book, "The Fundamentals of Top Management," has made a fine distinction between the two. He writes, "Administrative management is chiefly group management. Operative management is chiefly project management. The former is concerned largely with long time projections of the activities of Organisational groups. Operative management is concerned largely, with the short times actions in the execution of specific projects." Operative management is like a business mechanic who has learnt his executive trade chiefly in the school of "hand knocks" by the process of trial and error. Administrative management is like a professional executive who is trained in the art and science of management, decision-making and also equipped intermittently, who can adjust the management to maintain internal and external equilibrium and keep the Organisation stable and efficient.

### Using Multidisciplinary Approach

Decision-making is a complex process and is influenced by a number of disciplines—social sciences, physical sciences, pure sciences, mathematics and applied sciences. Health experts should understand the implications of all these aspects to arrive at sound decisions. Decisions for the health of people have not only to be logical but acceptable to the people also. We can represent the inter-disciplinary framework of decision-making with the help of the Chart 4.1

### Knowledge of Environment

Decisions in the domain of health affect and are affected by political, economic, social and cultural factors prevailing in the environment. Therefore, decision-making must be suited to the environment. The same decision may not be correct under two different sets of circumstances. A continuing situation of necessary interaction between an organisation and its environment introduces an element of environmental control in the organisation.[9]

CHART 4.1

**The Inter-Disciplinary Framework of Decision-making**

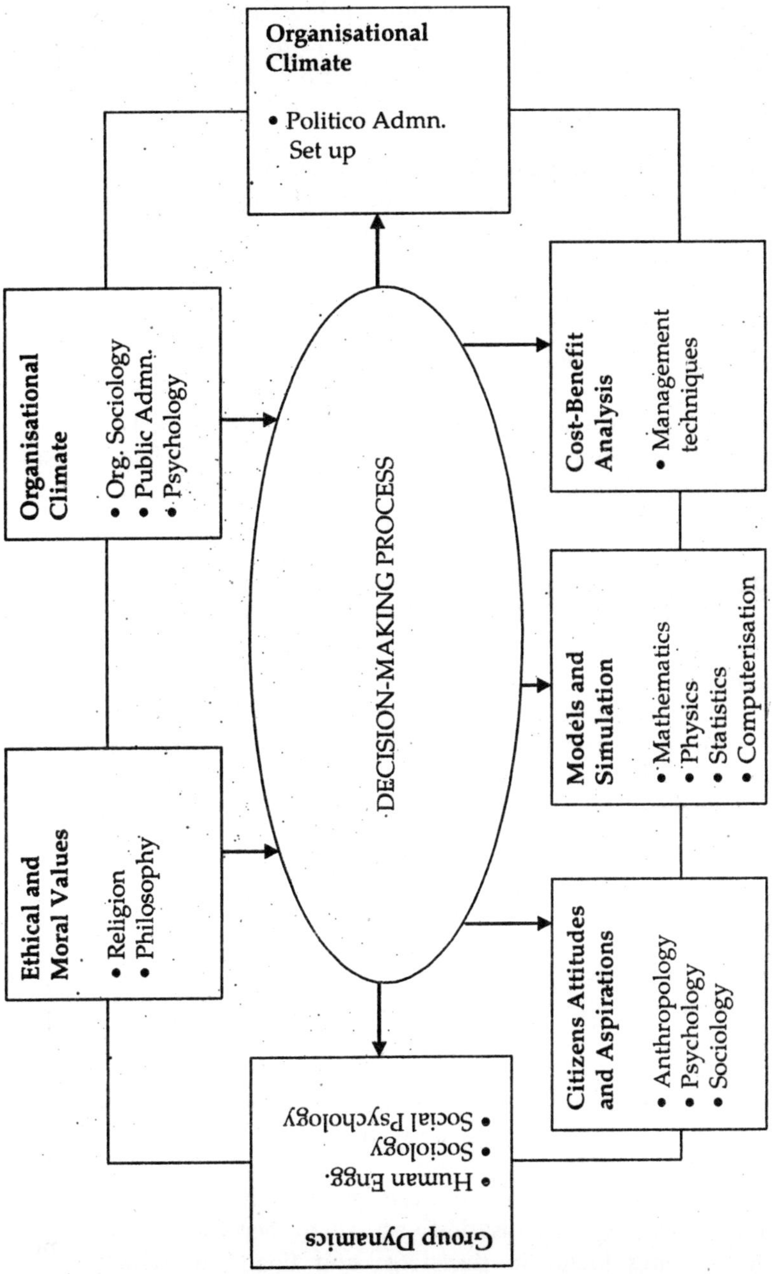

**Familiarity with the Aspirations of the Clients**

Decisions are the means and not the ends. Decisions affect the health care of the people directly or indirectly. Therefore, it is useful to consult the people interested in the decision, such as interest groups and the pressure groups, etc. Pt. Nehru had rightly said that the administrators should not retire in their cells but should mix with all kinds and conditions of people. From them, they will earn the things that are not in their files.

**Personnel and Organisational Requirements**

In a complex health organisation, there must be genuine goodwill between the superiors and the subordinates. This requires health leadership equipped with technical knowledge. Leadership must be innovative in taking decisions. We can sum up in the words of Simon who suggests that the process of decision-making includes three identifiable and essential phases. "The first phase of decision-making process searching the environment for conditions calling for decision. I shall call intelligence activity (borrowing the military meaning of intelligence). The second phase—inventing, developing and analyzing possible courses of action-I shall call design activity. The third phase-selection of a particular course of action from those available. I shall call, choice activity:[10]

**Data Base (Management Information System)**

Social, political and economic data are indispensable for decision-making. Information is the most important and crucial ingredient of the decision-making process. It is now well recognised that the decisions that a health executive makes today and the efficiency with which he discharges his functions and responsibilities, depend to a large extent on the quality of information which he is able to obtain, and the manner in which he uses this information. Decision-making in today's complex situation and environment requires scientific basis. With large number of variables some of them uncontrollable; more and more quantitative information is required to enable the health executives to take rational decisions. It is now less of imagination and personal judgment and more of quantitative analysis which is needed for providing the health executives with the different alternative courses of action, clearly bringing out the implications of following of each course of action, so that the executives may be able to take their decisions after considering all relevant aspects. In order to take right decisions they must get certain information—nothing more or nothing less—in the right form and at the right time. The aim of health administration is to develop an intellectual climate in which the non-rational elements are reduced to a minimum, in which, therefore, administrative organisation as such becomes less important as a determining factor in decisions; and finally in which the logic of the situation narrows the possible choice to one right answer.

### Knowledge of Management Techniques

There are many management techniques available which can help the health executives in taking quick and accurate decisions. The executives must learn these techniques so that the decisions made by them are sound. These techniques, wherever applied, have proved useful in good decision-making.

## PROCESS OF DECISION-MAKING

For health executives to make a wise decision, we must engage in five distinct steps as shown in Chart 4.2. These steps, however, are quite elusive and difficult for the average individual to follow in attempting to reach a wise decision. Most of us take a decision on the basis of emotions or hunch rather than logic. Therefore, it is necessary for the top-level and the middle-level health executives to take decisions on the basis of the steps outlined below. Let us analyze these steps in detail.

### Problem Identification

Diagnosing the problems is an essential step for rational decision-making. The ability of health executive to identify problems can be compared to that of a medical doctor diagnosing human problem. Sometimes, a decision-maker is led astray by identifying the symptoms as causes and when he subsequently treats the symptoms, he fails to eliminate the cause of the problem. Therefore, it is necessary that the problem is recognised and identified, and not simply the symptoms. In this step, the decision-maker must separate the relevant from the irrelevant; the material from the immaterial; the important from the unimportant. In this step, clear thinking and open-mindedness should prevail. Once the real problem has been identified and thus stated. The decision-maker enhances the chances of solving it to a large extent. The old proverb that 'a problem defined is a problem half solved is more than true in this situation'.

There are no definite steps in regard to problem identification. Handerson and Suojanen have indicated four main steps for the problem identification. In some situations, all of these may not be required. These are:

(a) determine expectation through present standards of performance,
(b) record actual performance by observation and measurement,
(c) observe differences between expected performance and actual performance, and
(d) identify the problem as to who, what, how and why of the observed differences.[11]

### Problem Analysis

Problem analysis is the next step in successful problem-solving.

CHART 4.2

**Decision-Making**

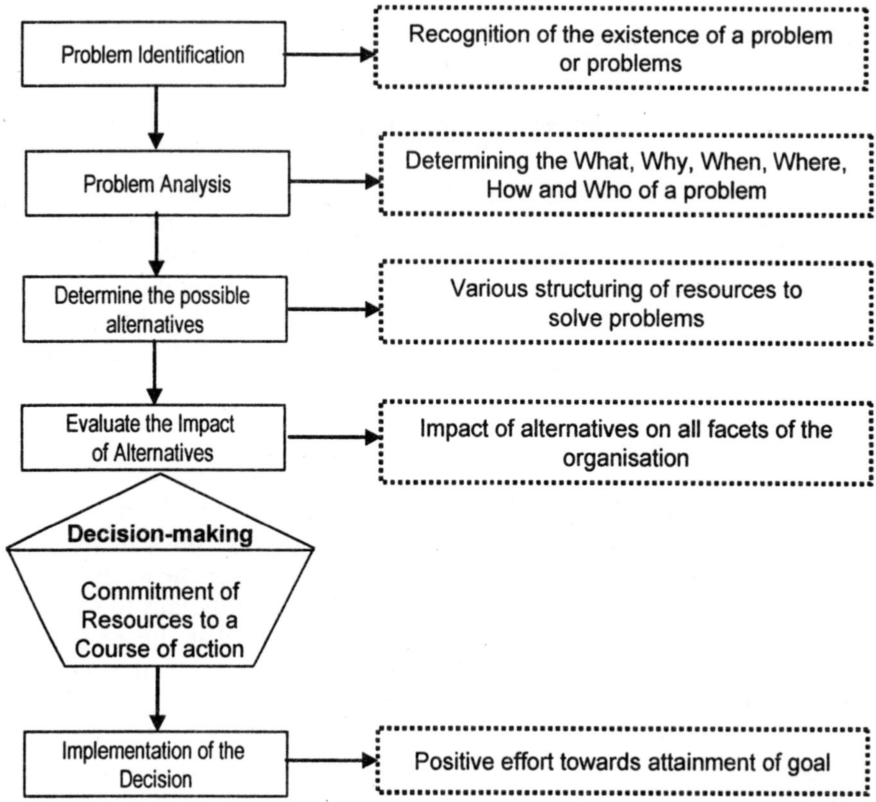


Henderson and Suojanen have suggested four steps to help problem analysis:[12]

(a) Classify the problem—separate symptoms from problems; describe the causes and nature of the problem. If it is too large, sub-divide it.
(b) Search for and gather data—combine additional information with what is known and determine their relationships.
(c) Analyse data—determine if the data is useful in isolating and describing the problem.
(d) Evaluate the data—relate the data to symptoms and causes for initial development of solutions.

**Determine Possible Alternatives**

This is a difficult step in decision-making. The decision-maker should keep in mind all logical solutions to the problem and not only those which tend to shape up his preconceived or pet solution. The emphasis should be to minimize the impact of previous solutions to the problem. There is nothing wrong to take into consideration the previous solutions but the thing to be avoided, however, is relying on these previous solutions as the only source of ideas. In trying to generate new alternatives, it is useful to list all and even the most remote alternative, one can think of on a piece of paper. Alternative solutions are in fact our only tool to mobilise and to train the imagination. Decision made without considering alternatives may have unfortunate consequences. Drucker makes this point succinctly in the following passage: "Whenever one has to judge, one must have alternative among which one can choose. A judgement in which one can only say 'yes' or 'no' is no judgement at all. Only, if there are alternatives can one hope to get insight into what is truly at stake. A decision without an alternative is a desperate gambler's throw, no matter how carefully thought it might be. If one has thought through alternatives during the decision-making process, one has something to fall back on, something that has been thought through, that has been studied, that is understood. Without such an alternative, one is likely to flounder dismally when reality proves a decision to be inoperative."[13]

**Evaluation of the Impact of Alternatives**

The decision-maker now takes into account each alternative solution to the problem and weighs it in terms of the parameters within which the decision must be made. In fact, the manager is here forecasting the impact of certain alternative, if it is implemented. If the decision is of national importance, then the views of public advisory committee, pressure groups and interest groups are also obtained. In brief, we can list four steps for determining possible alternatives and examining their impact.

(a) Identify resources—list everything available to assist in solving the problem.
(b) Develop alternative solutions—develop various combinations of resources leading to solutions of the problem.
(c) Test each alternative, analyse for:

Suitability will it solve the problem completely or partially, permanently or temporarily?

Feasibility—will it work? how much will it cost? can we afford it?

Acceptabilily—is it acceptable to those involved and responsible?

(d) List benefits, cost and risks associated with each alternative—is each alternative an improvement? can benefits and cost of action be weighed? what are the odds and successes of each alternative?

Drucker has rightly said that the right decisions grow out of the clash and conflict of divergent opinions and out of the serious consideration of competing alternatives.

**Selection of an Alternative**

This is the final stage of the decision-making. All the alternatives except the one chosen are cut-off. There are four important criteria for picking the best solution:

*(a) Measurement of Risks and Gains*

The executive has to weigh the risks of each course of action against the expected gains. He is to find out the ratio between the expected gains and the anticipated risks. The alternative in which this ratio is high may be selected as the decision.

*(b) Economy*

That course of action may be adopted which would give the greatest results with the least efforts.

*(c) Timing*

Decision concerning timing are very difficult to systematize. In an epidemic situation, as it recently happened in Orissa, Gujarat (during Disasters) the health experts must take immediate timely decisions before the diseases spread and take a mass toll of life and become uncontrollable.

*(d) Availability of Resources*

The most Important resources are the human beings, who will carry out the decision. No decision can be implemented efficiently without qualified people, who have to carry it out. Therefore, there is a need to find talented people either inside or outside the organisation, who have the capacity to implement the decision.

The selection of the alternative should be based upon the information collected and the judgement desirable to consider whether the selected alternatives will meet the approval of others, who will be involved in the implementation of the decision.

## TECHNIQUES OF DECISION-MAKING

The art and science of decision-making provides us a variety of approaches, methods, methodologies and techniques useful for taking high quality decisions. A decision-maker, in fact, stands between past and future events. Ideally, he finds a frequency pattern in the past that, projected into the future, gives hint of the probability of recurrence which is nearly all the precise quantitative knowledge he can obtain concerning the future. It is very difficult to discuss all these methods and techniques. We shall concentrate here in describing briefly some of the important methods:

1. Decision on the basis of past experience (Historical).
2. Experimentation.
3. Quantitative techniques.

Before we discuss these techniques, we must be clear that the quality of decision-making also depends to a great extent upon the attitudes of the personnel associated with the decision-making. P.R. Dubhashi has rightly said that decision-making, however is not a matter of mere formal system. If they are motivated by will to achieve, desire to deliver the goods, to show results, if they have a sense of urgency, a sense of function and commitment then they will look at everything positively and try to take decision rather than to delay them. If they only wish to play safe to shirk responsibility, and to pass on the buck to others, then they will make references which are not needed which results in delay and loss of public interest.[14]

### Decision on the Basis of Past Experience

Most of the decisions taken by the top health executives are generally on the basis of the past experience. The health managers can take care of the mistakes committed earlier perceptibly or impercepably. This is why most of the organisations while appointing top executives insist on some experience in the line earlier. This method is good, if it is applied to repetitive activities and changed conditions may be kept in mind. However, the past experience may not suit the situations which are entirely new, or there has been complete change in the organisational ecology. To quote Koontz and O'Donnel: "If experience is carefully analysed rather than blindly followed and if the fundamental reasons for success or failure are distilled from it, it can be useful as a basis for decision analysis. A successful programme, a well-managed company, a profitable product promotion, or any other decision that turns out well may furnish useful data for such distillation. Just as no scientist hesitates to build upon the research of others and would be foolish indeed to duplicate it, a manager can learn much from others."

We may keep the following facts in mind to make this technique as a valuable guide to rational decision-making:

(i) An effective record of the past experience must be kept so that it can be retrieved whenever needed.
(ii) Past experiences must be analysed in today's and future environment.
(iii) Past experience must be analysed critically to ensure their utility in the future.

### Experimentation

It is better to do experimentation wherever possible before taking a final decision. In most of the health organisations, we try the impact of the particular decision through a pilot project. After examining the impact of this pilot project, it is either extended to the entire area/field or stopped. Recently, the Ministry of Health and Family Welfare took decision to start reproductive and Child Health Services (RCH) in some districts of the states of the Indian Union. Based on the outcome of the results of this pilot project, it was decided to take up this project throughout the country and Ministry of Health and Family Planning has come out with RCH-11.

The difficulties with this technique are that it would require a lot of money, material and personnel resources to test the efficacy of a decision. It may also take a very long time before we ascertain the impact of that decision. As there would always be a time gap between the experimentation with the decisions and the ultimate decision, there is a possibility of future changes as future may not duplicate the present.

### Quantitative Techniques

In the words of Emory and Niland, "The Contribution of quantitative techniques to decision-making is largely in the appraisal step—the analysis of decision possibility. Quantitative techniques are unable to suggest hypotheses or to define problems or to suggest alternative.

These abilities remain in the domain of personality, experience and creativity. But, once alternatives have been defined, these techniques can be powerful tools for making quick and accurate appraisals:[15]

We must always keep in mind that quantitative techniques are only an aid to management for better decision-making. These are no substitute for better decisions. Many techniques would be discussed in separate chapters. We concentrate here on some of the techniques which can improve rational decision-making. We can classify these techniques as follows:

- (a) Techniques which can help the management in taking decisions under certainty or deterministic situations, e.g., cost benefit analysis, marginal analysis, network analysis, etc.
- (b) Techniques which can help the management in taking decisions under risk, but the decision-maker knows the probability of each risk. Here we can use techniques like operational research.
- (c) Techniques which can help the management in taking decisions under uncertainties. Here we can make use of the utility theory or preference theory and decision trees.

## GROUP DECISION-MAKING AND ITS TECHNIQUES

In today's world, a large number of decisions are usually taken by a group of people rather than an individual, e.g. in the health department, these are taken by its committees. We may distinguish here between policy-decision and day-to-day decision. Policy-decisions are generally taken by a group, while the individual decides on the pattern of day-to-day decisions, i.e. there is very little discretion vested in the individuals to avoid favouritism and nepotism. Group decision-making is a must in complex situations, dealing with multiple aspects, and to deal with such situations we generally appoint committees, study teams, task forces review panels, expert committees, etc. Group decision-making is significantly influenced by the climate and culture of organisations and the action profile of its members. Democratisation and dispersal of power are the basic ethos for effective group decision-making. In a health system, decision-making involves different specializations, therefore, group decision-making would enhance its value. For example, in All India Institute of Medical Sciences, we have Academic Committee, Administrative Committee, etc. to take group decisions.

## APPROACHES TO DECISION-MAKING

Broadly speaking, there are three widely held approaches towards the process of decision-making:

1. Rationalist Approach
2. Humanistic Approach
3. Integrative Approach

### 1. Rationalist Approach

This classical approach presupposes that a number of alternatives are available—based on mathematical analysis and logic. This approach considers reason as a superior source of knowledge and expands the ability of the manager to avoid unsought and undesired consequences.

A variant of this theory is the approach of March and Simon in viewing the organisation seeking a satisfying solution rather than an optimum one. According to this view, "The central concern of Administrative theory is with the boundary between the rational and the non-rational aspect of human social behaviour. Administrative theory is peculiarly the theory of Intended and bounded rationality of the behaviour of human beings who satisfy because they have not the wits to maximise."

The rationalist approach is recommended by Dror also. He mentions its five limitations as:

1. Too strong dependence on quantifications.
2. Impossible to deal with conflicting values.
3. Precise criteria indispensable.
4. Special characteristics of the political resources.
5. Inability to deal with large and complex system.

### 2. Humanistic Approach

The humanistic process is discussed by Chester Bernard in his book, "Functions of the Executives." He states that the ultimate decision may not be the result of logical processes, but may be determined by an approach developed within a framework of social and environmental conditions, past and present. Perceptions and past experience highly influence the decision-making in this approach. The basic elements of the humanistic solution to a problem are:

(i) The Social setting or environment of the decision-making.
(ii) The nature of the decision-making.
(iii) The goals of the decision.
(iv) The social impact of the decision.

### 3. The Integrative Approach

An integrative decision process combines both the rational and humanistic, the economic and social, authoritarian and the autonomous in such a way that all members of the work group feel better. This approach is most successful when decisions are made by those who do the work at the scene of the action rather than by those occupying executive offices, a long way from the firing line. Rational, ethical, economic and social considerations must be considered concurrently during the decision-making.

## Advantages of Group Decision-making

*Promoting Realistic Objectives*

Groups possess greater cumulative knowledge and facts as the member represent different specialisations and thus each can contribute from his angle and help in sharpening the decision to be made. The individual may take the decision in a hurry, while all the pros and cons are thoroughly examined by the member of a group.

*Developing Alternatives*

Since a group consists of many members there is a possibility of any alternatives before a decision is finalized. Individual may be biased in favour of one-sided approach while the group examines all the available alternatives before finalising.

*Participation and Support from Members*

Since the decision is taken with the help of members, therefore, they support it during implementation. They are ready to owe any responsibility for any lapse, etc. They are more satisfied with the decision and are more likely to support it.

*Group Cohesion*

Members of a group while deciding collectively develop certain common attitudes, beliefs and emotions. These feelings and beliefs, over a period of time, get strengthened and develop group norms.

*Promotes Action*

Member involved in decision-making understand all the limitations and, thus can be effective in implementing the decision effectively and economically.

*Promotes Effective Communication*

Members of the group develop better understanding through communication among them—a sine quotation for good decision-making and implementation.

*Promotes Satisfaction*

Members feel satisfied by contributing their viewpoints to the problem. This keeps the members happy and active.

*Promotes Interest in Risk Decisions*

It has generally been observed that groups generally are more prone to take riskier and difficult decisions than individuals. Four reasons are advanced for it:

(a) Risk-takers are able to persuade moderate member and prevail upon them to change their views on risk decisions.

(b) Members after becoming familiar with the issues feel more positive and confident to take risky decisions.

(c) Responsibility for decision-making can be shared, thus avoiding the fear of being pinpointed.

(d) Risk-taking offers an opportunity for group members to become the leader. Dominant and clever members generally occupy the leadership 'berth' in a group.

**Disadvantages**

Group decision-making has many drawbacks which may be mentioned here:

*1. Dominance of a few Members*

It has been seen in all plural decision-making bodies that few individuals usurp all the powers and whatever they decide is echoed by all.

This phenomenon was first discussed by Jains (1971). It refers to a mode of thinking in a group in which the seeking of concurrence among members becomes so strong and compulsive that it overrides any realistic appraisal of alternative courses of action. Members exhibit a tremendous desire for unanimity. In this, some individuals become mere showpieces. This phenomenon can be seen in most of the organisations. For example, Members of Parliament go by the decision of their party and thus lose their identity. Members of the group meet informally and chalk out the strategy to get the formal decision passed without much discussion. This is generally happening in most of the organisations. The personal experiences of the writer, as a member of the Board of Directors, Senate of a University, etc. clearly reveal that most of the members become ineffective or are made ineffective by some individuals who emerge as key persons and thus reduce the group decision-making to individual decision-making.

*2. Delays*

It takes a lot of time for all the members to find time and meet. Besides, it takes a lot of time in decision-making as all the members have their viewpoints and it becomes impossible to integrate them.

*3. Avoids Responsibility*

The group consists of many members and hence it becomes easy to pass the buck and avoid responsibility.

*4. Generates Conflict*

A final decision which does not incorporate ones viewpoint results in conflict and even sometimes rivalry.

## INFORMATION TECHNOLOGY AND DECISION-MAKING

In these high tech times, marked by a revolution in informatics and electronics, an effective administrator has to be a 'knowledge worker' in the service sector, which is 'knowledge' or 'information industry'. In such an industry, we receive information, process information and produce information as an output of decision-making. The time has come where there is hardly any scope of 'arbitary' and 'ego-based' decision-making. The behaviour of subordinates will be controlled not perhaps through the code of conduct rules but through better knowledge and information on the part of the boss. Hence, the information skill of the decision-maker in getting information, in storing information and using information is going to be the crux and future decision scenario.[16]

T.K. Rama Chandran in his Article, "Information and Systems Management in Government" in the Administrator, Oct.-Dec. 1997 rightly suggests the role of information system in decision-making. He says that millions of man hours and rupees are lost because right information is not available to the right person at the right time. Decisions are therefore, based on half-based information and is perhaps out of date; inaccurate or misleading. ....During a drought a few hundred bore wells were to be dug and a proposal to purchase some drilling rigs was put up for urgent clearance. When he asked as to how many bore wells were in existence, nobody seemed to know. Then he wanted to know how many rigs were already available and their locations. Again nobody knew however the purchase had to be made and there was no alternative but to go ahead with the order. Here was a case of decisions having to be taken without necessary and sufficient information being available with all the concomitant implications in terms of higher cost and inefficiency of resources use that the nation can ill-afford.

**Advantages and Disadvantage of Group Decision-making**

| *Advantages* | *Disadvantages* |
|---|---|
| 1. A group has more information than an individual. Members drawn from diverse fields can provide more information and knowledge about the problem. | 1 Groups are notorious time-wasters. They may waste a lot of time and energy, clowning around and getting organized. |
| 2. A group can generate a greater number of alternatives. It can bring to bear a wider experience, a greater variety of opinion and more thorough probing of facts than a single. | 2 Groups create pressures towards conformity and like group thinking forces members as to compromise on the least common denominator. |
| 3. Participation in group decision increases acceptance and commitment on the part of people who now see the solution as their own and acquire a psychological stake in its success. | 3. Presence of some group members, who are powerful and influential, may intimidate and prevent other members from participating freely. Domination is counter-productive; it puts a damper on the groups best problem-solvers. |
| 4. People understand the decision better because they saw and heard it develop; thus paving the way for smooth implementation of the decision. | 4 It may be very costly to secure participation from several individuals in the decision-making process. |
| 5. Interaction between individuals with varied view-points leads to greater creativity | 5 The group consists of several individuals and hence, it is easy to pass the buck and avoid responsibility |
| 6. Groups may also be able to capitalize on individual talents, allowing individuals to work on problems at which they most adept-specialization of labour. | 6. Disagreement over arriving at a decision may lead to conflict, resentment and ill-feelings between group members. |
| 7. Groups can accumulate more knowledge and facts. | 7. Groups often work more slowly than individual. |

| | |
|---|---|
| 8. Groups have a broader perspective and consider more alternative solutions. | 8. Groups are often dominated by one individual or a small clique, thereby negating many of the virtues of group procedures. |
| 9. Individuals who participate in decisions are more satisfied with the decision and are more likely to support it. | 9. Groups are often dominated by one individual or a small clique, thereby negating many of the virues of group procedures. |
| 10. Group decision processes serve an important communication function as well as a useful political function. | 10. Over-reliance on group decision-making can inhibit management's ability to act quickly and decisively when necessary. |

*Sources:* (a) J.L. Gibson, J.M. Ivanewich and J.H. Donnelly Jr. Organisation Behaviour, Structure and Process, Daltas, Business Publications, 1979, p. 117.

(b) R.A. Baron, Behaviour in Organisation, NY, Allyn and Bacon Inc., 1983, pp. 359-60.

## CONCLUSION

The decision-making process is a major function of management. The techniques the decision-making have been dominated mainly by quantitative models. New effective techniques applicable to the more basic decisions have not kept pace with the management science techniques. There are only a few creative techniques (brainstorming and synetics), and participative techniques which are not equal to the sophistication of the quantitative models. Yet, it is the basic, uncertain management decisions which are crucial for organisational success Irvin Summers and major David E. White in their Article "Creative Techniques—Towards Improvement of the Decision Process", Academy of Management Review, April 1976 have rightly concluded that exporting organisation assumptions and decision-making procedures inhibit organisations from attracting individuals with the most ability to provide unusual solutions. Implementation of explicit creativity techniques can attract these individuals to organisations and provide legitimacy and psychological safety for them. Creativity techniques do not replace management judgement in the risky process of decision-making. These techniques do have the potential to improve the process by improving the quality and quantity of inputs to those the must take the final decision. Techniques such as Delphi, nominal grouping, and heuristics offer some hope, but much more needs to be done in this important but neglected area of management decision-making. Besides, all these techniques have been experimented in the context of developed countries. Much more experimentation and application of these techniques are required in the developing countries like India, to ensure rational and acceptable decisions in complex organisations."

## NOTES AND REFERENCES

1. Fremont, A. Shull, Jr. L. Delbecq, Andre and L.L. Cummings, Organisational Decision-Making, McGraw Hill, New York, p. 31.
2. Ishwar Oayala. "Organisation for Public Policy in Government", Paper presented to the Indian Institute of Public Administration, Annual Conference, New Delhi, 20-10-1973.
3. C.William Emory and Powell Niland: Making Management Decision, Boston: Houghton Miffin, 1968), p. 12.
4. Clough, Donald J.: Concepts in Management Science, Prentice Hall of India, New Delhi, 1963, p. 51.
5. William, Newmann, H. and other, The Process of Management, Englewood Cliffs, NY. Prentice Hall, 1967, pp. 338-45.
6. Herbent G. Hicks, The Management of Organisation, McGraw Hill, New York, pp. 169-71.
7. W. Brookes Groves, Public Administration in a Democratic Society, Beston, 1950, p. 434.
8. Phillip, Marion. Developing Decision for Action, Taraporevala Publishing Industries, Homewood, Illinois, 1972, p. 212.
9. James D. Thompson and William J. McEwen, "Organisational Goals Environment", in A Sociological Reader on Complex Organisations, 2nd Edition, Amitai Etzion, Ed. Rinchan and Winston, New York, 1969, p. 190.
10. H.A., Simon, The New Science of Management Decision, New Delhi, 1990.
11. Richer I. Handerson and W. Soujanen Waino, The Operating Manager, New Delhi, 1975, p. 150.
12. *Ibid.*, p. 151.
13. Peter F. Ducker, The Effective Executive, Harper and Row, New York, 1967, p. 151.
14. P.R. Dubashi, "Expanding Decision-making in Public Administration", in *IJPA*, Vol. XXII, No. 1, 1976.
15. William E. Emory and Powell Niland, Making Management Decision, Houghton, Boston, 1968, p. 115.
16. N.K. Kulshrestha, "Management in Public Administration, The Decision Anatomy X-rayed", in *IJPA*, January-March, 1994, p. 45.

# 5

CHAPTER

# Supervision

> In the words of Halsey, it is "Selecting the right person for each job, arousing in each person an interest in his work and teaching him how to do it; measuring and rating performance to be sure that teaching has been fully effective, administrating correction where this is found necessary and transferring to more suitable work or dismissing those for whom this proves ineffective; commending whenever praise is merited and rewarding for good work and, finally, fitting each person harmoniously into the working group—all done fairly, patiently and tactfully so that each person is caused to do his work skillfully, accurately, intelligently, enthusiastically and completely."
>
> —*Halsey*

Planning, communication and supervision are the three main steps in the process of direction of health programmes and activities. Like every other aspect of organisation, supervision is also becoming very complicated and complex. The responsibilities of a supervisor have increased and a good supervisor is expected to have the qualities of head and heart besides his professional competence in his area of health activities. There is an old saying that "which is not inspected is not done." Hence, inspection, overseeing and supervision arise in response to the needs inherent in the functioning of an organisation.

Supervision is a compound word and its two parts are 'super' and 'vision', which means overseeing. In a hierarchical organisation, no one can claim to work without proper supervision. Generally, each officer is given certain powers and responsibilities and is supposed to be responsible to the officer above him for proper execution of the decision and use of delegated powers. Moreover, for proper functioning of an organisation, it is very essential that there should be proper coordination and link among different parts and organs of an organisation. It is also to be ensured that departments of an organisation do exactly the work which is expected of them. In common parlance, by supervision we mean direction accomplished by authority. In a broad sense, we mean superintendence and overseeing. Margarel Williamson has defined supervision as "a process by which workers are helped by a designated staff member to learn according to their needs, to make the best use of their knowledge and skills and to improve their abilities so that they do their jobs more effectively and with increasing satisfaction to themselves and the agency."

According to Millett, supervision entails two primary purposes. "One is to achieve coordination among the component parts of an agency. Since broad program goals are usually divided in operation among several different units of an organisation, management must make sure that the parts proceeded in a concerted and harmonious adjustment with each other. The second purpose is to ensure that each unit of an agency accomplishes the task each has been assigned." Williamson defines supervision "as a process by which workers are helped by a designated staff member to learn according to their needs, to make the best use of their knowledge and skill and to improve their abilities so that they do their jobs more effectively and with increasing satisfaction to themselves and the agency."

In the words of Halsey, it is "selecting the right person for each job, arousing in each person an interest in his work and teaching him how to do it; measuring and rating performances to be sure that teaching has been fully effective, administering correction where this is found necessary and transferring to more suitable work or dismissing those for whom this proves ineffective; commending whenever praise is merited and rewarding for good work; and, finally, fitting each person harmouniously into the working group—all done fairly, patiently and tactfully so that each person is caused to do his work skillfully, accurately, intelligently, enthusiastically and completely.

Health Officer and his team do supervision over the health institutions in the district. At PHC level, medical officer and Health Assistants are supervisors of sub-centres. Supervision is the most neglected area in the health departments. There is a lot of indiscipline in the field level institutions. These need be looked into during supervision and put the health system on sound footing.

## STYLES OF SUPERVISION

There are three styles of supervision:

(a) autocratic;
(b) anarchic; and
(c) democratic.

**Autocratic**

Here, the supervisors expect the subordinates to do what they have been asked to do. There is no choice with the subordinates. They have to follow the dictates of the supervisor right or wrong. Such style is very damaging, as the initiative of the subordinates is stifled. However, such a style may be used:

(a) to achieve consistency in operations;

(b) to deal with an emergency situation, like communal riots, epidemic, natural calamity, etc.; and

(c) to deal with subordinates with limited skills, capability and experience as well as with those who are not dependable.

**Anarchic**

Here, the supervisors are in practice non-existent, i.e. they tell the subordinates to do what they like. The workers have complete freedom. Such a situation is very dangerous and produce, very poor result.

This is a situation prevailing in many health departments in India. Every subordinate is becoming an island to himself with little supervision from above. Such a situation has developed as the supervisors have not been selected on the basis of merit.

**Democratic**

Here, the supervisor makes use of democratic or consultative method. i.e., he involves the subordinates. This makes the subordinates responsible and, thus. develops initiative in them. Such supervision is desirable, in general, and in particular:

(a) to deal with senior and highly qualified people, e.g., a Secretary Health to the Government of India supervising Joint Secretaries;

(b) to deal with responsible and reliable subordinates; and

(c) to deal with work needing creativity.

The style of supervision, thus, would depend upon the job factors (complexity, difficulty, creativity, quickness and consistent results) and personal factors (Skill, Reliability, Willingness, experience, etc.)

However, in normal circumstances, a democratic supervision can be said to be an ideal choice. "The supervisor on the lower levels secures cooperation and production by de-emphasising his own ego, stimulating group participation, and encouraging the maximum satisfaction of individual egos that is consistent with coordination.[1] Since health activities require uniformity as well as individual initiative, therefore, the supervision has to be tailored to the needs of the system.

**Essentials of Supervision**

For supervision to be effective, the following principles need to be observed:

*(a) Development of Agreed Work Standards*

Supervisors and subordinates may develop work standards and norms of performance against which supervision can be done. This would avoid the subjectivity of supervisor and subordinates. Such standards can be revised and appraised in the context of internal and external factors at a given period of time.

*(b) Developing Forms for Reporting*

Supervisors can design carefully the report forms which can help him in ascertaining the work of the subordinates. These procedures and contents of reporting can ensure smooth relations between the supervisor and the subordinate

*(c) Resolving Conflicts*

Supervisor should not allow any misunderstanding to continue among subordinates. These need to be resolved, otherwise the subordinates may paralyse the functioning of organisation. Supervisors must be prompt to remove all irritants either from top or from the colleagues to keep the subordinates functional and purposeful.

## CONTENTS OF SUPERVISION

It has been observed that supervisors in the health system conduct supervision superficially and intermittently, without any planning and follow-up. The result is the wastage of money on tour programmes and prevalence of poor condition of health services at field level. We mention here some of the ingredients of supervision, which need to be kept in mind by the supervisors to improve the performance at lower levels. These are: (a) knowledge of job contents, (b) administrative aspects, (c) relationships with the beneficiaries and the public, (d) personal interests, and (e) reporting and follow up.

**(a) Knowledge of Job Contents**

The first and foremost requirement of supervision is to ensure that the workers and supervisors understand their job. In this context, the supervisor has to be an expert as he is supposed to guide the health workers. It has been observed that the health supervisors in developing countries like India generally do not keep in touch with latest developments in their area of specialization as they are appointed on the basis of seniority. Younger elements, who work under the supervisors are more aware of the latest developments. Such a gap in supervisor's knowledge makes supervision superfluous. It is suggested that supervisors must be

CHART 5.1

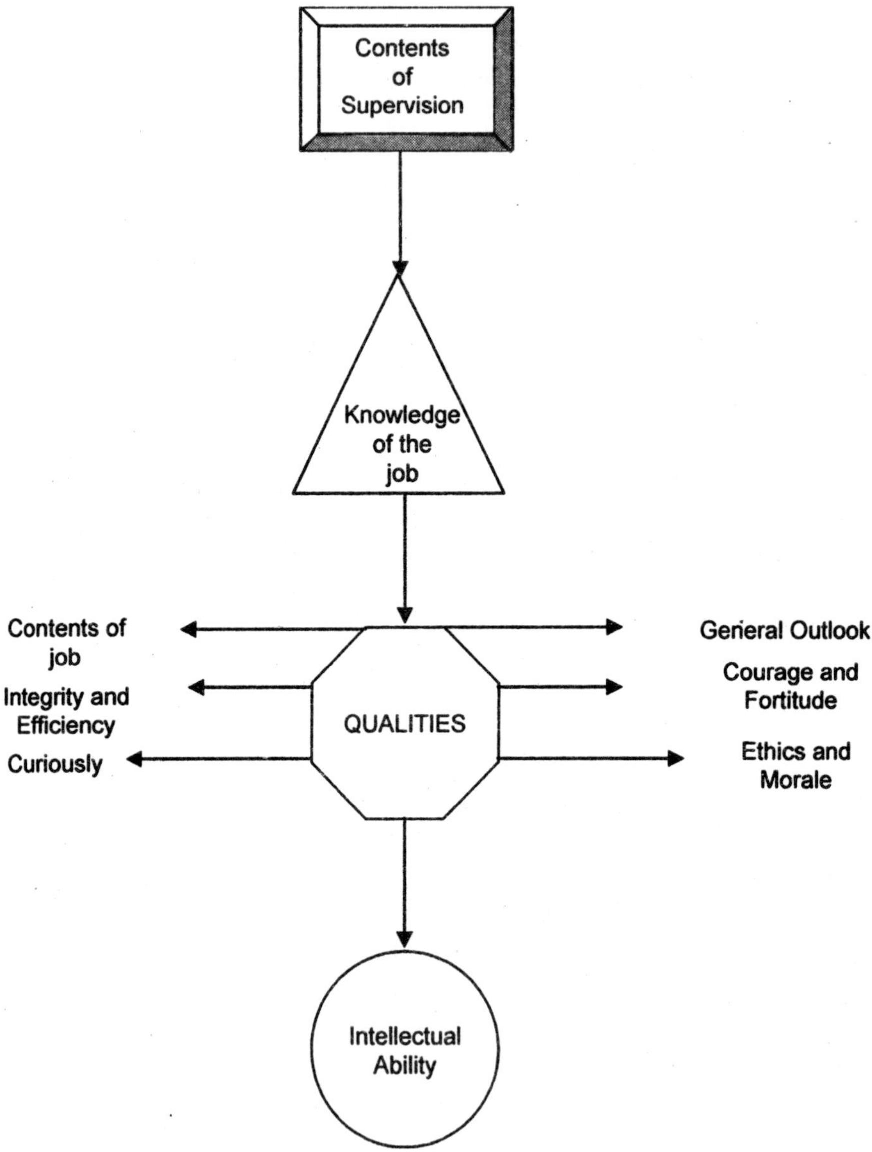


highly equipped in the field to check. Guide and motivate the subordinates. The multipurpose workers in District Ropar confided in the author and told Health Assistants are not well versed with their subject and cannot guide them in solving problems.

### (b) Administrative Aspects

Here supervision ensures proper upkeep of hospital equipment, records, etc. Supervisor is also to ensure that proper records of financial transactions are being kept and also that the equipment is being maintained. It has been seen that subordinates generally indulge in window dressing during the visit of the supervisor and this practice should be discouraged. Supervision should lay emphasis on improving the administrative system on a permanent basis.

To illustrate this with a personal observation, District Health Officer was to visit some PHCs where the author was also staying. The subordinates were extremely busy a week in advance of the visit of DHO to make the PHC tip-top from all angles. As soon as he left, the subordinates became callous.

### (c) Relationships with the Beneficiaries and Public

Administration has not merely to be good but it should be felt by the people as such. Supervisors need to know from the beneficiaries their reactions to ensure their participation. Supervisors should listen to the complaints/grievances of the people peacefully and instruct the subordinates to deal with the complaints. Such supervision would help in generating smooth relationship between citizens and administration.

### (d) Personal Interest

The supervisors should ensure the interest of subordinates in their work. There is a need of encouragement and morale boosting. The supervisor should have training in human relations, public relations and human dynamics. Supervision and control should ensure higher efficiency through clarification and encouragement by the supervisors. John D. Millett rightly observes: "Supervision is more than a process, it is a spirit which animates relationship between levels of organisation and which induces maximum administrative accomplishment, or when unsuccessful generates administrative paralysis. Effective management is concerned to realise the first and to avoid the second."[2]

### (e) Reporting and Follow-up

Supervisors need to prepare report of supervision, which can guide both the subordinates and the supervisor in future. Such reports can develop sufficient material for diagnosis and improvement. The remarks in the reports must be followed up to keep the subordinates alert. The test of the efficiency of supervision is the action on reports, i.e., the follow-up. Nigro has identified the following aspects of the supervisor's job.

(i) To satisfy their employee's desire for recognition.
(ii) To keep them informed.
(iii) To allow subordinates to make as many independent decisions as possible.

(iv) To avoid invading the specialist's bailwick.
(v) To keep the door open for conference and consultations with subordinates.
(vi) To accept the probability of being unpopular with at least a few subordinates.
(vii) To avoid over-optimism.
(viii) To assure the proper interpretation and execution of orders.
(ix) To abolish useless regulations.
(x) To recognise that assistants will sometimes be more intelligent than oneself.
(xi) To make no promises that cannot be fulfiled.
(xii) To expect loyalty, and give it, too.
(xiii) To avoid discrimination even in favour of a friend.
(xiv) To resist undue pressure and fight for the interests of subordinates.

Supervisory methods: These can be:

(i) Staff meetings.
(ii) Training seminars.
(iii) Review of Records.
(iv) Observation.
(v) Discussion with people.
(vi) Discussion with colleagues.

## QUALITIES OF A GOOD SUPERVISOR

Supervisors are the key persons in the health system of a Government as the success of the implementation of health policies depends to a great extent upon their ability, interest and experience. Supervisors can kindle interest into subordinates through their guidance and interest. According to J.M. Pfiffner[3] a good supervisor should possess the following eight qualities:

(1) Command of job content, i.e., expert knowledge of the work to be done;
(2) Personal qualifications like integrity; teaching ability, i.e. the ability to communicate his ideas to the workers and make them understand the management's point of view;
(3) General outlook, i.e., the supervisor should love his job and be absorbed in it and inspire those under him;
(4) Courage and fortitude, i.e., the ability to take decisions and assume responsibility;
(5) Ethics and morals, i.e., freedom from vices having social disapprobation;
(6) Administrative technology, i.e., the ability to manage;
(7) Curiosity, i.e., receptivity to new ideas; and
(8) Intellectual ability, i.e., intellectual alertness, etc.

Preparation of a check-list designed according to the health care services offered would ensure systematic supervision approach. According to Halsey, there must be an adequate and reasonably well balanced development of six qualities in a supervisor, viz., (1) Thoroughness, (2) Fairness, (3) Initiative, (4) Tact, (5) Enthusiasm, and (6) Emotional control.[4]

According to Chester Bernard, subordinates obey authoritarian command only when: (1) they understand what the order is and what purpose to achieve through their collective effort; (2) they feel in their cognition that the command is consistent with the organisational purpose and in obeying they are trying to be moral beings respecting a commitment; (3) they realise and understand that the command is the authority as issued and is compatible with their personal interests. If they see some gain or their personal interests are served in obeying the command, they generally accept it; (4) they know that they are qualified, competent and capable of complying with the orders. In other words, the nature of the command is such that they are mentally and physically fit to execute it.

Supervisors should possess personal and human relations quality. Professor Pfiffner has rightly summarised the importance of human characteristics of supervision in these words: "pattern of leadership desirable in supervisory positions is based upon behaviour emphasises co-operation, participation, consultation, and satisfaction for the egos of the rank and the file, even though the strong leader may have to subdue his natural desire for assertion and self-display." At another place he writes: "The supervisor on the lower levels secures cooperation and production by de-emphasising his own ego, stimulating participation, and encouraging the maximum satisfaction of individual egos that is consistent with co-ordination." The Hawthrone experiments (Elton Mayo group) and Michigan Studies have proved that employees can be most effectively motivated by people-centred and democratic leadership and by favourable institutional environment.

There is need for training supervisors in the art of successful supervision. In the words of Halsey:[5] "It has been demonstrated time and again that almost any person of normal intelligence and sincere desire to be of service to people, can acquire considerable skill in the art of supervising people, if he studies its principles and methods and apply them thoughtfully, conscientiously, and persistently. The personality of the successful supervisor of people is made up of a number of qualities and these qualities are made effective through the use of certain definite techniques. I believe, too that the qualities necessary to achieve success in supervising people can be developed and that the required techniques can be taught and skill in their use made permanent by practice. I believe that because I have seen it done by both old and new supervisors, and seen their department improve as they became better supervisors."

Besides, the qualification and qualities mentioned above, supervision should be mature enough to take timely action, based upon the given situation, rather than allowing the situation to deteriorate. For this, it is suggested that training programmes may be arranged frequently for supervisors to train them in the art and science of supervision.

The above conclusions definitely suggest that effective supervision depends in the final analysis upon "supervisors who understand people not just in groups but as individuals, different from one another, with varying interests and desires. Supervision means harnessing the productive energies of many persons into a common endeavor so that the desired output is realised to the fullest extent possible. No such objective can be realised without full attention to the peculiar characteristics of the people who make up any organisation.[6]

The ultimate purpose of supervision is to remove irritants from the path of field workers, provide them technical guidance where required and encourage them to serve better and in excellent way.

## Notes and References

1. J.M. Pfiffner, The Supervision or Personnel Human Relations in the Management or Men, NY, Prentice Hall, 1951, p 215.
2. John D. Millett, Management in the Public Service (New York; McGraw Hill Book Co., 1954), p. 98.
3. *Ibid.*
4. Halsey, G.D., Supervising People, p. 6.
5. *Ibid.*, p. 8.
6. Johan D. Millett, *op. cit.*, p. 122.

# 6

CHAPTER

# *Communication, Coordination and Control*

"Communication, coordination and control are the key for the efficiency and economy of the organisation. These are the lubricants of the engine of the Organisation. These are the life lines of administrative systems."

*—Author*

## COMMUNICATION

Barnard has viewed it as the means by which people can be linked together in an organisation to achieve the objectives of the programme.1 Health activities involve multi-dimensional aspects carried out by different functionaries. Therefore, it is essential to make all of them appreciate the intentions of health programme. Let us take the case of malaria control programme. It involves doctors, paramedical people, spray men, etc. To make the programme succelisful, all units communicate among themselves.

Communication is an integral pan of every function of health administration "and that is why it is said to be the bloodstream of an organisation." It is a two-way process between people. In communication a message is trar.smitted and received.[1]

| **TRANSMISSION** | ⇄ | **RECEPTION** |
|---|---|---|
| Message transmitted is the first half of the communication | | Message received and understood is the second half of the communication |

The art of effective communication is one of the key factors dictating the quality of human relations and also the professional performance level. Communication can be transmitted through audio-visual and audio-visual means. Communication plays the same role as the nervous system in a body. Norbert Wiener has rightly observed that communication is the cement that makes an organisation. Communication is central to the exercise of authority in an organisation.

In the words of Ordway Tead, "Communication is the touching of mind by mind, of person with person, whether it be one man, or a thousand. . . . It can include conversation, interview, dialogue, visual technique carefully used:"[2]

In the context of administration and management, William Scott defined communication as a process which involves the transmission and accurate replication of ideas ensured by feedback for the purpose of eliciting actions which will accomplish organisational goals.[3]

To quote Goddard: "Efficient communication are essential to all aspects of effective administration. Staff must be adequately and currently informed about plans, methods, schedules, problems, events and progress. It is necessary that instructions, knowledge, information be passed on for practical application to all concerned, and that they be so clearly presented as to make misinterpretation or misunderstanding impossible, proper and adequate communication is not just in one direction. It requires two-way passage. Administrators must be certain that they know and understand the problems of workers for whom they are responsible. Communication must flow from the bottom upwards, as well as from the top down."[4]

The most efficacious method of enhancing organisational effectiveness is bridging the communication gap between individuals and never allow the fog of misunderstanding to cloud human relations. Broadly speaking, communication is the means through which intentions of the programmes are translated to ensure fruitful results. It may even be looked upon as the means by which special information inputs are fed into social systems.[5] It is the means by which behaviours of the personnel engaged in the programme is modified; change is effected, information is made productive and goals are achieved." Barnard has viewed it as the means by which people can be linked together in an organisation to achieve the objectives of the programnk.[6]

Newman and Summer have viewed communication as an exchange of facts, ideas, Opinion, or emotions by two or three persons.[7] District health system communicates policy decisions to CHCs, PHCs and sub-centres for effective Implementation.

### Communication Management

Communication management means the designing of communication strategy, procedures and contents in advance, according to the nature and objectives of the organisation, to smoothen its operations and avoid misunderstanding and other complicated problems which could be generated out of the communication gap. The purpose is to function as a health team.

### Types of Communication Network

Communication network is of two types-formal and informal. Formal communication is authoritative and well defined as to who will communicate with whom, when and how. All the procedures are well laid out. Formal communication is effective in normal and routine situations. However, organisations cannot cope with rigid and inflexible communications to meet urgent and spontaneous needs. Informal channels develop network where formal channels are not well designed. Informal communication develops strong bonds. It may supplement, at times, formal channels of communication. Informal communication, however, sometimes carries rumour and distorted information which may damage the goodwill and prestige of the organisation. Thus, There is a need to make use of both the channels of communication as per the needs of the organisation. Since health is a service organisation and not based on the principle of hierarchy but specialization, therefore, informal channels may be encouraged for professional work.

Communication management is very weak in health care system and that is why the field staff do not take the contents of communication seriously. Communication needs advance planning and thorough evaluation of the possibility of acceptance of communication in true spirit by health personal at lower levels. Vague communication would confuse health workers and would retard the quantity and quality of the health programme.

**Direction of Communication**

The communication can flow through three channels, namely: (i) upward, (ii) downward, and (iii) lateral. Upward communication means the information submitted by subordinates to their superiors. Some of these are regular response monthly, quarterly, etc. while others are of temporary nature, that is when some special need arises. A survey of the most of the communication from lower to higher level would reveal that most of the information is not required at the top level resulting in a great wastage of time, money and effort. It needs to be streamlined.

Downward communication keeps the subordinates informed and thus helps in making the machinery of administration function. Such communication needs to be specific, clear and consistent with organisational needs so that subordinates can follow it and act upon It, However, it takes a long time to reach the subordinates because of the existence of many levels of administration.

According to Katz and Kahn, the downward communication system has five major objectives:

(1) To give specific task directive about job instructions.
(2) To give information about organisational procedures and practices.
(3) To provide information about the rationale of the job.
(4) To tell subordinates about their performance.
(5) To provide ideological information to facilitate the indoctrination of goals.

Lateral communication relates to the flow of communication between or within organisations at the same level. This is essential to achieve coordination and avoid delay. It is also called horizontal communication. This requires understanding among personnel at these levels.

Communication, takes a very long time to reach from upward downward and vice-versa as there are many channels through which the communication is to pass before reaching its final destination. Let me give a concrete example. Recently constituted health system corporations created to promote secondary health care are operating very rigidly. One Deputy Director Quality Control. a very efficient person. would send papers for approval to the Managing Director through Additional Director who would create unnecessary problems and would make the communication incomprehensible. Instructions issued about referral system have not been absorbed by the field staff. Hence, we may send communication directly to the persons concerned to ensure right communication and avoid distortions.[8]

## ESSENTIALS OF COMMUNICATION

The essentials of communication are:

### (a) Clarity of Thought

The first sine qua non of good communication is that the idea to be transmitted must be absolutely clear in the mind of the communicator. It must spring out from a "clear head." It should be understood by the personnel so that it may be fully appreciated and acted upon.

### (b) Importance to Action Rather than Words

In all communication, actions are more significant than words. Example is better than precept. An officer who is not punctual cannot succeed in enforcing the time-rules on the subordinates.

### (c) Participation

In this connection it is essential that both the parties (the communicator and the recipient) should participate in the communication. It is the only way to make the communication effective.

### (d) Transmission

The communicator must plan carefully what to communicate, with whom to communicate and how to communicate. How can the top personnel communicate with the workers when they themselves do not know or cannot understand all the facts about the new plans? Further, delegation of authority without responsibility breaks down the spirit of communication.

**(e) Keep the System Always Alive**

The system of communication should be kept open and alive all the year round. It is only by honest attempts that good communicative relations can be developed.

**(f) Cordial Employer-Employee Relations**

Effective communication requires good employer-employee relations which enable mutual appreciation of different viewpoints. According to Terry, eight factors are essential in making communication effective:

(a) Inform yourself fully;
(b) Establish a mutual trust in others;
(c) Find a common ground or experience;
(d) Use mutually known words;
(e) Have regard for context;
(f) Secure and hold the receiver's attention;
(g) Employ examples and visual aids; and
(h) Practice delaying relations.

According to Millet, seven factors make communication effective, it should be clear, consistent with the expectation of the recipient, adequate, timely, uniform, flexible and acceptable. In health care system, communication should be designed to promote health action in a few action-oriented words. Communication should be specific and fix the responsibility for results. What generally happens is that the communication is issued to the field staff without ascertaining the availability of resources. Such communication remains only on paper.

## DIFFICULTIES AND BARRIERS TO COMMUNICATION

These can be classified into three categories:

(a) Social and psychological,
(b) Organisational, and
(c) Mechanical.

**Social and Psychological**

People in an organisation come from different social backgrounds. The same problem may be viewed differently by different people. The messages are thus interpreted differently by different people. Information is distorted through adding and subtracting one's own ideas. Besides, the connotations of words are not properly understood. We can improve upon this through management by objectives (MBO) which can generate understanding about the true goals of the Organisation. Besides, the members of the Organisation may be encouraged to meet frequently to sort out differences.

**Organisational**

Organisation consists of many layers. The transmitted communication reaches the lower level through all the levels in between and vice versa. There is a danger of the information reaching the lower levels in a different context leading to friction, misunderstandings and distortion. It is suggested that the top personnel in the organisation must create an environment of trust and confidence. There is also a need of constant personal contacts of the top personnel with the subordinates to remove misunderstandings. Organisations generally transmit more information than required (overloading) which needs to be discouraged to ensure compliance.

**Mechanical**

These emanate from defective system of despatch and communication within the organisation, resulting in delays, etc. These may also result from the wrong use of media. It is suggested that a set procedure must be in vogue for smooth communication from upward downward, and *vice versa,* as well as horizontal. This would avoid overloading and ensure timely receipt of communication.

**New Developments**

There are now tools and techniques, both mechanical and electronic, which can help in improving communication system. This new technique is called MIS (Management Information System). "The purpose of a MIS is to raise managing from the level of piecemeal spotty information, intuitive guesswork and isolated problem-solving to the level of system insights, system information, sophisticated data processing and systems problem-solving. Managers have always had sources of information; the MIS provides a system of information. It is thus a powerful method for aiding managers in solving problems and making decisions."[9]

The following advantages can accrue from a good information system:

(a) Timely availability of information develops a high degree of confidence between top executives and the members of the management.
(b) Management does not have to resort to frequent meetings to sort out different issues.
(c) Executive time can be saved and devoted to critical issues.
(d) It helps in reviewing actual performance and devise corrective action.
(e) It helps in reviewing strength and weakness of an organisation, knowledge of which is most essential in formulating future plans and strategies.

## CONCLUSION

We suggest here some points which may be kept in mind while designing the communication system:

1. All the persons in the organisation should know the formal channel of communication so that they can report to the correct authority.
2. Communication need be as short as possible, otherwise there is danger of aberration of facts.
3. Communication source need be authenticated.
4. Connotation used must be familiar with the receiver as well as the sender.
5. Communication should be designed in such a away as to enlist support of the persons involved.

Effective communication among health functionaries can lubricate extra energy vital for the success of health programme. The holistic communication must involve the body, mind and soul to ensure effectiveness.

## COORDINATION

According to Mooney, coordination is the first principle of organisation and includes within itself all other principles which are subordinate to it and through which it operates. Coordination is the process of bringing activities or groups of activities into proper relation with each other to make sure that everything that needs to be achieved and that no two people are trying to do the same job.

Take the example of ward management in a CHC. Work is divided among different functionaries. However, nursing sister co-ordinates all activities to promote patient care.

Coordination is the means of distributing authority. Providing channels of communication, and arranging the work so

The right Thing are done . . . (what)
in the right place . . . (where)
at the right time . . . (when)
in the right way . . . (how)
by the right people . . . (by whom)

When an activity is coordinated, everything works well. A cooordinated activity is orderly, harmonious, efficient and successful.

According to Terry, co-ordination is the adjustment of the parts to each other and of the movement and operation of the parts so that each can make its maximum contribution to the product of the whole. According to

J.C. Charles Worth, "Coordination is the integration of the several pans into an orderly whole to achieve the purpose of the undertaking."[10]

Coordination implies the prevention of both duplication and overlapping so as to avoid administrative wastes of efforts, manpower and resources and to pool resources and experience in dealing with problems and achieving common objectives. Coordination—which is a means to an end and not an end in itself—must be considered in relation to its practical purposes which is to facilitate better performance and greater administrative efficiency in the system. To ensure efficient and economical functioning of an organisation, coordination is not only desirable but even essential. For the same reason, inter-organisation coordination is advisable, especially when the activities of the various organisation concerned are of a complementary nature.

Stressing the need for coordination, the UN Secretary-General stated at the 41st Session of the ECOSOC held in Geneva on July 5, 1966: "Apart from the continuing need to avoid overlapping and inconsistencies, coordination is more and more conceived in a positive and dynamic sense and aimed at providing an agreed direction and a framework for action and at ensuring not only that activities dovetail into one another but there is a full measure of forethought and harmony in the carrying out of our responsibilities."[11]

"Among all administrative activities, coordination is the most fascination and, sometimes, the most delicate intellectual exercise. No organisation can attain its goals without adequate coordination among its units and their functionaries. . . .

Coordination is, indeed, the administrative manifestation of Creativity, may be with an all-pervading effect on the organisation as a whole. . . . It aims at an inter-linking between one experience and another with an emerging synthesis.[12]

Coordination is distinct from the hierarchical process of authority, command and control. Unless coordination procedures are observed, satisfactory programming and implementation are impossible. Co-ordination may be achieved through collaboration in working for the same cause, or cooperation in the sharing of a joint task by two or more parties; often it includes both modes of action.

Coordination may lead to one organisation performing services or attacking a problem on behalf of all organisations in the system. It may also lead one or more parties, on the basis of information and consultation, to refrain entirely from participation in a given activity so as to avoid duplication of efforts. Coordination in such circumstances is accomplished by separation of functions rather than by a decision to work in concert.

A distinction needs to be drawn between administrative and programme coordination. The object of administrative coordination is economical and efficient house-keeping. It is advocated primarily for fiscal reason or the desire to achieve maximum efficiency at minimum cost. It deals with such problems as common services, common standards of employment and common budget presentation. It does not itself achieve coordination of programmes but facilitates such coordination. Programme coordination is concentrated on activities best suited to priority issues.

**Methods of Achieving Coordination**

These can be formal and informal. Formal methods of coordination would differ according to the purpose to be achieved. We may divide the purpose into three aspects:

(a) Programme Coordination,
(b) Administrative coordination, and
(c) Procedural coordination.

**Programme Coordination**

It can be achieved through:

(i) representation at each other's meetings on all appropriate occasions;
(ii) early consultation when one organisation felt that the other might be interested or involved in an activity;
(iii) creation of standing or 'ad hoc' joint committees whenever circumstances warrant; and
(iv) full and continuous personal contact among the experts and officials of the organisation. However, care should be taken that time may not be wasted in meetings.

**Administrative Coordination**

Coordination relating to personnel and financial matters may be achieved through personnel department/establishment section and budget section. Personnel and financial administration can help in coordinating the personnel and financial resources.

**Procedural Coordination**

Such coordination can be achieved by devising suitable manuals detailing procedures. Such manuals need to be kept uptodate. Informal methods are more productive. Co-ordination can resecured through informal methods such as:

(a) Instilling dominant objective among the members of the group;
(b) Developing generally accepted professional standards and norms making it easier for employees to work with one another enthusiastically; and
(c) Promoting informal contacts to supplement formal communication;
(d) Encouraging upper echelons to maintain close contact with personnel working under them; using group methods for informal exchange of ideas and views.

In programme co-ordination, health experts must forget their status and should concentrate on the requirements of the programme and promoting the efforts of all to programme delivery.

**External Coordination**

Besides the internal coordination, there is a need of external coordination. The chief executive should see that his organisation develops environmental linkages. Linkages are points of interactions with the environment. These can be classified into four categories 'enabling', 'functional', 'normative' and 'diffused'.

The enabling linkage ensures and protects the organisational authority to operate its access to resources and its power to achieve results (political). This would ensure effective coordination with political wing—ministry, legislature, board, etc.

Functional linkage is to link the programme with the task environment. Such coordination would avoid duplication and overlapping and promote the unity of purpose among allied agencies. Diffused linkages "life enlighten movement", mean to reach the clients through mass media, It is the duty of the chief executive to keep the members adequately informed of the affairs of the Organisation, arrange for their education, encourage their participation, ensure sound relationship between staff and members, give necessary and prompt attention and consideration to complaints and suggestions.

This visualizes the need for effective public relations. This would result in cordial, equitable and, therefore, mutually profitable relations between the administration and their beneficiaries.

Nonnative linkages mean as what ought to be done. This requires that the chief executive must pay proper attention for getting the researches done either in the Organisation or outside to find out the best methods to achieve the maximum output. He can seek the collaboration of the experts from the universities and training institutions.

Since, health departments from the top to the bottom are linked with many other departments, there is a need of developing effective linkages. For example, the buildings of health centres are constructed, and maintained by PWD, therefore, health department must maintain co-ordination with PWD.

According to Gulick, some of the difficulties arise from (a) the uncertainty of the future—as to the behaviour of individuals and of people; (b) the lack of knowledge, experience, wisdom and character among leaders and their confused and conflicting ideas and objectives; (c) the lack of administrative skill and techniques; (d) the vast number of variables involved and the incompleteness of human knowledge, particularly with regard to man and life; and (e) the lack of orderly methods of developing, considering, perfecting and adopting new ideas and programmes.[13] To these are added four more by Seckler-Hudson. These are the "size complexity personalities and political factors, the lack of leaders with wisdom and knowledge pertaining to public administration and the accelerated expansion of public administration to international dimensions.[14]

## CONCLUSION

Coordination is becoming complex in the health system as the quantitative operations of the health organisations are increasing at a very fast rate without making changes in the administrative structure and procedures responsible for coordination. Therefore, there is a need of advance planning and decision-making to achieve effective coordination. There is also need to create structures to strengthen district health system. Coordination is not a simple process but is directly linked with the total management. Until and unless all the principles of the orgnisation like planning, objectives, span of control, unity of command, authority and responsibility, etc. are not well defined, co-ordination becomes impossible and impracticable. A good organisation leads to prompt and good coordination and good coordination makes a good organisation.

### Control

Control is essential for good health administration. According to Newman and Summer, "The aim of control is to assure that the results of operations conforms as closely as possible to established goals."[15]

Hemi Fayol says that "control consists in verifying whether everything occurs in conformity with the plans adopted, the instructions issued and principles established. It has for its object to point out weakness and errors in order to rectify them and prevent recurrence."[16]

### Objectives

The objectives of control are as under:

(a) to ensure that the health work has been accomplished according to stated objectives within budgetary and time limits;

(b) to enable the health administration to identify the causes of work deficiencies;

(c) to enable the health management to suggest remedial action;

(d) to improve upon the health system; and

(e) The ultimate purposes is to achieve decent health care to the people.

### Essentials of Good Control

For control to be effective. it must be:

(a) *Timely*—Control needs to be exercised timely, otherwise there can be additions in problems.

CHART 6.1

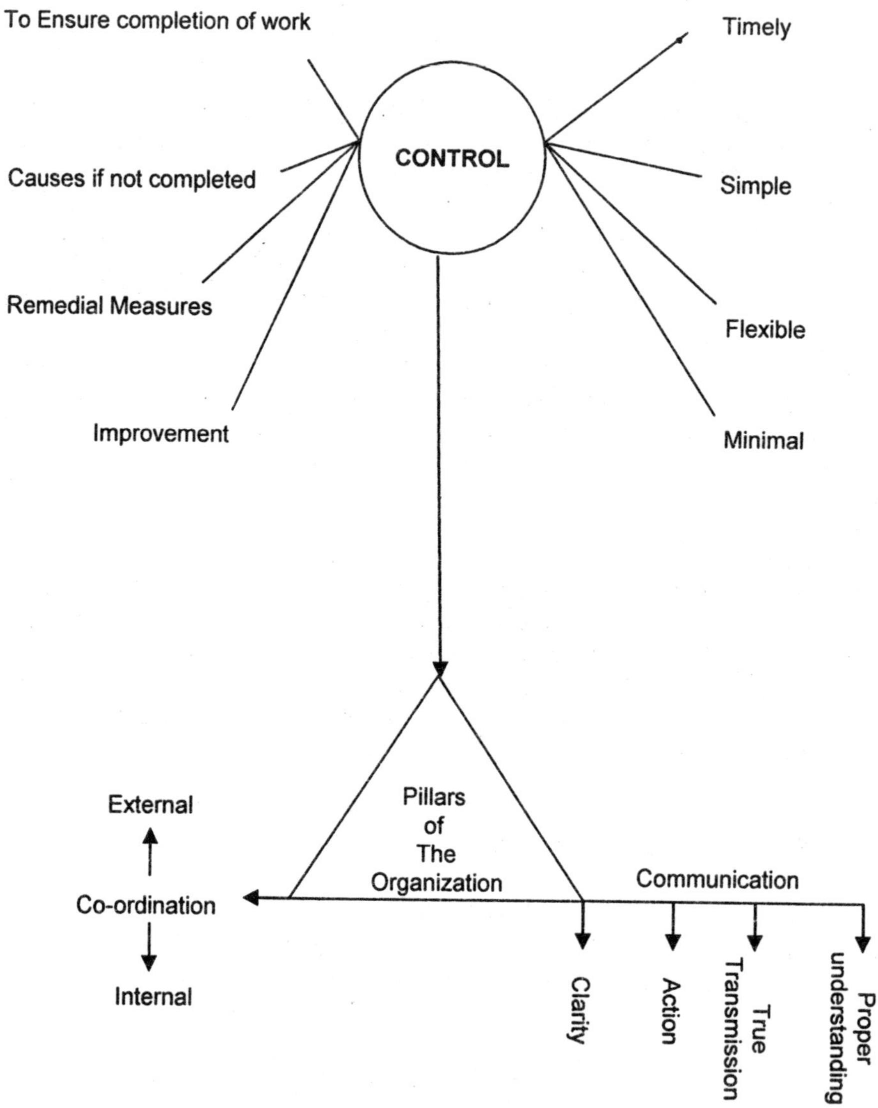


(b) *Simple*—Control mechanism should be simple so that it can be easily adopted to make amends.

(c) Flexible-It should be flexible as too rigid control may be self-defeating.

(d) Minimal—Control must be exercised rarely but must be thorough.

Whenever, it is done. all aspects need to be diagnosed.

## Control Process

*(a) Establishment of Health Standards*

It is very important to set health standards for control mechanism as actual performance has to be compared against such standards.

Such standards in physical sciences are set with certainty and can easily be compared with actual. However, in social situations, it is very difficult to lay down standards. In spite of the availability of modern management techniques it has not been possible to lay down standards. There are large variations. For example, how much load of work should a doctor undertake in a PHC ? How many patients would a doctor examine? Because of the difficulty of laying down standards, control becomes difficult.

*(b) Measurement of Performance*

It means measurement of performance in units in which standards were laid. Such measurement must be reliable and intelligible. Measurement must be objective.

*(c) Compare between Performance and Standards*

After measurement of performance, we may compare performance with standards set. Generally, there would be difference—either there may be more achievement or less achievement. In the Indian context, it is generally less as can be seen from our Five Year Plans.

*(d) Determination of the Reasons for Difference*

There is a need to analyse the reasons for this deviation. We may isolate the reasons in different categories—personnel, financial, procedural, structural, etc.

*(e) Correction*

Based upon the causes, we may bring about the necessary correction. We may involve experts in O & M if the problem is large, otherwise, we may introduce minor corrections. Control for example, to check spread of communicable diseases is essential. otherwise diseases can spread in geometrical progression. All the National Health Programmes provide for control measures. Control may not necessarily cover all aspects of primary health care, but should include the following criteria, effectiveness, equity. efficiency, and impact:

- *Effectiveness* is an expression of the degree of attainment of the pre-determined objectives and targets of a programme, institution, or activity seeking to reduce a health problem or improve an unsatisfactory health situation. This factor depends on whether the various activities and measures undertake work (efficacy) and the degree to which they are accepted by those for whom they are intended.

- *Equity* considers the coverage of population groups and geographical areas, distribution of resources and facilities, and effectiveness of services in different areas. Equity in the distribution of health care depends on the extent to which different geographical areas and population groups, according to age, sex, or wealth, have access to essential services.
- *Efficiency* is an expression of the relationship between the results obtained from a health programme or activity and the efforts expended in terms of human, financial, and other resources, health processes, technology and time. The reason for assessing efficiency is to improve implementation and gain a better idea of the progress made.
- *Impact* is an expression of the overall effect of a programme, service, or institution on health and related aspects of socio-economic development. The assessment of impact thus aims at identifying any necessary change in the direction of health programmes, so as to replan primary health care accordingly and its contribution to health and overall socio-economic development.

Thus, the health department must plan in advance the processes of communication, co-ordination, and control to execute the health programmes in right spirit. The failures of these processes result in bottlenecks, low performance, interpersonal jealousies and miss the objectives of health care-decent health for all in 21st century to lead a healthy prolonged life.

## Notes and References

1. Barnard, Chester I, The Functions of the Executive, Cambridge: Harward University Press, 1968, pp. 226-27.
2. Ordway Tead, The Aim of Administration, New York, McGraw-Hill, 1951, p. 45.
3. William, G. Scolt, Organisation Theory, Richar D. Irwin, Homewood Ltd., 1967, p. 153.
4. A Goddard, Principles of Administration Applied to Nursing Service, World Health Organisation, Geneva, 1958, p. 85.
5. Koontz, Hand C., O'Donnel, Principles of Management: An Analysis of Managerial Functions, London, McGraw Hill, Kogakusa Ltd., 1972, pp. 538-40.
6. Chester I. Barnard, The Functions of the Executive, Cambridge Harward University Press, 1968, pp. 226-27.
7. H.H. Newman, C.E. Summer, The Process of Management: Concepts, Behaviour and Practice, Englewood Cliffs, NJ, Prentice Hall, 1961, p. 59.
8. Daniel, Katz and Kahn, Roben L.: The Social Psychology of Organisation, Wiley, New York. 1966. p. 239.
9. R.G. Murdich, Information Systems for Management, Prentice Hall, 1985, p. 14.

10. G.R. Terry, Principles of Management. Richard D. Irwin., Inc., Illinois, 1956, pp. 33-34.
11. UN Secretary-General quoted by David Owen Coordination of Development Assistance Among the International Agencies, Robinson, (Ed.), *op. cit.*, p. 165.
12. M.A. Muttalib, 'The Theory of Coordination Re-Discovered and Re-Formulated', Vol. XXIV, No 2, *77th Indian Journal of Public Administration*, p. 238.
13. Gulick and Urwick, L., Papers on the Science of Administration, p. 40.
14. Fayol, Henri, General and Industrial Management, p. 107.
15. Newman and Summer, The Process of Management, p. 561.
16. Henri Fayol, Henri, General and Industrial Management, p. 107.

7

CHAPTER

# Headquarters and Field Relationships

## MEANING

Headquarters means the apex organisation of an enterprise wherein policy is developed and review understanding. In the Union and State Governments, the Secretariats Health of respective Governments are headquarters organisations. This is also termed as top-management.

For coordination, control and communication, there are State Directorates. District offices and Block offices which serve as field offices for top management but headquarters for the field agencies operating under them. This is called middle management. Thus, headquarters and field office are a relative term. The offices providing concrete services at the lower level are actual field offices. A field office may be merely an outpost of the headquarters with no authority, or it may be an agency with adequate authority and responsibility delegated to it. For example, District Health System is a field office for state health department at headquarter and divisional level while District Health System is headquarter for CHC, PHC, SC and voluntary health workers.

Field offices are created mostly on the basis of geography. The conventional methods are locating offices in already carved out geographical areas—district, blocks, etc. However, some agencies, like Electricity Boards, Railways have their own functional systems. It is suggested that geographical approach may be adopted as it is more convenient and useful from both citizens and administrative view points. In health, geographical approach has been adopted.

## NEED

Field health agencies are essential to provide services to the people in an economical and efficient manner as near to them as possible, eighty per cent of the health problems of the people are local in nature which can be settled by field agencies. Only very few activities need the attention and concern of headquarters. Brian C. Smith mentions: 'There are a number of social, economic, administrative and political factors which make some measure of deconcentration, both a desirable and inevitable feature of systems of Government."[1]

Let us examine the factors which are responsible for the growth of field offices.

**(a) Social**

Many field offices come into existence where close contact between the health system and the people is essential and useful. Social communication is very important in many programmes like ICDS. Under CDS, Anganwadis have been created in every village or a combination of 2-3 villages. A sub-centre for health services has been established for a population of about 5,000 people. Such field offices can help in promoting social change and health development.

**(b) Economic**

Field health offices can be set-up to save the costs of persons which they would incur on travelling.

**(c) Professional**

Professional efficiency and convenience lead to the establishment of field offices. For example, the field offices of health utility services are created to promote professional efficiency and economy as diseases are based on local situations.

**(d) Political**

Political decisions based on political considerations lead to the creation of field offices. For example, health institutions are set-up in the constituencies of ministers. There may be other reasons as well, like scientific and technological developments, making regulatory mechanism effective, people's participation, etc.

## ESSENTIALS FOR A FIELD OFFICE

While creating field offices, we may keep the following essentials in mind.

**(i) Cost of Creation**

The creation of field office means extra budget and extra level for the headquarters. Headquarters would require more personnel to control extra field agencies. Therefore, the total cost involved in the creation of field offices may be kept in mind *vis-a-vis* the benefits.

**(ii) Viability**

Field offices need be created when there is sufficient activity and resources for them. For example, many sub-centres created by health department have become unviable. The Government of India is actively considering winding up of the unviable sub-centres as a part of structural reforms in the health sector to equip them fully.

**(iii) Administrative**

Field offices may be created when administrative efficiency can be enhanced because of deconcentration.

**(iv) Technical**

Fields offices may be created to meet technical requirements. For example, the field offices of health system are created nearer to the families to facilitate control of communicable diseases.

## METHODS OF COMMUNICATION, COORDINATION AND CONTROL BETWEEN HEADQUARTERS AND FIELD AGENCIES

Regardless of the degree to which field operations are deconcentrated geographically, the headquarter has to maintain continuous supervision over such operations. There are number of methods by which the headquarters exercise control over the field offices. Some of these are inherent in the powers vested in the top administration at headquarters. e.g., (i) prior approval of the programmes to be implemented, (ii) allocation of financial resources, (iii) appointment and transfer of personnel from one agency to another, and (iv) laying down rules and regulations, etc. In doing these, the following methods are used:

**System of Reporting**

Reporting on pre-designed forms at different intervals of time is an essential requirement of field agencies for the knowledge of the headquarters. Besides, there are many points on which reports are required from time to time to formulate and review policy measures. The frequency of reports would differ from organisation to organisation. Let us explain with an example of a reporting system in World Health Organisation at regional level. The country offices of World Health Organisation send four reports every year to the regional office. The WHO representative submits four reports each year, three quarterly reports and a quarterly-*cum*-annual report known as *The Country Reviews* by April 1, June 1 (2 months report), in the last week of October and January 1, respectively. He has also to send field visit reports. Sub-Centres send the reports to primary health centres. These after compilation by PHC are sent to District Health Office. District Health Office after consolidation sends these to the state headquarters. The purpose of reporting is to:

CHART 7.1

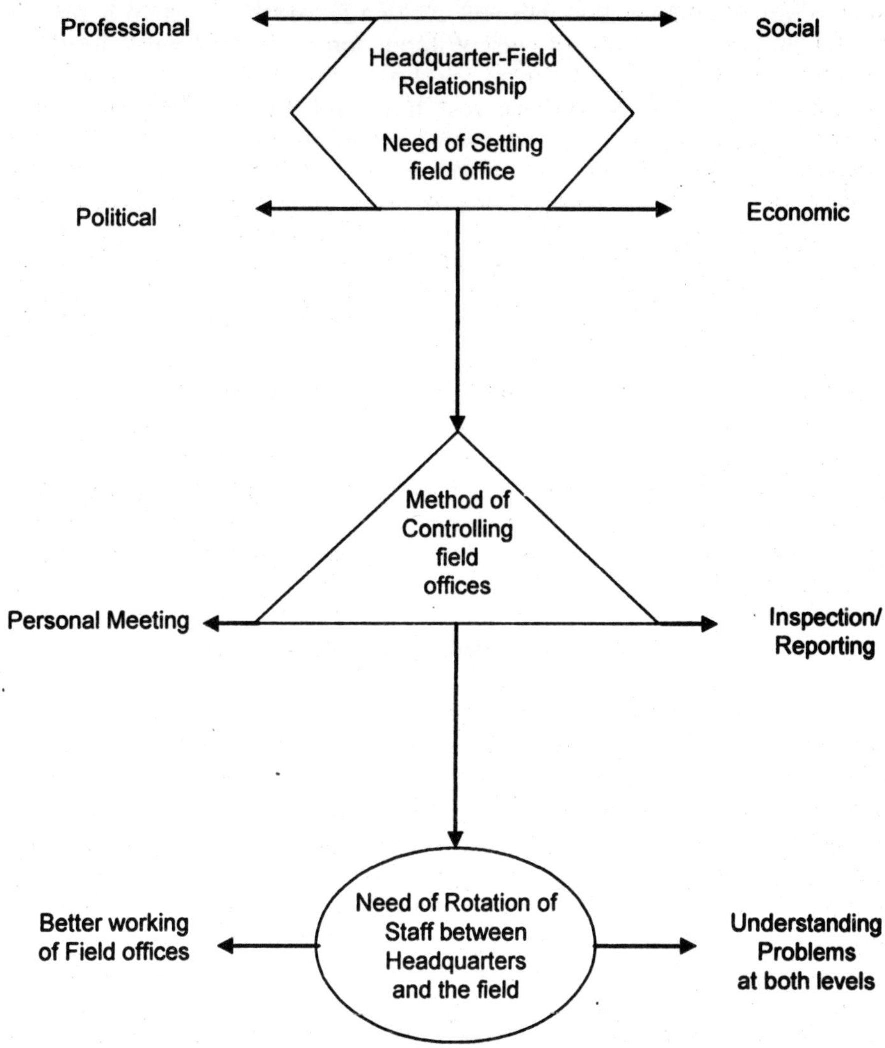


(a) Measure the progress in the field.
(b) Locate problems in the field.
(c) Confirm that the arrangements for implementation of policies are adequate.
(d) Guide the field staff in future on the basis of past developments.

However, in practice, it has been seen that formats for reporting are nor properly designed, resulting in confusion. There is a need for definite guidelines for the preparation of field reports to facilitate the comparability of reports on related matter and reduce, as far as possible, the element of subjectivity. We may keep in mind that many organisations do not send genuine reports; information that will evoke a favourable reaction is played up and the lapses are glossed over. Without some standard guide forms, it is all too tempting for reporters to inject extraneous bits of information.[2]

Reporting and its analysis cost time and money. Therefore, only standardized, authenticated and useful reporting may be used to have genuine field control and field development. For this purpose, there is a need of designing and installing Management Information System to suit the needs of the organisation. This would hasten the exchange of information between headquarters and fields. Besides, it would help in improving efficiency in operational functions, controlling Organisational performance, and supporting intelligent planning by providing such information to the decision-making which is most relevant, accurate, complete, concise, timely, economical, reliable and efficient. In addition, the use of electronic gadgets can speed up the flow of information. In this context, district information centres set-up by the Government of India can serve as an effective link between headquarters and the field agencies. Recent info-revolution can help in developing suitable software for effective reporting for health, especially epidemics and spread of communicable diseases.

## FIELD OBSERVATION AND INSPECTION

In addition to formal reporting, observation and inspection are indispensable if field operations are to be kept under effective control and the mistakes made in one field are not to be repeated in another. The inspection should not be conducted for isolated activities as is the practice in most of organisations, but should combine together all the issues needing attention at the field level. This combination of aims is necessary partly because travel costs have to be kept within the limited budgetary allocations and also to economize the use of staff time.[3]

Let us mention the problems of inspection in the Indian context:

(a) Inspecting officers do not prepare the review points on which inspection is to be conducted, resulting in adhocism.
(b) Inspection reports are not prepared and if at all prepared are in skeleton form leading to wastage of inspection efforts.
(c) Inspections are planned with ulterior motives resulting in the wastage of money and time of the Government.
(d) No use of inspection report is made in policy-making, planning, decision-making and control of health services.

The inspection tends to be too short and hurried to be of much value in producing realistic judgments on operational problems. The Study Team of the Administrative Reforms Commission of state level. Administration also recommended that "the provision relating to periodic and other prescribed inspections by the inspection and supervising officers at various levels should be meticulously carried out and any laxity in this regard should be severely dealt with." In spite of all these handicaps, the cumulative insight gained by the headquarters over field offices through observation and inspections helps in developing good relationships between headquarters and field agencies, as well as in effective evaluation.

## PERIODIC MEETING OF THE FIELD ADMINISTRATORS

Reports and inspections are used independently for each field office. When all the field offices are needed to act simultaneously and consistently, meetings are arranged. We observe that the Director of Health Services frequently calls the meetings of District Health officers of all the districts and in turn the DHO often calling the meeting of all PHC officers in the district, etc. A World Health Organisation Manual rightly suggests that, for a formal committee the agenda should make the purpose clear. But it is worthwhile to write a brief summary of the purpose of a meeting, stating what is hoped to achieve.[4]

Some meetings are called to communicate information, others to exchange views and ideas, and others to make decisions about plans or activities. The success of any meeting depends on the quality of communications.

If the purpose is to pass on information or to explain some things, the speaker should find out if this has been done successfully, e.g., by allowing questions and discussion which will show whether the subject has been understood.

If the purpose is to seek the views of members, the chairman or secretary should summarize the view expressed or put them in different words to obtain the agreement of those present about what has been said.

Quarrels and shouting at meeting do not help. They are often the result of poor communication. There are fewer disagreements when people understand each other clearly. It has been seen that such meetings are called without advance planning, resulting in the dislocation of field work. The members attend the meetings without adequate facts and information with them, resulting in wastage of money and time.

## PROBLEMS OF HEADQUARTERS AND FIELD RELATIONSHIP

The success of administration depends upon the effective functioning of the field agencies. Field agencies are the points of contact between citizens and Health Administration. Therefore, the headquarters need to devise ways and means to keep the field offices functional, efficient and responsive. However, we find that people have lost faith in field administration. They are highly dissatisfied. Improper handling of field problems by the headquarters is also responsible for the problems in the field. Let us discuss some of the problems of field agencies and suggest remedies.

**(1) Viewpoints of the Field Agencies not Appreciated by the Headquarters and vice-versa**

Most of the field offices complain that the headquarters do not understand their viewpoints relating to the urgency of the field situation as they have to face the concrete situation and give results to the people. Headquarter's people, on the other hand, feel that the field office do not understand the constraints of the head office and are mostly asking for one resource of the other, i.e. putting forth their difficulties rather than utilising the local resources efficiently. Pfiffner and Presthus have put it thus. It has been said that there is both a headquarters and a field way of life, the two groups often viewing each other with smugness and suspicion. Field workers insist that headquarters does not understand their problems; a person transferred from field to headquarters soon loses his touch with the field. There is much drudgery in field brought about by headquarters directives, the utility of which field worker questions.[5]

To overcome this, the following is suggested:

(a) A regular rotation among field and headquarters staff needs to be followed with definite rules and regulations.
(b) A good communication needs to be designed to keep both the agencies well informed of each other.
(c) A clear-cut demarcation of duties and responsibilities between the two may be laid out to avoid confusion and constant references.

**(2) Field Staff not equipped with the Necessary Authority and Resources to Discharge Responsibility**

Fields offices are to provide services to the people and therefore, they may be equipped with necessary authority and resources. The headquarter does not release the finances and other materials in time to field offices, causing many hardships to them. The heads of these field offices waste their time in approaching the headquarters' frequently. To quote Pfiffner and Presthus, "A flourishing complaint among ambitious and mobile personnel in the field is that they do not have sufficient authority to make operational decisions. They must refer even routine matters to some higher echelon, which often delays action for weeks, while some communications are never answered. The inevitable result is a feeling of frustration on the part of field units. It is suggested that the field offices must be equipped as per their need with necessary resources and authority so that they can concentrate in the achievement of objectives. A stitch in time saves nine."[6]

**(3) Communication to the Field Staff not effective**

Field agencies complain of poor communication resulting in

inactivity. Communication may be designed scientifically to make the actions result-oriented. It should also done in very clear and specific language.

### (4) Political Interference in Locating Field Agency

Many field organisations are created purely on political grounds. For example. many Governments set-up primary health centres at places which are not convenient to a large population.

## Notes and References

1. Brian, C. Smith, Field Administrative: An aspect decentralization, Routledge, London, 1967, p. 6.
2. Waller, R. Sharp, Field Administrative in the United Nations System, The Carnegie Endowment for International Peace, London, Slovens and Sons, 1961, p. 226.
3. *Ibid.*, p. 253.
4. WHO: On Being Incharge, Geneva, 1980, pp. 101-2.
5. Pfiffner and Presthus, *op. cit.*, p. 211
6. *Ibid.*, pp. 218-19.

8

CHAPTER

# Organisational Analysis for Health Services

"Organisational analysis is a technique to ensure the achievement of maximum results with minimum costs, in terms of human and material resources of the organisations. The objective of organisational analysis is to improve pattern of relationships between persons in an organisation and to create harmonious arrangement of work with reference to its main objectives. The need for the design of sound organisational structures for an enterprises and their continual evaluation in terms of suitability through organisational analysis has been recognized as an effective means to promote improvement in corporate performance. "Good organisation structure does not by itself produce good performance just as good constitution does not guarantee great Presidents, or good laws a moral society. But a poor organisation structure makes good performance impossible, no matter how good the individuals may be."

*—Peter F. Drucker*

After the formulation of the plan, the health organisation is designed to implement the plan. Even the best machine gets rusty without timely maintenance. Many aspect of the working of an Organisation have to be examined, to evolve a modified design for an organisation, in order to ensure their efficiency. Development in information technology requires further dramatic organisational restructuring through organisational analysis. National competitiveness will increasingly depend on flexibility requiring fast responses from a government that is enabling rather than providing the directions for change. This includes details about the levels of supervision, the chain of command, the accountability and transparency in the functioning of an organisation and finally the criteria for evaluation. Organisation Building is extremely important in the field of Public Administration. No administrative performance is possible without a suitable organisation.

We have discussed the structure and functions of health organisations from the Union level to state level and down to Sub-centre level in the first volume. Before we discuss the meaning, significance and techniques of organisational analysis, let us understand the meaning of the term organisation.[1]

From these definitions, we can draw inferences for designing health system. According to Dimock and Dimock. "Organisation is the systematic bringing together of Interdependent parts to form a unified whole through which authority, co-ordination and control may be exercised to achieve a given purpose. Organisation is both structure and human relations."[2]

According to Mooney, organisation is the forum of every human association for the attainment of a common purpose.[3] Harbert A. Simon has concluded that organisation affects the people who work for it, in five different ways:

(i) The organisation divides work among its members; by giving each employee a particular task, it limits and concentrates his attention on that task;

(ii) The organisation establishes standard practices; by working out, detailed procedures, it relieves employees of the need to determine such procedure, each time they use crossways;

(iii) The organisation transmits authoritative decisions: by despatching such decisions downward, upward and crossways;

(iv) The organisation provides a communication system; and

(v) The organisation trains and indoctrinates its members by providing for the "internalization" of influence relating to knowledge, skills and loyalties; training enables employees to make decisions as the organisation would like them to be made.[4]

It would therefore. be of utmost significance to stress that organisation is not merely a structure; in fact, it embraces a structure as well as the human beings who man and run it in order to realise the pre-conceived objective.

P.R. Dubhasi has rightly said that Organisation Building is extremely important in the field of Public Administration. No administrative performance is possible without a suitable organisation. Building of an administrative organisation is, therefore, the starting point of any administrative performance.

Organisation can be formal and informal. According to Simon, formal organisation means, "a planned system of co-operative effort in which each participant has a recognised role to play and duties and task to perform. The key to the whole process is effective co-operation among the persons engaged in the operation."[5]

But, the actual working of any organisation is not according to the formal plan. The informal relationship of the persons working in the organisation may be different from the formal expected relationship. It is better to encourage informal relationships among personnel in an organisation.

Keith Devis has enumerated the following five practical benefits which can be derived from informal organisations which may be kept in mind by the management:

1. It blends with the formal organisation to make a workable system for getting the work done;
2. It lightens the workload of the formal manager and fills in some of the gaps of his abilities;
3. It gives suggestion and stability to work groups;
4. It is a very useful channel of communication in the organisation; and
5. Its presence encourages the manager to plan and act more carefully than he would otherwise do.[6]

Likert has called this general principle, 'the principle of supporting relationships', in which decision-making. Leadership, motivation. communication and control move together. He states, "the leadership and other process of the organisation must be such as to assume a maximum probability that in all interactions and all relationships with the organisation each member will. in the light of his background values, and one which builds and maintains his sense of personal worth and importance.[7]

Likert mentions the following concrete attributes (Likert. 1967, pp. 13-17).

(a) Superiors are supportive of subordinates and have high performance goals for the Organisation:
(b) There is a mutual trust and confidence between superiors and subordinates and consensus on Organisational goals;
(c) There is a high level of accurate communication upwards and downwards and laterally within the Organisation;
(d) Goals setting and control is done within work groups rather than on a man-to-man basis or simple downward communication of orders;
(e) There is high degree of co-operation within and among work groups in the Organisation; and
(f) Overall this produces an Organisation matched by a high degree of participation of all members at all levels in each of the Organisation.

Joseph L. Massive defines Organizatiion "as the structure and process by which co-operative group of human beings allocates its tasks among its members, identifies relationship and integrates its activities towards common objectives."[8]

Amitai Euioni states, "Organisations are social units (or human groupings) deliberately consturcted and reconstructed to seek specific goals."[9]

W. Richard Scott: "Organisations are defined as collectivities that have been established for the pursuit of relatively specific objectives on a more or less continuous basis."[10]

Robert V. Presthus defined Organisations as "system of structural interpersonal relations . . . individuals are differentiated in terms of authority, status and role with the result that personal interaction is prescribed. Anticipated reactions tend to occur, while ambiguity and spontaneity are decreased."[11]

A careful analysis of these definitions would reveal different emphasis put by different scholars. Some regard it as a mechanism to achieve certain objectives (classical theory).

Here emphasis is on the structural framework in which grouped activities are assigned to people, authority relations established, individual efforts properly co-ordinated and responsibilities fixed. The structure is created to help accomplish enterprise goals more effectively. The major implications of this theory are specialisation, scalar, authority, span of control, and structural relationships of functions. There are others who regard it as a system. The system approach looks at the organisation as a total system comprising a number of interacting variables. Under this approach organisation is viewed not merely as a formal arrangement of superior and subordinates or a social system, comprising informal organisation and people's influences on each other, but as a total system of formal organisation, individuals, social system, the physical setting (man-machine systems) and environment, all constantly interacting with each other. The systems approach studies the organisation as an integrated whole encompassing many sub-systems, and considers each system as a part of a still larger system.

The structure of Health Organisations at the state and district level is in utter chaos. One of the contributory factors to this hopeless state of affairs is the lack of managerial knowledge since most of them occupying senior positions have been promoted from their professional and technical posts. It is very difficult to achieve much from such organisations in the new millennium which need a dynamic health system to incorporate new health care schemes and accommodate technical and scientific revolutions. The need of health organisations is to improve their structure and functioning through organisational analysis.

Health Organisations are mostly designed on Weber's model and are like other government organisations. These are totally unsuitable for decent health care delivery system. We have to design health organisation keeping in view flexibility, urgency and seriousness. Hence, we must combine various theories to design good health Organisations.

## ORGANISATIONAL ANALYSIS

Organisational analysis is a technique to ensure the achievement of maximum results with minimum costs in terms of human and material resources by the health organisations. The objective of organisational analysis is to improve pattern of relationships between persons in a health organisation and to create harmonious arrangement of work with reference to its main objectives. The need for the design of sound organisational structures of an enterprise and their continual evaluation in terms of suitability through organisational analysis has been recognized as an effective means to promote improvement in health institutions performance. Peter F. Drucker has rightly observed; "Good organisation structure does not by itself produce good Performance— just as good constitution does not guarantee great presidents, or good laws or a moral society. But a poor organisation structure makes good performance impossible no matter how good the individuals may be."[12]

## NEED FOR ORGANISATIONAL ANALYSIS

Organisational Analysis is needed in all the health organisations whether old, new or proposed. Many health organisations have become dead woods and are unfit to deliver good health services. It should be a continuous activity and should be used at regular intervals of time to ensure that the structure and functions of the health organisations are in tune with their objectives ensuring decent health care to the people. Its purpose is to weed out those activities which impede the performance of an organisation. There are. however, critical situations which warrant immediate intervention of this technique. Let us mention these critical situations:

### (a) Change in the Objectives of the Health Organisations

It is not unusual to find health organisations continuing a traditional organisation structure long after its objectives, plans, and external environment have changed. We find the changes in the patterns of diseases. More non-communicable diseases are coming up at a fast rate. We cannot cope with these diseases with the existing organisations. Such mistakes occur when health organisation fails to plan properly towards a future substantially different from the past or present. The organisational analysis would help the management to determine as to what kind of organisation structure will best serve future needs and what kind of people will best serve the Organisation.

### (b) Change in the Method of Work

The changes in science and technology produce the changes in the methods of work, e.g., introduction of new techniques for the promotion of health would change the working patterns of health personnel. This automatically requires a different type of organisation, e.g. introduction of highly sophisticated machines for tests.

**(c) Over-organisation**

The existing health organisations become complicated over a period of time. Over-organizing results from complicating undue levels of structure and procedures. In such an organisation. people are busy in the meticulous application of rules and regulations rather than performance. Such a situation immediately calls for organisational analysis to avoid frustrating results. Tertiary health care institutions like PGI, Chandigarh, AIIMS, New Delhi, come under this category.

Besides, the need of organisational analysis is felt under many conditions. Let us mention some of them:

1. Failure to clarify relationships resulting in friction, politics and inefficiencies.
2. Failure to delegate authority.
3. Confusion of lines of authority and of information.
4. Excessive rigidity in the Organisation resulting in operational difficulties.
5. Lack of proper co-ordination.
6. Absence of systematic groupings of related activities.
7. Maximum layering.
8. Authority without responsibility and *vice versa.*
9. Lack of clear-cut demarcation between line and staff functions.
10. Lack of judicious span of control and unity of command.

Thus, these and many other deteriorating signs can warrant the need of organisational analysis to keep health organisations efficient. Madhukar Shukla in his article, "Harnessing Personal Creavitity" in *Business India,* February 9 to 22, 1987 has rightly said that:

> "Managerial functions are no longer confined merely to routine control and co-ordination of activities. Rather, the manager often has to deal with unforeseen situations, where the earlier practices are no longer appropriate. While most managers are potentially capable of coping and responding to situations creatively and of generating new alternatives, very few actually do so. One major reason for this is their own conception of how an organisation functions and their own role in it. Most executive think of the organisation as being a systematically designed and highly efficient giant machine. They see themselves as the implementers of organisational plans and policies by involving logical procedures and applying rational techniques. . . It is this kind of 'hardware' view of the managerial role and personality that deter most managers from being creative. Such a self-image reduces the individuals capacity to play around with ideas, toy

with apparently absurd solutions (all innovative ideas look absurd in the beginning), and to take the intellectual risk of imagining far-fetched, though desirable, alternatives."

## TECHNIQUES OF ORGANISATIONAL ANALYSIS

1. Organisation charting.
2. Organisational manuals.
3. Checklists of the principles of an organisation.
4. Job Analysis.

### I. Organisation Charting

The organisauonal chart is a simple form of depicting the various functional groups or departments which have been set-up to achieve the objectives of a health organisation. The organisauon chart conveys the basic information such as flow of authority and communications, responsibilities of various units, line and staff relationships, categories and number of personnel, grades of personnel, etc. Terry defines chart as: "a diagrammatical form which shows important aspects of an organisation including the major functions and their respective relationship, the channels of supervision, and the relative authority of each employee who is in-charge of each respective function."[13]

McFarland describes an organisational chart as the formal organisational relationships which executives intend should prevail.

#### *Chart Contents*

Charts may show individually or in various combinations, such information as:[14]

1. Basic organisation structure and flow of authority.
2. Responsibilities assigned to units and individuals.
3. Line and staff relationships.
4. Name of components.
5. Positions and incumbents.
6. Number of personnel.
7. Present and/or proposed structure.
8. A venues of promotion.
9. Management development requirements.
10. Salary data.

Too many details should be avoided in the chart. It should be easy to understand and simple to follow:

#### *Advantages*

Hicks feels that "without a chart, many people might view the organisation as just a group of people, parts, or activities." The organisation chart provides us with a picture of the structure. The chart is a means through which we can better understand the organisation as a whole, the components of the organisation, and the inter-relationship among these different components.[15] He compared organisation charts to a road map and opines that just as the road way is not the system of roads itself, an organisation chart is not the organisation itself.[16]

### *Limitations*

On the limitations of organisation charts, Kast and Rosenzweig write as follows: "The organisation chart is usually simplified, abstract model of the structure. It is not an exact representation of the reality of the structure and has many limitations. It shows only a limited number of the relationships, even in the formal organisation, and none of these in the informal organisation. It does not, for example, indicate the degree of authority which a superior has over a subordinate. Does the superior has the right to hire and replace the occupant of a subordinate position ? More importantly, it does not indicate the interactions between equals or the lateral relationship between people in different parts of Organisations."[17]

Inspite of their shortcomings, charts of the official organisation are worthwhile. The fact that laws are not obeyed in their every detail is not considered a sufficient reason for abolishing the rule of law in human affairs.

Kast and Rosenzweig feel that "inspite of these limitations, the organisation chart provides a useful starting point for the investigation of structure. It gives some indication of the hierarchical nature of positions and indicates the major activities performed. It prescribes certain patterns of formal interaction among positions. Thus, the chart communicates some important attributes of the structure."[18]

### *Suggestions Regarding Drawing and Increasing the Usefulness of Charts*

The following suggestions may be helpful in drawing a good chart:

1. The chart should be simple and easy to comprehend.
2. Chart should be given clear title, date and number.
3. It would be better if solid lines are drawn to indicate flow of formal authority and dotted lines to show informal relationships.
4. Sufficient details should be given for clarity.

### *Classification*

(i) Skelton, functional and personnel charts;

(ii) Vertical, horizontal and concentric charts; or

(iii) Master and supplementary charts;

*Skelton Charts*

A skelton chart is only the graphic presentation of the essential hierarchical framework. It contains the principle sub-units, usually depicted as hollow squares or rectangles. These are arranged in levels of echelons of hierarchical status, connected by lines suggesting different types of authority. The line of command is usually indicated by solid black line, while broken or hatched lines represent functional relationships.

*Functional Charts*

Functional charts usually apply to sub-units, with the boxes showing smaller breakdowns into divisions, units or sections. Sometimes they go down far enough to depict every first line supervisor. Each box contains a write-up of the duties, activities or functions of that particular, sub-unit, executive or supervisor.

*Personnel Charts*

A personnel chart is of the same graphic design as the functional chart, but the boxes contain personnel information. This may consist of the job title of the supervisor and each subordinate and in some cases the names of the incumbents are listed.

*Vertical Charts*

It shows the organisational structure in the form of a pyramid, the lines of command proceeding from top to bottom in vertical lines. This is the most common type of chart and is simplest to understand but cannot accommodate details of any magnitude.

*Horizontal Charts*

It follows the pattern of a tree drawn sideways. It is more compact than a vertical chart and can show a large number of posts and their grouping. It is comparatively easier to prepare. An organisation chart may be built up using both the vertical and horizontal pattern. In such a combined chart the top structure is shown vertically while the subordinate posts are shown horizontally.

*Concentric Charts*

It depicts the pivotal position of the top executive in the centre of concentric circles. Position of successive levels of subordinates extend in all directions outward from the centre.

*Master Charts*

Its shows the entire organisational structure, without the necessary details. A departmental chart is devoted exclusively to a department and given details to the relationships, authority and responsibility within the department. Thus, one master chart may be supplemented by several departmental charts, to understand the picture of the organisational as a whole.

The writer carried out a study of about 20 health organisations through their charts. It was revealed that these charts are used only as decorative pieces in the offices of the top executives without any practical use. These chart can help us in taking corrective action whenever there is expansion in the organisations. There is no consciousness among the top executives to make use of the chart to improve organisational structures. The writer suggested many changes in the organisational structures as per the examination of charts and these were welcomed by the top executives. It must be obligatory to review the charts every year like physical verification of inventories, to keep the chart up-to-date and functional. A study of some District Health Offices of some states revealed poor organisational set-up.

Simple studies of organisational chart can thus help in improving the structures of the health organisations resulting in the efficiency of health care operations.[19]

**2. Organisation Manual**

Organisational manuals are either non-existent or outdated in health organisations. These are used only for negative purposes like disciplinary action, etc., but not for positive purpose to promote better understanding of the health system and the rôle of the specific individuals in it.

An organisational chart provides a graphic illustration of the organisation. Where a detailed description of organisational relationships are desired to promote understanding of basic organisational structure by means of descriptions of the various jobs that may be depicted only by title on the charts, manuals are used. These ordinarily are made up of organisational chart accompanied by descriptions of the different position charted. A common break-down of headings in organisation manuals is by general function. responsibilities and authority, and relationships with others. Such manuals are generally kept in loose leaf form to facilitate revision.

They have come into wide use, particularly in large organisations. A detailed study of the manuals of a large number of health organisations revealed the following shortcomings which need the attention of the health chief executives to improve performance:

(i) Most of the manuals are out-dated. These were designed decades ago and were never revised to accommodate changes.

(ii) The language of these manuals is more oriented to legal frame-work. It becomes difficult to interpret the correct meanings.

(iii) In many organisations. these are kept only by the Chief Executive and are not distributed to all. New incumbents are not provided with these manuals.

(iv) Manuals are generally prepared by the top executives. It is essential to associate staff associations in reviewing the existing manuals or designing new manuals.

(v) We can thus conclude by saying that the manuals can be useful only if these are properly worded, reviewed intermittently, easily understood, and put into use by the staff in an organisation.

### 3. Work Distribution Charts

One of the newest and most promising tools in organisational analysis is the work distribution chart designed for the study of work assignments and job content within any single unit or work group. It shows who does what and for how long. The chart provides useful information pertaining to the ways in which employees spend their time.

In a work distribution chart the vertical column on the left lists the major activities for which the entire unit is responsible. The other vertical columns are assigned to the employees of the unit in descending order of job rank, from left to right. For each employee, the separate tasks performed and the number of hours devoted to each task during a standard time period are entered. The tasks are classified by the major activities in the left handed column and totalled by major activity.

The work distribution chart lays out work assigned. In a form that facilitates critical questioning of the existing distribution. It does not provide solution but it makes finding them a great deal easier. Work distribution charts are non-existent in health organisations and that is why it leads to inter-personal conflicts. Proper distribution of work can promote harmony and avoid interpersonal problem and thus add to the efficiency of health system.

### 4. Checklists of the Principles of an Organisation

Another technique of organisation analysis is that of systematic checking of present and proposed arrangements against accepted principles of health organisation. This will provide a fairly comprehensive audit of the organisational arrangements. Such a checklist may be valuable and when used in conjuction with charts and manuals of organisations.

#### *Guiding Principles of Organisation*

Several writers have tried to offer principles of organisation aimed at its smooth functioning of business operations with a minimum effort. Here we acquaint ourselves with the principles offered by a few writers.

S. Avery Raube in his paper, "Principles of Good Organisations", offers the following principles:

(i) There must be clear lines of authority running from the top to the bottom of the organisation.

(ii) No one in the organisation should report to more than one line supervisor. Everyone in the organisation should know to whom he reports, and who reports to him.

(iii) The responsibility and authority of each supervisor should be clearly defined in writing.

(iv) Responsibility should always be coupled with corresponding authority.

(v) The responsibility of higher authority for the acts of its subordinates is absolute.

(vi) The number of authority should be kept at a minimum.

(vii) Authority should be delegated as far down the line as possible.

(viii) The work of every person in the Organisation should be confined as far as possible to the performance of single leading function.

(ix) Whenever possible, line functions should be separated from staff function, and adequate emphasis should be placed on important staff activities.

(x) There is a limit to the number of position that can be co-ordinated by a single executive.

(xi) The organisation should be flexible, so that it can be adjusted to changing conditions.

(xii) The organisation should be kept as simple as possible.[20]

Most of the personnel working in health organisations are not clear about their duties and responsibilities. Inspite of massive changes and our advancing to new millennium shortly, we find that most of the health personnel need re-examination of their duties in the changed context.

**5. Job Analysis**

A job is a collection of tasks, duties, responsibilities which, as a whole, is regarded as the established assignment to individual employee. Job analysis is the procedure by which the facts with respect to each job are systematically discovered and noted. It is sometimes called Job Study, suggesting the care with which tasks, processes, responsibilities and personnel requirements are investigated. Job information provided by Job Analysis is used in:[21]

1. Organisation and integration of the whole health workforce in organisational planning.
2. Recruitment, selection and placement.
3. Transfer and promotions.
4. Training programmes.
5. Wage and salary administration.
6. Settlement of grievances.
7. Improvement of working conditions.
8. Setting production standards.
9. Improvement of employees productivity through work simplification and methods improvement.

Job analysis would help us to find the utility of the personnel in an organisation. It also helps us in identifying job relationships and skill required for effective performance.

According to Fulmer, there are three basic charting techniques which can be employed in the analysis of an informal organisation.

1. The Sociogram/Sociometry.
2. The Interaction Chart.
3. The Influence Chart.

**I. The Sociometry**

The pattern of liking and disliking among group members is termed the friend sociometric structure. It was devised by Moreno in 1934:[22] "Sociometry has been defined as a method for discovering, describing and evaluating social status, structure and development through measuring the extent of acceptance or rejection between individuals in groups."[23] J.G. Franz defines it, "as a method used for the discovery and manipulation of social configurations by measuring the attractions and repulsion between individuals in a group."[24] Let us illustrate with the help of a diagram which indicates the social interaction among six members of an organisation.

The figure given below is a Sociogram Depicting patterns of attraction in group of six persons. Each circle represents a group member. Solid arrows represent attraction, broken arrows represent rejection. Reciprocated attraction occurs where the arrows represent rejection. Reciprocated attraction occurs where the arrows go in both directions. Person A is a 'star', who is attracted to all others. Person 0 is a reject. Persons D and F are isolates. Persons A, B and E form the nucleus of a clique.[25]

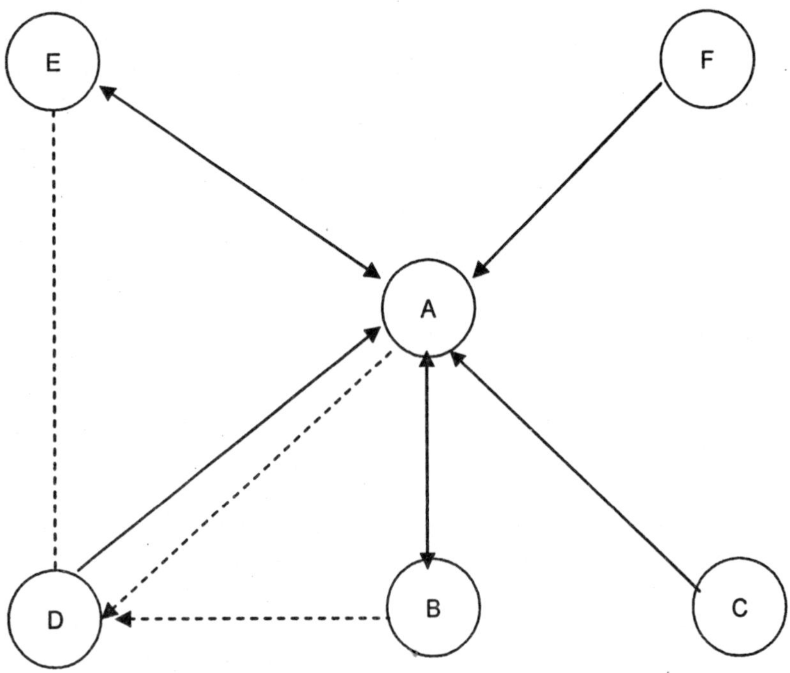

What is the significance of this charting from the point of view of organisational effectiveness. Friendship or attraction among some members, may be for passing the time together, resulting in the wastage of time. It is for the leader to diagnose it and use this Information to break this clique to make them work-oriented. Its advantage can be to Information pertaining to organisational behaviour, if we understand this clique.

**2. The Interaction Chart**

Another attempt at charting the informal organisation has been made by Robert F. Bales who developed what is called as Interaction Process Analysis."[26] Interaction patterns in a group functioning can be understood by observing who talks to whom about what, and how frequently. While socio-grams uncover possible friendship groups, interaction charts point at actual friendship groups. For example, let us explain with the help of 8 persons in a Group A, F and B form the close knit group indicated by their mutual attraction. A, B and C also form a friendship group as A moderates between B and C, H is a social isolate. This information can be of great use to the top leaders to produce desirable changes as they can understand whom to contact.

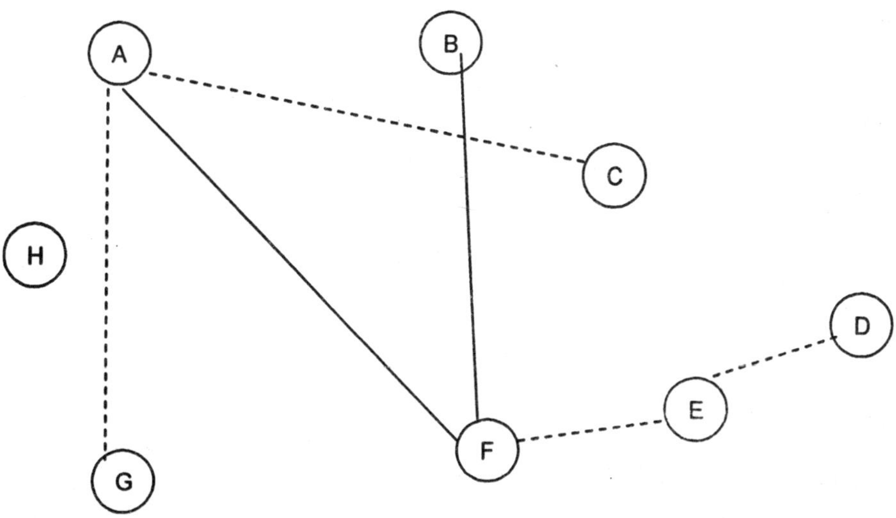


**3. Influence Charts**

These are used for charting problem-solving networks and for identifying individuals who are most commonly asked for help. Let us explain some categories of influence charts:

*(a) Power Structure*

The structure is the distribution of authority and influence within the group. Power is important as it determines a member's status, estimated worth and prestige. It has been found that the more powerful members of the group receive a greater number of messages or communication and are more frequently consulted than others. We can locate such persons, who enjoy power structure, through the charting of influence.

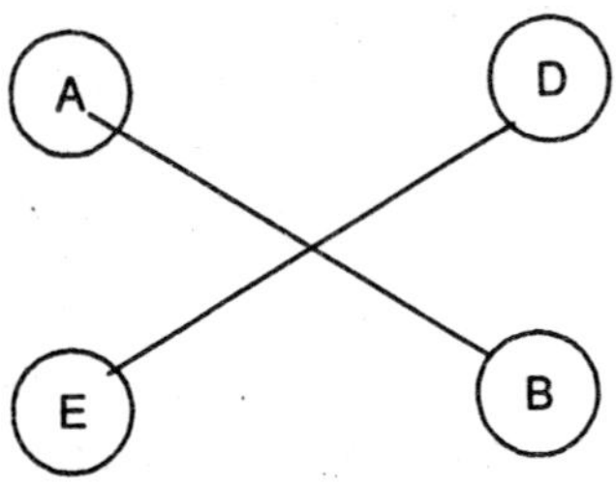


**Wheel**

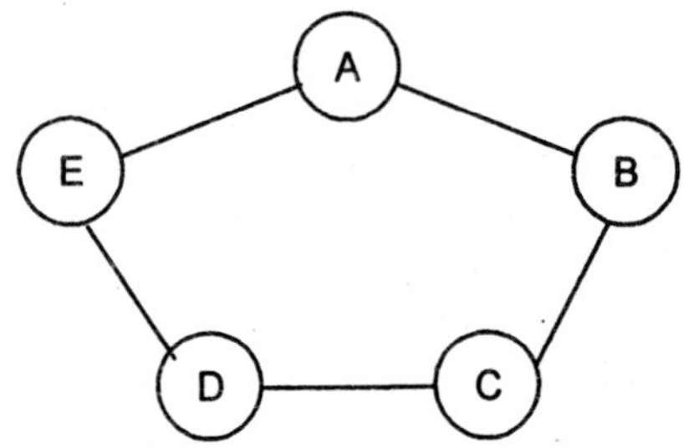


**Circle**

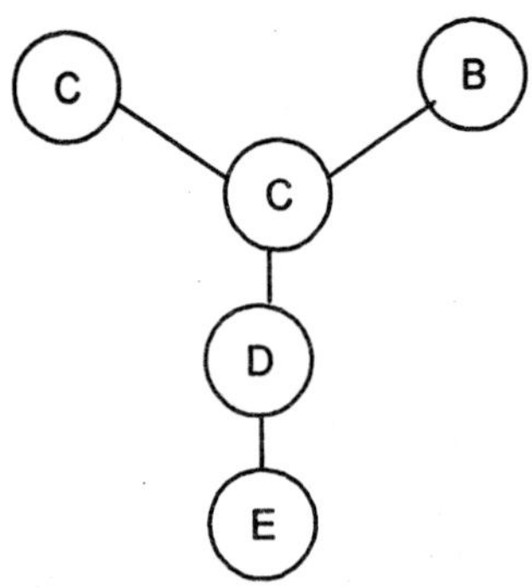


**Chain**

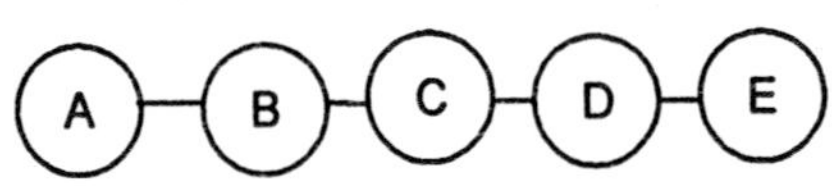


**Line**

*(b) Communication Structure*

The communication structure refers to the network or pattern of communication channels between group members. The number, capacity and distribution of communication channels affect group functions, especially in problem-solving, information distribution and the development of organised way of working.

Leavitt (1951) had carried out a classic study in which he compared different communication networks in groups and observed their effect on group behaviour. The communication nets studied by him varied in degree of centrality. Those who work in the network were found most satisfied as they participated equally.

*(c) Role Structure*

The role or work structure is the pattern of member's tasks and responsibilities in the group It is the group's division of labour or distribution of roles. This can help in distributing work according to the linking of the members in a group. Besides these, there are also other techniques to diagnose and improve the functioning of formal organisations.

**4. Role Analysis (See Chart 8.1)**

Role is the point where the organisation and the individual meet. Role means the pattern actions expected of a person in activities involving others. Role analysis aims to decode the actions expectation from the individual and the individual's expectations from his action with the organisation; and brings into focus where these can meet so as to ensure performance and effectiveness. When expectations of role are materially different or opposite, a person tends to be in role-conflict. This generates psychological reactions—low self-actualisation, low self-esteem, job, tensions, job disenchantment/alienation, job dissatisfaction. Role analysis may be used to define a role more clearly to pave the way for effectiveness. The purpose of role analysis exercise is to help the role occupant to clarify his role to reduce role ambiguity, so that he may become more effective.

Organisational effectiveness follows from the effectiveness of the individuals in their respective roles. Our efforts should be to maximise the effectiveness of each individual in his role so that we can maximise contribution of each individual. The ultimate goal of role analysis should be to ensure integration of the goals of management, employees and the organisation

There are also many other techniques which can be helpful in understanding of the functioning of the organisation. Let us mention their names only:

(a) Information systems that supply cognitive inputs on all sides of conflict issues;
(b) An open communication system that is transactional insofar as areas of disagreement or conflict are concerned;
(c) Individual counselling and therapy services for persons voluntarily participating individual-development programmes;
(d) Use of peers as an influence system;
(e) Laboratory-training groups;
(f) Planned study sessions on conflict issues;
(g) Use of survey-research feedback techniques;
(h) Group therapy for organisation units including adaptations of encounter where feasible;
(i) Face-to-face collaborative meetings with parties to conflict issues; and
(j) Simulation sessions preparatory to confrontation. Other techniques discussed separately.

CHART 8.1

**Organisational Analysis**

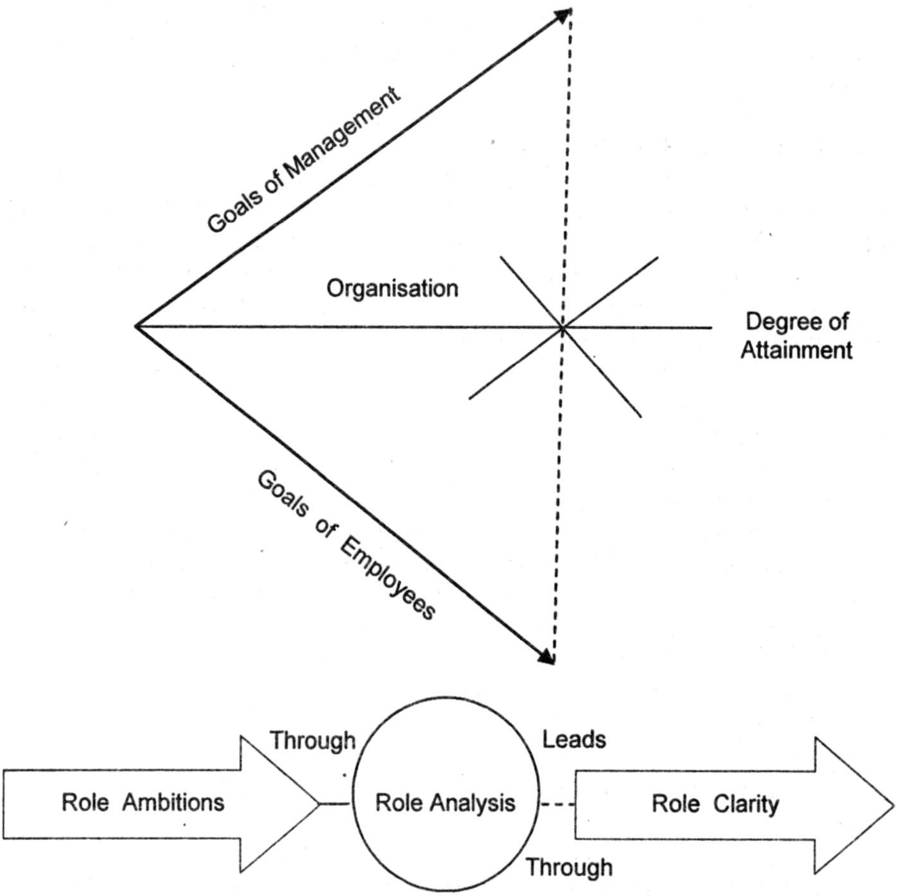


Management cannot ignore the understanding of informal relationships, if efficiency is to be achieved. An analysis of an informal organisation would help the management to maintain a conducive atmosphere, resulting in the achievement of organisational goals as well as helping in the fulfilment of individual goals. The purpose of both formal and informal organisation should be to integrate the individual with the organisation, using both formal and informal mechanism. This means that the individual has to be willing to include a great deal of himself in the organisational life. Shri P.R. Dubhashi,[27] in his Article on "Organisation Building" has rightly said that "an Organisation must emphasis team work and group work rather than a rigid hierarchical system, inappropriate to tasks which require flexibility and co-ordination of different agencies." Commitment cannot be obtained by coercion. It can only be ensured when the objectives and modes of behaviour of the organisation match his own goal and value, otherwise, he is alienated and alienated members do not perform upto their level of optimum capacity.

The explicit objective of organisational development effort is to increase the capability of organisation, as also the groups and individuals participating in them, to learn and apply new ways of dealing with complex internal and external relationships and processes and to view and manage change as an integral and normal function. There is also a need to regard organisational development as a long range and continuous effort. This implies that planned changes in one or more of the sub-systems of the organisation should be such as to build flexibility and adaptability into the system to cope effectively with turbulent and complex external environment, while maintaining its own dynamic equilibrium.[28]

The task facing managements of today is skilfully to blend together the formal organisation with the informal in order to minimise conflict and to encourage healthy adjustment and co-ordination. This can be achieved by managerial recognition of the importance that informal groups have upon individual attitudes and morale. The supervisor should encourage the formation and growth of informal groups; he should recognize their leaders and assign them jobs that reflect their group position; he should see that they are properly informed about policies and procedures. If proper encouragement is given to informal groups they will respond in positive rather than negative ways.[29]

We can thus conclude bys saying that we must synthesize the merits of both formal and informal groups to get a proper understanding of the nature of an organisation. Keith Davis has rightly said that "the informal organisation needs to be strong enough to be supportive, but not strong enough to dominate."[30] In short, we can say that we must try to synchronize formal and informal goals.

We can conclude that the structure of health care system must be kept to suit the requirements of the health system. We must introduce administrative reforms to inject changes to avoid lag between health organisation structure and the requirement of health system.

## Notes and References


1. Following studied carried out by the writer can be studied to understand the practical application of organisation analysis:
   (a) Organisation on and working of the South-East Asia, Regional Office of WHO, Sterling Publishing, New Delhi, 1977.
   (b) Organisation and Managerial Problems of Apex Co-operative Organisation with special reference to MARKFED, Co-operative Perspectives, Vol. 2, No. 1, June 1977.
   (c) Organisation and Management of Co-operative Organisation; *Indian Co-operative Review*, Vol. XIV, No. 2, New Delhi, January 1977.
   (d) Organisation and Administration of Family Planning Field Work; A Case Study of Haryana PEN, A Magazine of Family Planning Associated of India (Haryana Branch), 27, August 1975.

2. Dimock and Dimock: Public Administration, p 104.
3. J.D Moony: Principles of Organisation, I.
4. H. Simon: Administrative Behaviour, p. 30.
5. H. Simon: Public Administration, p. 5.
6. Keith Davis, Human Behaviour at Work, 4th Edition, McGraw Hill, New York, 1972, pp. 257-59.
7. Earnest Dale Management—Theory and Practice, 1973, Tokyo, McGraw Hill, p. 149.
8. Joseph L. Massive: Essentials of Management, Prentice Hall, Englewood, N.J. Cliffs. 1964, p. 64.
9. Amitai Elzioni: Modern Organisations, Prentice Hall, Englewood, N.J. Cliffs, 1964, p. 64.
10. W Richard Scott, "Theory of Organisation" in Robert E.L. Fairs, (ed.) Handbook of Modern Sociology, Paul McNally & Co., Chicago, 1964, p. 488.
11. Robert V. Presthus: Foreward: A Theory of Organisational Behaviour, *Administrative Science Quarterly*, June 1958, p. 50.
12. Peter F. Drucker: The Practice of Management, Heinemann, London, 1955, p. 225.
13. Terry, Geroge, Principles of Management, Richard D. Irwin Inc., Homewood, 1972, p. 378.
14. Harry L. Whyl, Office Management Hand Book, ed. by Harry Whyl, 1958, p. 225.
15. Herbert G. Hicks: The Management of Organisation: Systems and Human Resources Approach (2nd ed.), New York McGraw Hill, 1972, p. 259.
16. *Ibid.*
17. Kast and Rosenzweig. *op. cit.*, p. 175.
18. *Ibid*
19. *Indian Co-operative Review*, Vol. XIV, No. 2, Jan. 1977, p. 163.
20. Reprinted in Max D. Richards and William A. Neilander: Reader in Management, Bombay, D.B. Taraporevala, 1971, pp. 692-700.
21. Dale Yoder: Personnel Management and Industrial Relations (5th ed.), New Delhi, Prentice Hall, p. 281.
22. J.L. Maroeno, Who Shall Survive, Washington Publishing Co., 1969, p. 29.
23. Urie Bronfeabrenner: "A Constant Frame of Reference for Sociometric Research", Sociometry, VI, pp. 363-72.
24. J.G. Franz, "Survey of Sociometric Techniques with an annotated Bibliography", *Sociometry*, II, pp. 76-90.
25. L. Mann: Social Psychology, John Wiley and Sons, Inc., New York, 1969, p. 29.
26. Robert, F. Bales: Interaction Process Analysis, Cambridge, Man Addison, Wesley, 1950.
27. P.R. Dubhashi, Organisation Building, *IJPA*, Jan.-March, 1980.
28. *Management Quarterly*: The Post-Graduate Committee of the Institute of Chartered Accountant of India, Vol. 2, 1 June 1976, p. 61.
29. Hyneryager and Heckmann: Human Relations in Management, 1967, p. 415.
30. Keith Davis: Human Behaviour at Work, New Delhi, Tata McGraw Hill, 1972, p. 272.

9

CHAPTER

# Method Study and Work Measurement

Health Organisation is a service organisation and thus, in order to be effective, must conduct its business quickly and efficiently. This would depend upon the choice of right procedures and methods. However, health system is suffering from red tapism and outdated methods hampering the success of the health care delivery systems. Primary Health Care set-up with all earnestness could not make much headway, as the wrong methods and procedures created bottlenecks.

A study conducted by National Institute of Health and Family Welfare found that patients have to wait for 3-4 hours in OPD before getting their turn. Even to get a room in Private ward means too much of formalities, both at the time of admission and discharge. Methods and procedures in a hospital are so complicated that the attendants of patients get exhausted even before the admission of the patient. Wrong methods, practices and procedures hamper the functioning of health care system. How can we come out of this chaos? How can we remove these irritants? The only answer is to introduce method study as a continuous exercise to maintain health care system alive, functional and dynamic. Let us now discuss the meaning, scope and utility of method study.

Method study is one of the techniques of work study to improve on 'How' of doing work. It is a technique to improve method of work, with a view to increase efficiency and effectiveness of resources—men, money and material. In common parlance, 'Method' stands for the means of accomplishing an end, while study means application of mind to a problem or an exercise. Method Study then traces the cases responsible for poor administrative and clinical performance, so that appropriate remedial action may be taken. In broad terms, it may be said that the Method Study approach can help in successfully grappling with a view to find solutions to all problems, which face the working of a health organisation. In sum, we can say that the Method Study is like an autopsy aimed at eliminating the disease rather than the symptoms of ailment. The scientific and technological advancements are affecting the functioning of health machinery and thus there is a corresponding need to adjust the methods of Public Administration to suit the changing conditions for optimum performance. Method Study can be of immense value to the health administrators through its help in adjusting the procedure of work to the changed conditions. Method Study is a continuous activity to ensure that the methods of work in a health organisation are in tune with its objectives and are helping in accelerating the progress of the health organisation, rather than retarding it. Method Study must be use when a new organisation is created or when an alteration is made in the existing organisation or when some problem arises in the existing health organisations.

While organisational analysis deals mainly with the division of work and responsibility for the efficient fulfilment of objectives, the method study deals with the way the work is performed. British Standards Institution defines Method Study as the systematic recording and critical examination of existing and proposed ways of doing work, as a means of developing and applying easier and more effective methods and reducing costs.

According to Indian Standards Institution, the Method Study is the systematic analysis and improvement of work methods and systems through the application of innovatory techniques to achieve better utilization of resources.

According to an ILO document, Method Study has been defined as the systematic recording, analysis and critical examination of the existing and proposed ways of doing work and the development and application of easier and more productive methods.

Russel M. Currie says that Method Study is a systematic and analytical approach to problems which will enable all the relevant factors to be evaluated so that decisions may be made. An analysis of these definitions would reveal that the Method Study must be systematic and analytical and should be directed to the existing or potential problem to promote efficiency.

## NEED OF THE METHOD STUDY

Method Study is a continuous activity and must be used at definite intervals of time to ensure the good health of an organisation, as we know that prevention is better than cure. However, there are certain health organisations, which may need the immediate use of Method Study to improve their adverse conditions. The sick organisation can be identified from the symptoms which presage the need for the Method study in an existing work situation. Let us mention here some such symptoms whose presence can warrant the need for an immediate application of Method Study:

1. Dissatisfaction among the clients/beneficiaries about poor health services.
2. Escalating operating costs.
3. Low morale of the staff.
4. Lack of discipline among the employees visible through late-comings, not available during the office hours, etc.
5. Work not being done to maintain time schedule.
6. Competition among the personnel.
7. Low equipment utilization.
8. Lack of co-operation and co-ordination among the different sections of an organisation.
9. High wastage of contingent material.
10. Existence of bottlenecks.
11. Inconsistencies in quality.

## OBJECTIVES OF METHOD STUDY

Method Study is basically interested in finding better ways of doing things, resulting in better performance. To quote R.M. Currie, Method Study is essentially concerned with finding better ways of doing things and it contributes to improved efficiency by getting rid of unnecessary work, avoidable and other forms of waste. It makes the efficiency possible through:

(a) Improvement of existing obsolete processes and procedures.
(b) Improved layout of office and working environment.
(c) Economy in human effort.
(d) Suggesting the best use of money and material.
(e) Improved design of the goods or services provided by the organisation.
(f) Improved quality.
(g) Job satisfaction.
(h) Improved flow of work.
(i) Standardisation of processes and products.

In brief the Method Study aims at optimization of resources which are:

*Manpower*: Brain, Skill, morale and effort.
*Materials*: Inventory, Quality, Standards.
*Equipment*: Design and Operation.
*Services*: Communication and Information systems.
*Space and Building*: Availability, design, utilization.

## ESSENTIALS OF METHOD STUDY

We must always keep in mind that Method Study is only an aid to better methods. Its success pre-supposes a number of essential elements. Let us mention some of them:

(a) An urge and desire on the part of the personnel in the organisation and the Method Study Team to find better methods.

(b) Requisite skill, attitudes and ability in the persons engaged in Method Study.

(c) Proper rapport between the method Study team and the key personnel in the organisation.

(d) Involvement of the personnel of the organisation being studied to get a lot of unwritten information and for understanding the dynamics of the organisation.

(e) Need of suggesting the introduction of only such methods which can be implemented by the organisation without much cost and resistance. Besides, the need of technical considerations may also be kept in mind.

(f) Making all the employees in the organisation to understand the implications of new methods through seminars, lectures or any other method to thwart the potential fears amongst the employees of the proposed changes.

Joseph Prokopenko in his Article, "Management Approaches to Productivity Improvement" in Management in Government, April-June, 1995 suggests the following essentials based upon experiences in developed and developing countries.

Highly successful productivity programmes have been carried out at national, regional and local levels in many countries (i.e., Singapore, Japan, Hong Kong, Philippines, South Korea, some European countries, United States and Canada). Experience suggests that productivity promotion in public services at the micro-level typically follows certain directions. For example:

- changes in managerial styles and practices;
- awareness raising, management training and development;
- action-oriented productivity improvement;
- group activity and participation of various types;
- introduction of productivity incentive schemes; and
- development and strengthening of productivity improvement institutions, including international networking activities.

## ASPECTS OF METHOD STUDY (See Chart 9.1)

A Method Study investigation involves generally all the steps of a scientific method. There are seven essential steps in the application of a Method Study. Strict adherence to their sequence, as well as to their content, is essential for the success of an investigation. They are shown as below:

| | |
|---|---|
| SELECT: | The work to be studied. |
| RECORD: | All the relevant facts about the present method by direct observation. |
| EXAMINE: | Those facts critically and in ordered sequence using the techniques best suited to the purpose. |
| DEVELOP: | The most practical, economic and effective method, having due regard to all contingent circumstances. |
| DEFINE: | The new method so that it can always be identified. |
| INSTALL: | That method as standard practice. |
| MAINTAIN: | That standard practice by regular routine checks. |
| REVIEWING: | Locate discrepancies between the authorized procedures. |

The ultimate purpose of method study should be the aim of Integrating it into normal management process so that search for Improvement becomes a matter of accepted practice in an organisation.

*Applications*

Some Examples:

1. Method of Registering a patient.
2. Method of calling patients for examination.
3. Method of allotting wards.
4. Method of payments of hospital dues.
5. Method of collecting laboratory reports.

Bermolak has suggested 10 points method study for successful productivity improvement programmes:

(i) Clear objectives and an integrated productivity plan.
(ii) Continuing productivity activity.
(iii) Central point of responsibility.
(iv) Measurement of results.
(v) Top level interest and commitment.
(vi) Role and importance of management approaches.
(vii) Manager accountability for productivity improvement.
(viii) Raising productivity awareness throughout the organisation.
(ix) Communication and training.
(x) Employee involvement and incentives.

CHART 9.1

**Procedure of Method Study**

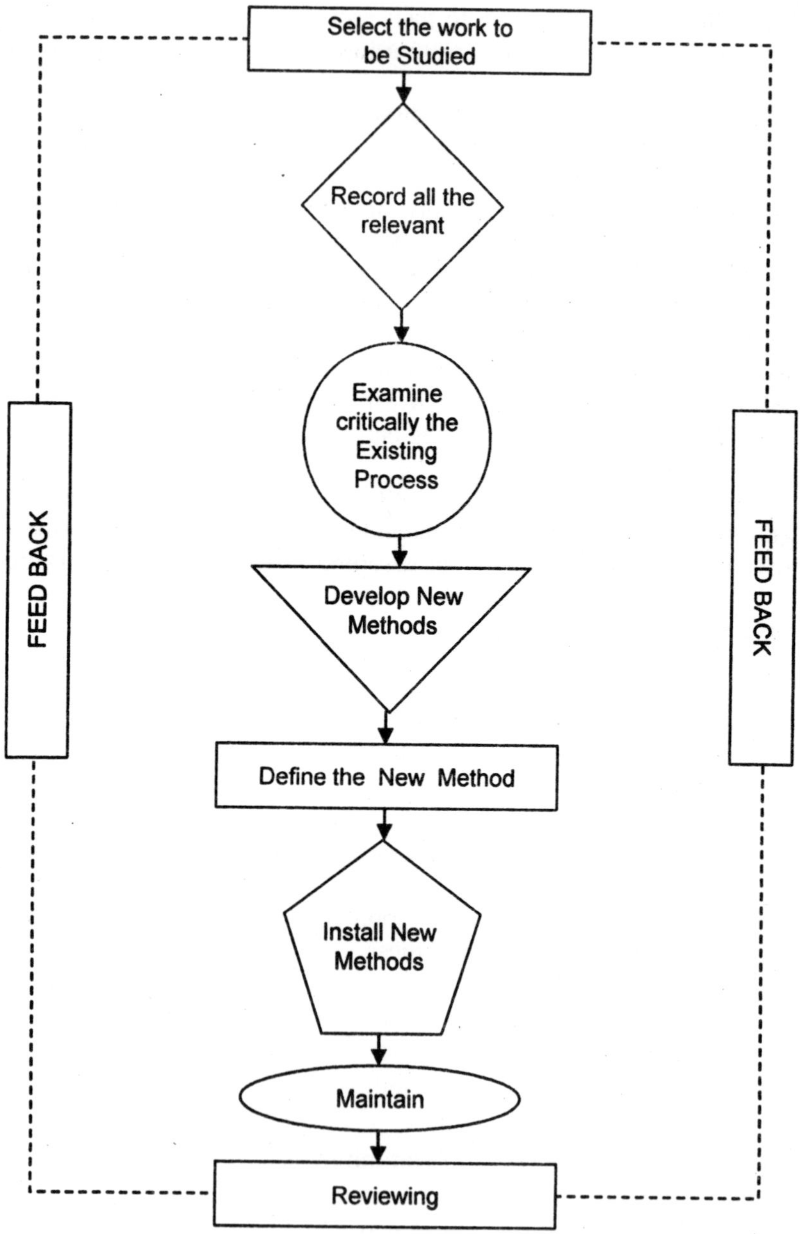

Proficiency by an individual is not creative until it transforms into efficiency, the means to act diligently, with your heart in your work, with a gusto to improve, a spirit to outshine your own present abilities. This spirit of challenging yourself by yourself is the secret of self-improvement and personality unfoldment.

—*Chinmaya*

## WORK MEASUREMENT

Today, there is a widespread feeling in the public about the inefficiency in health administration. As health organisations grow in size and complexity, they become difficult to manage. In most of the organisations, health administration is run by hit and trial methods, i.e., without any yardstick to measure the individual and collective performance. The measurement of human work has always been a problem for management. The plans for the provision of goods or services at a predetermined cost are often dependent on the accuracy with which the amount and type of human work involved can be forecast and organized. While it has commonly been the practice to make estimates and set targets based on past experience, these too frequently prove a rough and unsatisfactory guide. Without measurement, the organisation operates in darkness with hardly any basis for comparison or control. Before, we discuss the techniques of work measurement, let us discuss its meaning and need. Most of the health activities have no standards in terms of output and time! How can we allocate human resources without knowing these standards? That is why in most of the health organisations, there is lot of mismatching and some health organisations are over-staffed while others are under-staffed. All these problems can be solved if we introduce the concept of work measurement to ensure effective planning, implementation, control and supervision.

Work measurement can improve the functioning of preventive, promotive and curative, health services. In curative health services, planning can be done acurately for OPD, operation theatre, ICU Nursing services, etc. to provide decent health care. This technique is easy to apply. provided it is done from time to time to introduce desired changes.

### Meaning

Work measurement is concerned with the determination of the amount of time required to perform a unit of work. The time required for this task is commonly referred to as the standard or allowed time.

Thus, work measurement is to provide a yardstick for human effort which can help in efficient manning, improved planning and control. sound and effective schemes.

As stated in an I.L.O. Publication:

"Work measurement is the application of techniques designed to establish the time for a qualified worker to carry out a specified job at a defined level of performance."

The Work Study Report of the Secretariat Training School, Ministry of Home Affairs, defines it as:

"Work measurement is the application of techniques designed to establish the work content of a specified task by determining the time required for carrying it out at a defined standard of performance by qualified worker."

Work measurement is thus a device for estimating more precisely the amount of time it should take or will take to perform the assigned work. Work measurement has both a negative and positive role. Negatively, it locates the existence of ineffective time, positively it sets standard times for the performance of work. Since Method Study is a technique for reducing work connot, therefore, it is necessary that Method Study should precede work measurement. In short, work measurement is interested in investigating, reducing and subsequently eliminating ineffective time.

It is very easy to apply this technique to highly repetitive operations. It is said that it is very difficult to apply this technique to work of key administrative posts; who work with unpredictable results and whose special requirements impose personnel needs not necessarily related to work volume or time. However, we must try to use this technique even under such situations through establishing norms or standards of performance which may be less precise but rational. This technique would make even such persons accountable and responsible rather than they make their own kingdom within the organisation.

## OBJECTIVES OF WORK MEASUREMENT

Work measurement is concerned with investigating, reducing and eliminating ineffective time. Besides, it also helps setting performance standards, which connote the optimum rate of output that can be achieved by a qualified worker as an average for a working day or shift, due allowance being made for the necessary time required for rest. The following advantages would result through the application of work measurement in an organisation:

### 1. Comparing Alternative Methods

There are generally many methods to perform a given job. Where two alternative methods seem equally good and suitable. the one which consumes less lime for completion will be better. The techniques of Work Measurement offer the best means of making this choice.

**2. Correct Manning of Work**

Staffing is an important area of management. Work Measurement can help us in making the Public offices staffed by persons in right quantity and quality. Most of the Committees and Commissions have reported that health departments are over-staffed to a great extent but they have not offered any method by which to assess and curtail the staff.

**3. Effective Planning and Scheduling of Operations**

Effective planning and scheduling of operations require the exact estimation and availability of resources—men. money and material. All these can be made possible through the technique of Work Measurement as the information generated by this technique form a reliable basis for planning and forward loading the men and material for the administrators to utilize them to their best advantage. The main cause of the failure of the planning in India has been the lack of any accurate measurement of work. Unless the work has been measured, it cannot be planned and scheduled with any assurance that a promised operation can be met.

**4. Effective Means of Control**

Once the operations have been planned, these are to be implemented. At the stage of implementation, management is interested to know how close this is to actual field realities. There is a need of control by the management to ensure the pre-designed output. Maintenance of proper records for all types of activities plus a knowledge of the performance, which is maintained while work is being done, form a reliable basis for control.

**5. Helpful in Cost Estimation**

Standards are helpful determining the cost of the work performed. This is helpful to management in preparing budgets and in measuring the effectiveness of forecasts. By knowing what the cost should be and comparing them with budget figures. it is possible to ascertain the reasons for the difference. This may mean that there is a need for devising more efficient procedures and setting new standards to conform to them. Thus, standards help in reducing costs.

**6. Better Staff Morale**

It creates better morale in the staff through their perception of what is expected of them in terms of quantity and quality. The efficient workers can be separated from the poor workers and thus the work of efficient workers can be recognized. This is also helpful in installing incentive wage system.

**7. Measure of Efficiency**

Standards as a basis for measuring the effectiveness of any organisation by indicating the achievements as compared with the standards.

**8. Better Management**

On the basis of the standards, managerial functions can be predicted and discharged more effectively.

**9. Direction to Future Research**

**10. Improving Quality**

Quality is magical. Quality passion has magical effect on our thinking patterns. We start seeing "Q" in every object. Standards give clue to the problem areas where research may be carried out to solve the problem.

## BASIC PROCEDURE AND TECHNIQUES

As enunciated earlier, there are fundamentally eight basic steps in performing a complete work study. Some of these are relevant for work measurement. Isolating those steps which are necessary for Work Measurement, the basic procedure could easily be formulated. Depending on the ultimate use for which the Work Measurement is to be put will determine as to whether all the eight steps are necessary. The essence of work measurement, would depend on selecting the requisite unit of measurement. A standard unit of measurement should be comparable, exact and stable. The measurement of all work done in an organisation could be carried out through measuring by any of the three ways—measuring individual output, measuring groups on routine work and groups on special work.

## BASIC STEPS (Chart 9.2)

*Select*: The work to be studied.

*Record*: All the relevant data relating to the circumstances in which the work is being the methods and the elements of activity in them.

*Measure*: Each element in terms of TIME over a sufficient number of cycles of activity ensure that a representative picture has been obtained.

*Examine*: The recorded data and element times CRITICALLY to ensure that unproductive or random elements are separated from productive elements; the recorded times, each element and determine a representative time for each.

*Compile*: A time for the operation which will provide a realistic standard of performance and will include time allowances to cover suitable rest, personal needs, contingencies, etc.

*Define*: Precisely the series of activities and method of operation for which the time has been allowed and issue the time as standard for the activities and methods specified.

CHART 9.2

**Health as Management Tool for Development**

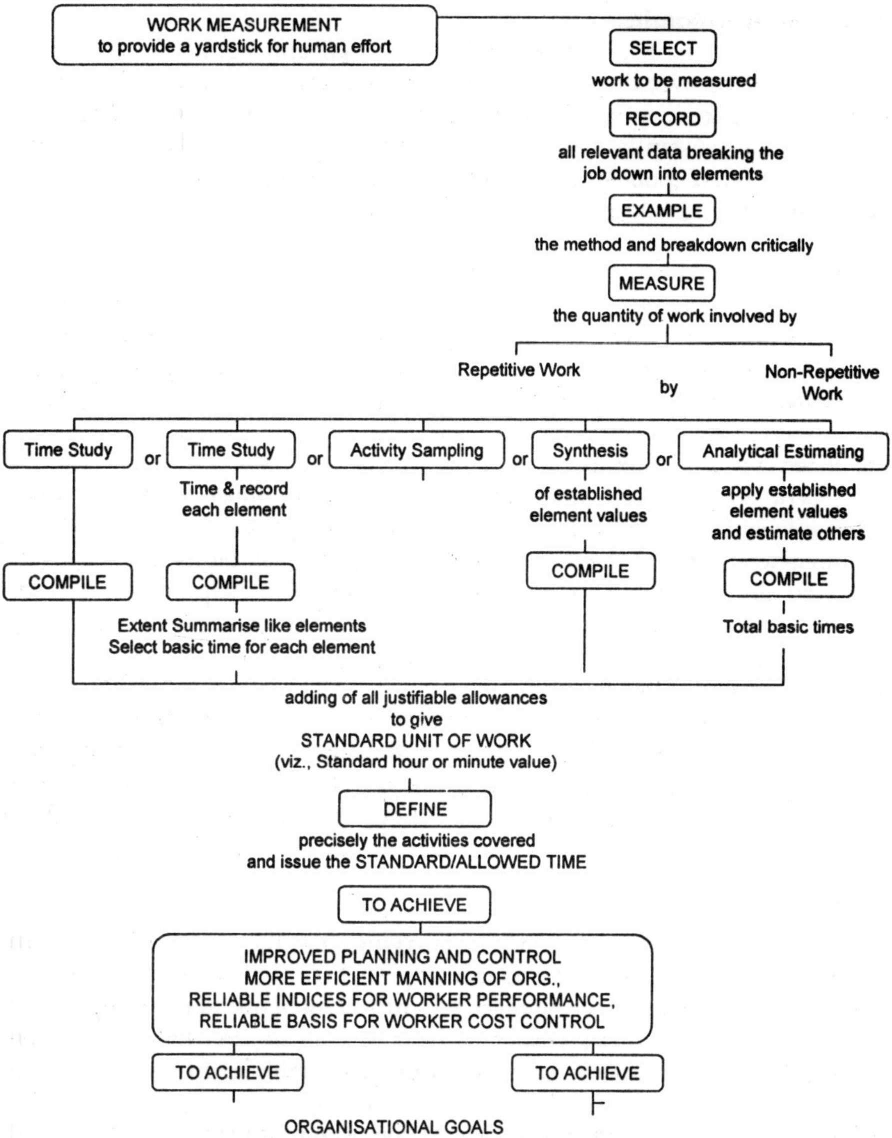


## ESSENTIALS OF WORK MEASUREMENT

Besides the competence, the Work Study men must ensure the congenial environment within the organisation where work improvement programmes are being installed. Work Study men must possess commonsense, imagination, patience, enthusiasm, tact and above all a pleasing personality. Let us mention some of these factors, which may be kept in mind by the Work Study men and the top management, to ensure the best results:

**I. Cordial Relationship**

Work study team must establish cordial and equitable relationship with the person working in the organisation being investigated. This would generate harmonious relationship advantageous to both sides. The study team should constantly endeavour to dispel the impression that they would devise anti-staff policies and measures. There should be mutual trust, sincerity, devotion, loyalty and an open attitude.

**II. In-built Reliability, Consistency and Uniformity**

The work study team should not make superficial suggestions but should see that the standards meet the criteria of reliability, consistency and uniformity. The organisation must provide the coercive measures in case of deviation so that the system can operate well.

**III. Incentive Opportunity**

The management must ensure incentive to those who can ensure more efficiency and productivity as compared to the standards framed. This would encourage the keen workers to progress fast rather than allowing them to get frustrated. Such individuals can also help in the ultimate raising of their own standards through their own examples.

**IV. Participative Management**

Before enforcing the new standards, we must ensure their acceptance by all the employee in the organisation through participative management or management by objectives. There is a fear that the employees may resist and even resort to strikes, etc., if not taken in confidence. Such standards would be accepted whole-heartedly and would produce best results.

**V. Cost Benefit Analysis**

A huge cost is incurred in carrying out the Work Measurement programmes and ultimately maintaining such programmes. As a result of such an investment there should be certain benefits and saving over a period of time. The initial costs may tend to increase, but they should soon level off to a point where savings should inevitably crop up.

**VI. Careful Selection of the Work Measurement Team**

The success of the measures of work measurement programmes depends to a great extent upon the right skill and attitudes of the personnel associated with the team. Only properly trained and experienced personnel in the relevant field should be chosen. Measurement is a practical job and it requires a competent and experienced person.

## TECHNIQUES OF WORK MEASUREMENT

Let us discuss some of the techniques of Work Measurement:

### 1. Subjective Judgement

Work measurement involves here the subjective judgement of the management, i.e. experience and guess work. This is generally known as rule of thumb standards. It is very difficult to apply these standards universally and in large scale organisations. Moreover, cannot be justified on scientific grounds.

### 2. Record of Past Performance

These represent what is rather than what should be. Standards thus arrived are indicators of work and time requirement and can be used for controlling the operations. It may be calculated as follows:

Staff members Minutes per unit:

$$= \frac{\text{Total number of staff members considered} \times \text{Minutes in work week}}{\text{Weighted number of units completed}}$$

This method is not suitable to improve the performance of organisation as standards are measured based on past performance and not what ought to be.

There are many scientific methods. Let us mention some of them. These are:

(i) Time Study
(ii) Pre-determined Motion Time Systems (PMTS)
(iii) Activity Sampling
(iv) Analytical Estimating
(v) Synthesis.

### (i) Time Study

Time study is the most important technique of work measurement. It is concerned with the direct observation of work while it is being performed. Let us define the concept of the Study as applicable to work measurement. As stated in I.L.O. Publication, "Time Study is a work measurement technique for recording the times and rates of working for the elements of a specified job carried out under specified conditions and for analysing the data so as to obtain the time necessary for carrying out the job at a defined level of performance."

In a document issued by Secretariat Training School, Ministry of Home Affairs, New Delhi, it is stated that, "Time Study is a technique for determining as accurately as possible from a limited number of observations the time necessary to carry out a given activity at a defined standard of performance",

According to J.A. Larkin, Time Study is "a work measurement technique for recording the times and rates of working for the element of a specified job carried out under specified conditions, and for analysing the data so as to obtain the time necessary for carrying out the job at a defined level of performance."

**Basic Steps**

The basic steps in the Time Study Procedure have been depicted as follows:

CHART 9.3

**Basic Steps for Time Study Procedure**

**Survey Job Content**
(Correct method, operating conditions and quality, Assess Nature of constituents to be measured)

|

**Plan**
(The programme by which all the constituents can be measured economically and accurately)

|

**Define Elements**

|

**Measure**
(Recording the rate and time for each element repeated in sufficient volume to provide reliable data covering all expected conditions)

|

**Extend**
(To obtain the basic time for each element by the calculation observed time × observed rating)
(standard rating)

|

**Collate Data**
(To establish representative basic time for each element in the task)

|

**Determine Relaxation Allowance**
(For each element in the task)

|

**Allow**
(For other relevant factors, and summate to establish)

|

**Standard Time**
(For the defined job)

|

**Applications**

The answers to the many questions like those given below would help health institutions in better planning, implementation and evaluation of health services. This would also help in weeding out unwanted activities to provide decent health care to all in the new millennium. This would also promote transparency. Accountability and good management. These techniques would help the health system in locating the reasons of non-utilisation of health services by the people inspite of their availability and accessibility. This would promote better health manpower planning and drugs and equipment management.

1. How many patients can be examined by a doctor in a given time?
2. How many operations can be done in different specialities in a given time?
3. How many X-rays can be taken out per hour?
4. How many ECGs can be taken per hour?
5. What is the utilisation time of different categories of health workers?

## CONCLUSION

The health administration is facing shortage of Personnel and equipment. However, we are not utilizing the existing equipment and personnel. We can get answers to many problems in health administration through method study and work measurement.

10

CHAPTER

# *Management of Inter-personal Relations*

Whenever two people meet, there are really six people present. There is each man as he sees himself, each man as the other person sees him, and each man as he really is.

—*William James*

"Management effectiveness depends to a great extent upon the human factor, as we know that human rather than capital is key to development. If we can diagnose the causative factors affecting human behaviour, we would be able to sublimate those factors and put them to constructive use. This techniques can even help the manager to diagnose his own behaviour. This understanding can provide him kinetic energy to influence, direct and therefore condition the behaviour of the people in his organisation."

—*Author*

## INTER-PERSONAL RELATIONS AND RESOLVING CONFLICTS

Health system consists of different categories of workers. There is no operation which can be handled singly by a lone health functionary. It requires the co-operation and support of different categories of personnel to achieve the goals of health. Let us take an example of an operation of an ENT patient. It requires the co-operation of nurses, anesthesia expert, medicine specialists, ward boys, etc. However, what we find in practice is that there are no cordial relations among them. This results in inefficiency and bad delivery of health care and ultimate harassment to patients.

All the health functionaries need an education in understanding the inter-personal relationships and their management to ensure the insulating of health institutions from internal behavioural disturbances. W.C. Schultz (The Interpersonal World, 1966) maintains that there are three inter-personal needs, (i) inclusion-the need of Interaction and association, (ii) control—the need for authority and power, and (iii) affection. The developing of successful inter-personal relations in the context of organisational goals is a challenging task and a slow process. It requires a deep psychological understanding of oneself as well as of others, with whom one comes into contact in various organisational capacities. In India, since most of the positions are occupied by virtue of merely the academic, professional and seniority qualifications, without any regard for proficiency in inter-personal relations. Therefore, many of the persons on these jobs cannot handle the health institutions efficiently. One of the important qualifications for any assignment is true understanding of inter-personal relations, which play greater role than other factors.

Based upon personal experience, research and observation, it can be said with certainty that, those who understand the socio-psychological make up of their colleagues prove to be very successful and get most of the work done through them in spite of other hurdles. However, with the best of organisations, managers, lacking in understanding of inter-personal relations are not able to handle even routine organisational functions. That is why we define a leader as a person who does not do the things himself but gets the things done by colleagues.

## METHODS TO UNDERSTAND AND IMPROVE INTER-PERSONAL RELATIONS

### Model of Johari Window

Let us explain in brief the model of Johari Window, which helps us in understanding inter-personal awareness. The Johari Window is a theoretical model for studying inter-personal relations. It was developed by Joseph Luft and Harry Ingham (the name Johri combines their first names). This model depicts how people expose themselves to others and receive feedback from others in their interpersonal relationships. The analysis of the model shows that the Johri Window has four parts; Arena, Blindspot, Closed and Dark. Arena depicts the "Public Self" that is known to the self and others. The Blindspot area known to others, but not to the self. The closed area is the private self which is known to the self but not to others. The Dark area is neither known to self nor to others.

**JOHARI WINDOW**

| | |
|---|---|
| ARENA | BLIND SPOT |
| CLOSED | DARK |

The examination of this model suggests that if the Arena is very Small, there is very less spontaneous interaction. On the other hand, the larger arena enhances the chances of participation in any relationship to make correct perceptual judgements about each other. This helps them to develop realistic mutual expectations and increases their level of trust and influence. As the Arena expands, the closed area of private self becomes less and it becomes less necessary to hide things one knows or feels. The Blindspot takes longer to reduce because self-concept protection mechanisms are involved.

We may learn from the Johari model that a genuine and permanent relationship can prosper only if it revolves around the needs or aspirations or they may be convinced of the desired changes. A close inter-personal relationship is maintained by building trust, acceptance and support. All these would lead to the development of faith among themselves. Faith is contagious and if developed once, is sure to have positive influence on the organisation development.

**Transactional Analysis (I am OK, You are OK)**

The term "Transactional Analysis" was first used by Dr. Eric Berne in 1957. This technique gained further momentum after the publication of his two books, i.e. (i) Transactional Analysis in Psychotherapy (1961), and (ii) Games People Play (1964). Thomas A. Harris developed the concept further in 1967 through his book I am OK, You are OK.

Originally, TA was basically a method of Psychotherapy. Later on, it was used in improving inter-personal relationships and communication. TA concentrates on the rational and analytical side of human behaviour which is observable. TA is concerned with transactions between people—both Verbal and non-verbal, Physical and emotional, implicit or explicit.

This technique presupposes the existence of three ego states—Parent ego state; Adult ego state; and Child ego state; acquired by an individual since childhood. Each ego state is a distinct source of particular behaviour. However, one does not stay in only one ego state; instead, a person switches occasionally from one to another, as can be noted through observing behaviour and listening to what is said and how it is said.

**Three States of Personality**

| C | CHILD EGO |
|---|---|
| A | ADULT EGO |
| P | PARENT EGO |

*(I) Parent Ego*

The parent state is the collection of recordings in the brain of the childhood experiences which are unquestioned and imposed external events. The little boy feels that his parents are strong and forceful while he is small and weak. He is forced to accept the advice of the parents and take them as fundamental truths.

*(ii) Child Ego*

The child in man is the recording of internal events which are responses of the little person to what he sees and hears. Most of the reactions in this category are the feelings of tear, relgion, anger, hurt, happiness, laughter and creativity.

*(iii) The Adult Ego*

The adult in man is the data processing computer which makes decisions after compiling the information obtained from different sources. This comes out of the experiences of analysing and comparing the facts and figures. It is the rational aspect of personality. No one ego state is ideal for all the situations. Problems usually occur when an ego state that is not approximate for a situation becomes a source of behaviour.

The recording of the parent, child and adult—all take place in the early childhood. Recording of the parent and child starts in the few months after the birth. The adult is recorded after the child is in a position to move and see the things himself and decide about course of action. This usually starts when he is 10 months old. At this stage he begins to verify the truth of what parents say. Although by doing so, he may not be able to erase the recordings in P and C. Depending upon the early experiences of life, one of the four life positions may be developed in a man. These are: (a) I am not OK, you are OK; (b) You are not OK, I am not OK, (c) You are not OK, I am OK and I am OK, you are OK.

Let us now discuss the implications of these four positions. In the first position, "I am not OK, You are OK", the managers have little confidence in themselves, take little initiative and generally follow the orders of others, whom they consider OK. In the second life position, I am not OK, you are not OK. nothing gets done and the organisation functions in disarray. The third position "I am OK, you are not OK" can be seen in organisations when health managers have no faith in their subordinates. Such managers generally behave rather arrogantly in their relationships with the subordinates. However, in the fourth situation "I am OK, you are OK", there is very co-ordinal relationship between health managers and subordinates.

The basic question which needs answering is what is the use of this analysis? What would we get out of it to improve individual health worker and organisational efficiency? The answer is very clear in that this analysis helps in understanding the present personality of an individual. The goal transactional analysis is to help a person through various methods like leadership, congenial environment, counseling to achieve the fourth situation, "I am OK, you are OK."

Let us discuss the important characteristics under each category:

**A. I am not OK, you are OK**

(i) Lack of self-respect and self-confidence.

(ii) Feeling of inferiority and negative approval.
(iii) Servile and non-asserting.
(iv) Lack motivation and strive to progress.
(v) Dominated by situations and lacking initiative.

*Implications*

Managers in this category generally follow the orders of those whom they consider OK. They can never lead the organisation to excellence.

**B. I am not OK, you are not OK**

(i) Low opinion and lack of self-confidence.
(ii) No trust in others, rather always suspicious.
(iii) Negative feelings of thoughts about self and others.
(iv) Not straight forward.
(v) Depressed and de-motivated.
(vi) No faith in colleagues and No delegation.
(vii) No initiative believes in *status quo*.

*Implications*

The organisation having such people can never achieve its goals, as people work at cross purposes creating chaos and anarchy.

**C. I am OK, you are not OK**

(i) Lack of trust and confidence in colleagues.
(ii) Feeling of superiority and power.
(iii) Blaming his colleagues.
(iv) Don't allow others to participate.
(v) No interest in feedback.

*Implications*

Such managers are arrogant and are unable to harness the creative potential of their subordinates or team members. The organisation either stagnates or perishes.

**D. I am OK, you are OK**

(i) Respect for self and others—High Self Esteem.
(ii) Interested to provide democratic leadership.
(iii) Honest and sincere in work and with colleagues.
(iv) Initiative to do new things and an attempt to move himself and colleagues to excellence.

*Implications*

Cordial relationship between superiors, subordinates or team mates ensures a vibrant, progressive and competitive organisation, which has edge over others.

In developing countries, most people belong to the first category "I am not OK, you are,. as the atmosphere in the home and the school is influenced by parents and teachers, who are authoritarian. The situation is different in developed countries, where the children in home and schools are encouraged to be independent. The second situation " I am not OK, you are not OK" is available among such persons, where the persons in their childhood have been neglected and not provided the necessary love and care. It may be psychological, i.e. internal family problems that economic or social. In the third category, "I am OK, you are not OK" we find the persons who have been derived love and affection during their childhood. They think that whole world is their enemy and except them all are wrong and do not know anything. The fourth category "I am OK, you are not OK", is an ideal situation. There are very few fortunate people who get such atmosphere where they can bloom.

The above analysis helps in understanding the present personality of an individual and the goal of transactional analysis is to help a person achieve the fourth situation, "I am OK, you are OK" . Although it is a challenging task to erase various negative impression registered during childhood, but a determined and conscious efforts may help in moving towards the ideal situation.

Although it is challenging as it is a very difficult task to erase the various impressions registered from childhood, but a determined and conscious effort may help in moving towards ideal situation.

## ROLE OF TRANSACTIONAL ANALYSIS IN MANAGEMENT

It is very important for the key personnel or health managers to understand their subordinates intimately through the records of their personal profiles and intercourses. What is happening today in complex organisations is that relationships are too formal and as a result the health managers never find time to understand their colleagues or subordinates or team members. They allocate work to them and expect results from them like machines, with utter failure. Therefore, the important task of the leader is the art of the co-ordinating and motivating the individuals. Through proper understanding of their colleagues, the leader can help them to improve and achieve excellence through Transactional Analysis.

S.R. Desai in his Article, "Transactional Analysis—A new way to Managerial Effectiveness", in *Lok Udyog*, has listed his experiences. Some of the experiences enlisted are:

1. T.A. enables the managers to become aware about their ego states for the first time.
2. Based on this awareness, they do feel the need for shifting ego states as per the demands of the situations.

3. It helps them to become aware of the effects of their communication (transaction) with others and why and how it breaks or builds.
4. They become aware of the need and efficacy of positive strokes and disfunctional effect of negative strokes.
5. Time structuring is one of the most important insight of T.A. through which a manager is able to understand how he is using his time of life and what changes he should introduce in his time planning which would not only make him an effective, manager but also a happier human being.
6. T.A. concepts help them to reduce work tensions and increase harmony in working with people.
7. We spend a lot of time and energy in worrying about the conduct and behaviour of others. Even if half of this time is devoted to peeping into ourselves it would totally transform us and our surroundings.
8. T.A. develops capacities of awareness, spontaneity and intimacy.

Let us now discuss the four positions and the role of management in each position. The health manager with a life position—I am not OK, you are OK is too much populous-oriented. He is more concerned with getting things done. His feelings and emotions guide his actions. He may be a popular leader but may not be effective.

In such situations, the managers may be given the executive development programme where they may be given training to make themselves really effective, assertive and attend to business rather than simply running the administration. This training must be repeated and must be managed by well trained so that they can generate required change in managers through lecture method, group discussion, syndicate method, role playing, etc.

Managers may be left in a free and open environment in which they may analyse their roles. The purpose of this is to provide managers with increased awareness of their own behaviour and how others perceive them. Effective leadership is an essential ingredient for organisations to succeed in the dynamic complexity of our society in the decades ahead. These leaders, who are not so fortunate, must comprehend the multitude of variables that affect leadership effectiveness and carve out unique personal styles for followers satisfaction and organisational successful performance.

One who has developed a life position. "I am OK, You are not OK" may be too much task-oriented. He will not care for the feelings and emotions of his people and will thus earn their displeasure. He may be effective, but unpopular with his people.

In such situations, the manager can extract work temporarily and may not be able to create permanent efficiency and self-sustained effectiveness. Subordinates may work only because of the fear of punishment and may not be inclined whole heartedly. Therefore, here again, identified manager of this category may be given training in the art and science of motivating their subordinates as well as cultivating good relationships with the employees, which is essential for efficient organisations.

The Manager should try to use the techniques of management like decentralization, delegation, MBO, etc. Centralization of powers may be highly fascinating to authoritarian leader but the subordinates do not enjoy working under this atmosphere. In delegation, the subordinates respond by developing a constructive sense of responsibility. Delegation, thus, improves the behavioural climate in the organisation and paves the way for efficiency. Koontz and O'Donnell, have given some necessary personal qualities that can contribute to successful delegation. These are:

(a) give other people's ideas a chance;
(b) allow subordinates to take decisions independently;
(c) be patient counsellor and not a hovering hawk;
(d) response confidence and trust in subordinates; and
(e) know how to use controls judiciously.

The need for delegation is felt more in case of those colleagues who show a tendency to depend on authority than be independent. Managers should, therefore, thoroughly identify the weaknesses, develop potential and positive attitudes conducive to accepting and successfully using the delegated authority. Training in delegation should be supplemented by counseling and performance appraisal.

US President, Ronald Reagan advised practising managers (*Fortune*, September 15, 1986): "Surround yourself with the best people you can find, delegate authority and don't interfere." In locating such individuals, one should understand that each individual is unique, with different instincts, emotions and sentiments and, therefore, he has different potentiality. Therefore, there is a need for recognizing, understanding, appreciating and nurturing subordinates' talents rather than merely condemning them. The leaders can make all the colleagues OK, provided they are properly understood and directed.

A manager with the life position: I am not OK you are not OK is neither relations-oriented nor task-oriented. He will neither be popular nor effective. In such situations, organisation development techniques must be introduced to stimulate both the manager and the employees. Besides, separate training courses may be arranged for them. It is also advisable that some managers from good organisations may be imported to improve the situation. It has been observed that changes at the top level made in such situations turn out to be very good. Besides, we must observe organisational principles to discipline everybody such as:

(a) *Objective*: Each group of tasks must have an objective that contributes to the objectives of the organisation as a whole.

(b) *Definition*: Each group of tasks must be clearly defined so that everyone knows what the tasks are.
(c) *Command*: Each group of tasks must have one person in charge, and all concerned must know who this person is.
(d) *Responsibility*: The person in charge is responsible for the performance of the people in his group.
(e) *Authority*: Each person in charge of a group of tasks must have authority equal to his responsibility.
(f) *Span of Control*: No person in charge of groups of tasks should be expected to control more than six to ten other people.
(g) *Balance*: The person in charge of several groups must see the groups balance. For instance, case finding must not be so extensive that more cases of a disease are found than can be treated.

It is only with the life position. I am OK and you are OK, that a leader becomes both popular and effective as he is concerned with good relations with his people as well as his services. The manager can build a strong adult by recognizing the child in him, controlling his own feelings and emotions on the one hand, and understanding and appreciating the views and feelings of others. We should promote such situations so that these may be imbibed by others. Special prizes may be given to such organisations, so that structure is highlighted. Where managers recognize their responsibility towards employees and are willing to play a positive role in building an atmosphere of mutual trust and confidence and there are positive responses from the employees, these would encourage the development of a goal system, i.e. a group of interrelated but separate elements working towards a common purpose. This would help generate co-ordinated efforts towards accomplishing goals. The tempo of such developments can be maintained through the building up of morale.

Transactional analysis has made a major contribution to the study of job satisfaction and employee motivation by helping managers in clarifying the source and consequence of the three ego states: Parent, Child and Adult behaviour discussed earlier in this chapter. It also helps in understanding the origin of bad feelings and their relationships to stroking. A stroke, according to Dr. Eric Berne is an intervention, a unit of recognition, a word of welcome, word of praise or a gesture of liking such as a pat on the back or a hug. A stroke may be positive or negative.

Likert and his associate emphasized that TA, may be used to move the Organisation towards system 4, which can ensure the ideal situation, "1 am OK, you are OK." Table 10.1 contrasts System with System 4 and shows the corresponding concepts in Transactional Analysis. An analysis of the Table would reveal the utility of TA in generating System 4 management.

Where managers recognize their responsibility towards employees and are willing to play positive role in building an atmosphere of mutual trust and confidence, it encourages the development of a group of inter-related but separate elements, working towards a common purpose.

The tempo of such developments can be maintained through the building up of Morale. L.D. White has defined Morale as an index of both a sound employment situation and a positive means of building up an efficient organisation. Alexander Leighton defined morale as the capacity of a group of people to pull together persistently and consistently in pursuit of a common purpose. In order to ensure the situation "1 am OK, you are OK", constant efforts must be carried on for building morale both on the intellectual and emotional plane. Intellectually morale has to be built on communication between the employees, their participation in planning and decision-making processes. Emotionally, morale has to be built up by sound relationship, team spirit and indoctrination.

TABLE 10.1

**The Analysis of Transactions in Managerial Systems**

| | *System*<br>*Exploitative Authoritative* | System 4<br>Participative Group |
|---|---|---|
| 1. Leadership | Superior has no trust in subordinates; their ideas are not sought. Superior operates from his P, often the Critical P. Subordinates do not feel free to talk to boss. Subordinates are expected to respond from their. Their suggestions are seldom taken serious. Bossss often assumes that he is OK—but not subordinates. Little delegation. Subordinates follow instructions, they develop no healthy self-concept. | Superior has great deal of trust in subordinates. Their ideals are sought and they feel free to talk to their boss. Transaction are on the A-A' basis: subordinates are expected to develop their own ideas. Boss and subordinates feel OK about each other. Superior is a member of a team with emphasis on competence, not authority. There is a great deal of delegation subordinates feel accountable for their actions and they feel OK about their accomplishments. |
| 2. Motivation | Superior operating from P uses especially fear, threat, punishment and occasionally rewards. The boss wants dependent subordinates in their C. This is what he gets. No participations, no involvement, low satisfaction. Subordinates do not feel responsible for achieving organisational goals. Superior reminds them that they are not OK, not conducive for team work. | Great emphasis on involvement based on group action and team work, interaction is based on A. Responsibility is shared with a great deal of individual is shared with a great deal of individual commitment to organisational results. Great deal of cooperation by members who are OK and also consider others OK. |

| | | |
|---|---|---|
| 3. Communication | The boss, from his P, gives orders, which are viewed with suspicion by subordinates. They also do not dare to level with their boss, who considers himself OK but not the employees. Consequently, upward communication is inaccurate and the boss is not answer of what is going on in the enterprise | Free communication flow in all directions. Since communication is primarily in the A mode, it is very accurate. This means superiors are well informed about problems facing subordinates. The focus is on objective problem-solving, not on finding, scapegoats for difficulties. Superiors and subordinates consider each other OK—a pre-requisite for genuine communication. |
| 4. Decision-making | Decisions are made by the top managers who view others are not OK. Subordinates are hardly ever involved in decisions related to their work. They operate in their C, follow orders, but are not motivated to contribute. | Decisions are made at all levels of the organisation. Decisions are made objectively, based on A ego state. Problem and their causes are identified and alternative courses of action are evaluated. The best course is selected after objective analysis. Subordinates are involved in this process which reinforces their OK lie position |
| 5. Goals | Organisational goals are established at the top in an autocratic manner in the superiors P ego state. Although subordinate. | Organisational and personal development goals are set at all primarily through group actions. Subordinates based on their A ego state, set a goals primarily themselves and discuss them with the superior. There is a great deal of participation and individuals set high performance goals. The sense of direction makes superiors and subordinates feel OK and enhances their self-image |
| 6. Control | External, rigid controls are concentrated at the top. The boss, driven by his P, tries to control everything. Since subordinates are considered not OK, they cannot exercise self-control. Subordinates in their C ego state, try to meet control standards—even if inappropriate—instead of speaking openly to the superior. There is considerable hidden resistance to control. | Review and control is shared by members of the organisation. Subordinates based on their A, execises self-control and self-guidance. Controls are used for feedback, not to put blame on individuals. Analysis of deviations from plans is objective. Emphasis is on forward looking controls to prevent deviations. Measurements of performance is in a positive environment in which superior and subordinates adopt an OK position. |

*Note*: P = Parent ego state; A = Adult ego state; C = Child ego state.
*Source*: *Journal of System Management*, July 1980, p. 33.

Transactional analysis has played a major contribution for studying of job satisfaction and employee motivation by helping managers in clarifying the source and consequence of the three ego states: Parent, Child and Adult behaviour discussed earlier in this chapter, it also helps in understanding the origin of bad feelings and their relationships to stroking.

A stroke, according to Dr. Eric Berne, is an intervention, a unit of recognition, a word of praise or liking gesture such as a pat on the back or a hug. A stroke may be positive or negative Managers differ in their ability to give positive and negative strokes. Those with insight into human problems observe the organisational climate carefully, before giving a particular type of stroke. In a 'gamy' organisation, for instance, even good ideas are treated otherwise. The effectiveness of managers, thus, depends to an extent upon the organisational climate itself. Management should, therefore, discourage the behaviour pattern and the activities which are harmful to the organisation through appropriate stroke at different occasions.

The ability of managers to choose right types of strokes can certainly be developed by training them in understanding the three ego states and the impact of positive and negative strokes on employee motivation and job satisfaction in different situations. It may also help them in analysing their own behaviour, liberating them from the assumptions which are unfounded, utilizing their time in constructive work rather than game playing or pastimes and making desirable change in their attitude towards the subordinates. It thus assists in establishing an efficient management.

Managers differ in their ability to give positive and negative strokes. Those with insight into human problems observe the organisational climate carefully before giving a particular type of stroke. In a 'gamy' organisation, for instance, even good ideas are treated otherwise. The effectiveness of managers, thus depends to an extent upon the organisational climate itself. Management should, therefore, discourage the behaviour pattern and the activities which are harmful to the organisation through appropriate strokes on different occasions. Table 10.2 gives the four life positions and how to use them to improve organisational efficiency. The analysis of the table suggests that we must first understand the existing status of the employees and then try to modify their behaviour, to ensure organisational efficiency and dynamics.

## CONCLUSION

Managerial effectiveness depends to a great extent upon the human factor as we know that human rather than capital is the key to development. If we can diagnose the causative factors affecting human behaviour, we would be able to sublimate those factors and put them to constructive use. This technique can even help the manager to diagnose his own behaviour. This understanding can provide him kinetic energy to influence direct and therefore, condition the behaviour of the people in his organisation.

TABLE 10.2

**How Life Position Influences Employee Behaviour**

| *Life Position* | *Communication* | *Delegation* | *Growth* | *Handles disagreement by* | *Solves problems by* | *Attitude* | *Feelings to others* |
|---|---|---|---|---|---|---|---|
| I'am OK You're OK | Openly shared | High | Indepen dently | Mutual resolution | Consulting others trusting himself | Initiative | Equal |
| I'm not OK— You'are OK | Defensively shared | No | By coaching | Perceiving differences in opinion as evidence of his inadequacy | Relying almost completely on others | By praise or admonition | Inferior |
| I'm OK— You're Not OK | Aggressively shared | Delegation not accepted | Learning is blocked | Placing blame on others | Unilaterally rejecting other's ideas | When forced | Superiors |
| I'am Not OK— You'are Not OK | Abruptly shared | Confusion | Withdraws and repeats errors | Escalating the conflict involving a third party | Succumbing to Problems | By reprimands threats | Despondent alienated |

This technique provides clues to motivational behaviour, which is influenced by internal likes and dislikes. The work of eminent psychologists like Douglas McGregor, Maslow, Likert, Argyris and others suggest that external techniques like threat or temptation for monetary benefits are unscientific. The real motivations can come only from those strokes/factors, which influence one's egoistic need: A stroke, according to Dr. Eric Berne, is an intervention to mould the behaviour of the members of an organisation. Such a situation would provide a healthy environment which can provide the ideal situation to achieve maximum organisational efficiency as well as promote happiness among individual members. Such a situation would provide identity between the organisational goals and the individual goals. Thus, the technique promotes managerial effectiveness, as it offers a wide range of alternatives (strokes) for correcting and controlling the behaviour imperfections of the members of an organisation. The need is therefore to train the top executives in the theory and practice of this technique

Based upon personal observation of a number of health institutes in Haryana, Punjab, Himachal Pradesh and Karnataka, the author feels that most of the top personnel in health system at state, district and block levels have no understanding of inter-personnel relationships. They are mostly in a position of "I am OK, You are not OK." This attitude is creating inefficiency in health system. The Government should arrange good training courses for senior health functionaries so that they can be made OK and in turn influence others. Besides, the environment should post only such persons to top positions, who have the ability to understand inter-personnel relationships.

# 11

CHAPTER

# *Motivation and Morale*

> "Motivation represents unsatisfied needs which creates a state of tension or disequilibrium causing the individual to move in a goal-directed pattern towards restoring a state of equilibrium by satisfying the needs."
>
> —*Herzburg*

Motivation is a tendency which keeps a person attentively and purposefully engaged to achieve his formulated goals. Thus, a sense of commitment occurs only when the enterprise becomes a perpetual vehicle for the satisfaction of the dominant needs of the employees, so long as the employee strives fully to achieve the goals of the enterprise.

It has been noticed that the performance of medical and health personnel, either as individuals or members of a group, is less as compared to their capabilities in terms of skills, abilities and capacities. Finer, for example, states that demonstrated performance generally never exceeds more than fifty per cent of individual's ability to perform.[1] This is one of the main reasons for the failure of our health system not fulfiling the commitment of Health for all enunciated in 1976. Most of the primary health care institutions have become defunct in the practical sense. Most individuals tend to balance their efforts around an assessment of relative cost (time and energy) and benefits.

The basic question arises as to why medical and health personnel feel alienated from the organisational goals. Why most employees do not utilize their potential skills and capabilities into kinetic skills and capabilities to achieve the goals of health? Why do most employees feel frustrated in discharging their duties? Why do we discern cleavage between the management and employees? Why do the employees of one health organisation work with more efficiency than another. Why do some employees become indolent and inefficient resulting in decreased efficiency and lower morale? What are the factors which lead to the pollution of organisational environment? Which are the factors and conditions which impel individuals to achieve excellence? These and other such questions can be analysed, if we understand the meaning, scope and utility of motivation in improving professional efficiency. It is quite obvious that the mere possession of knowledge, skill and ability will not ensure best results, as performance depends upon motivation as well. It is only when the employees are properly motivated that they will use their skill, knowledge and ability to ensure best results. The most important task of the health department must be to give abundant and constant evidence of its belief that personnel in the health organisation are the key to provide decent health care.

This requires the proper motivation of employees. Motivation is of utmost importance as it constitutes the base for the management functions of planning and organizing. The state health department must devote considerable time and effort in planning for and achieving high levels of motivation and morale. We may safely lay down that the tone of an organisation is a reflection of the motivation from the top.

The concept of motivation is used by the psychologists and sociologists as means of answering two basic questions concerning human behaviour. Why is man impelled to act? Or what determines the direction of his actions? Like many other concepts in Psychology, motivation is a variable, which is characteristic of the organism, not directly observable, and therefore, only to be inferred indirectly from the behaviour of the organism.

The term motive is derived from the Latin word 'emovere', which means 'to move'. In fact, without motivation, man would be stagnant creature, never moving, never acting. Psychologists view motivation as the force which impels or incites all living organisms to action.

Motivation is a tendency which keeps a person attentively and purposefully engaged to achieve his formulated goals. This, a sense of commitment occurs only when the enterprise becomes a perpetual vehicle for the satisfaction of the dominant needs of the employees, so long as the employees strives fully to achieve the goals of the enterprise. From the above discussion, it is clear that motivation as such cannot be observed, rather it is a concept derived to cover a number of relationships having their immediate point of origin within the organism.

## MOTIVATION CYCLE

Three elements—needs, drives and goals—interact in motivation. Each may also thought of as a stage in a cycle, for the first leads to the second, the second to the third and the third to the first. The first stage of the motivational cycle can be referred by three names: need, drive or motive. These are almost but not entirely synonymous. Need refers to a desire within the individual. Drives are the intra-organic activities for a particular type of behaviour. The third stage in the motivation is called the goal. Every behaviour is directed towards a goal and when the goals are attained, the need, drive or motive is satisfied. In practice, this chain is more complex than it appears to be.

CHART 11.1

**Health as Management Tool for Development**

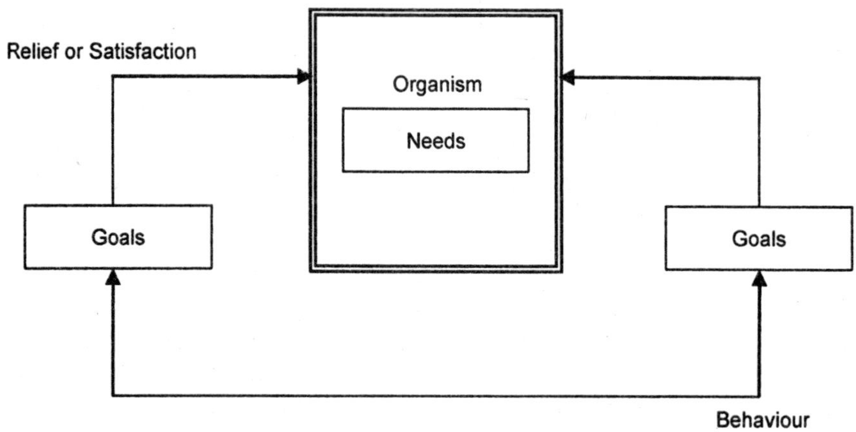


## METHODS/THEORIES OF MOTIVATION

There are many theories which provide insight into human behaviour and the factors which can help in changing the given behaviour, to promote organisational efficiency. Let us discuss some of them.

### 1. Monistic or Economic Theory of Motivation

This theory is based upon the notion that the people feel highly motivated when rewarded with more money. F.W. Taylor, the father of scientific management, believed that people would work harder if paid more money. Even today, the financial incentives can add a great deal to the efficiency of the personnel. We cannot say that financial incentives are everything but we can definitely say that in today's world, money counts a lot. According to Peter F. Druck, "The carrot of material rewards has not, like the stick of fear, lost its potency." Medical personnel are paid non-practising allowance to encourage them.

Gellerman too regards money as an important motivator when he states, "money may well turn out to be the costliest motivator of them all, but money may also prove to the most potent motivator of all, at least in certain circumstances, and when used on a sufficient scale." However, to assume that financial awards are the only sources of motivation would tentamount to over simplification. To quote Barnard (Functions of the

Executive), "..... material rewards are ineffective beyond the subsistence level excepting to a very limited proportion of men; that most men neither work harder for material things, nor can be induced thereby to devote more than a fraction of their possible contribution to organized efforts. The opportunity for distinction, prestige, personal power, and the attainment of dominating position are much more important than material rewards in the development of all sorts of organisations including commercial organisations." Thus, the Executives in the organisations must look after the material welfare of employees so that they can contribute their best.

**2. Expediency Theory of Motivation**

This theory is based upon the idea that health and medical personnel have certain built-in-expectations from the jobs they are performing. They are motivated if they find their expectation satisfied. Victor Vroom in his book, 'Work and Motivation' has indicated that,

$$\text{Valence} \times \text{Expectancy} = \text{Motivation}$$

where Valence is the strength of an individual's preference for a particular outcome and it can be negative or positive. Expectancy refers to the probability that the desired outcome will really be brought about by his action. The organisation can be benefited with the ideas of this theory, if expectations of the employees are integrated with the organisational goals through various approaches like Management by Objectives, Organisational Development, etc. The Management must try to fulfil the individual expectations of its staff members.

J.B. Miner (Theory of Organisational Behaviour, pp. 160-61) has rightly said, based on research, that "these research tests have now yielded sufficient theoretical support so that it seems safe to conclude that expectancy theories are on the right track. They certainly do not explain all motivated behviouar on all types of Works Organisations, but they do explain enough to be worth pursuing future. Inspite of its apparent complexity, the model provides a very useful tool for understanding, predicting and influencing behaviour and attitudes in Organisation."

**3. Equity Theory of Motivation**

According to this theory, an employee relates his own input/output ratio to that of some other person or persons with whom he compares himself. This theory reflects the meaning contained in the proverb 'A single sinner sinks the boat'. Most of the employees become slow, less active and even sluggish when they see that their fellow workers have no interest in their work. This theory suggests that the organisation should either remove or improve workers, otherwise this contagious disease may permeate the entire organisation, resulting in its collapse. In most of the organisations, few off-members encircle the top management and develop cliques. These individuals get undue favours, both financial and non-financial, without merit, skill or hard work. Such developments are highly resented by other staff members, resulting in the pollution of the organisational environmental. We even notice a turbulent and charged atmosphere in these organisations. Such an atmosphere lowers the motivation of real workers to perform their work efficiently.

**4. Maslow's Theory of Human Needs (See Chart 11.2)**

Abraham Maslow identified the hierarchy of needs, which can explain the dynamics of human motivation. His theory states that there are five types of human needs arranged in a particular order from the lower to the higher. These can be depicted as given below.

CHART 11.2

**Maslow's Hierarchy of Human Needs**

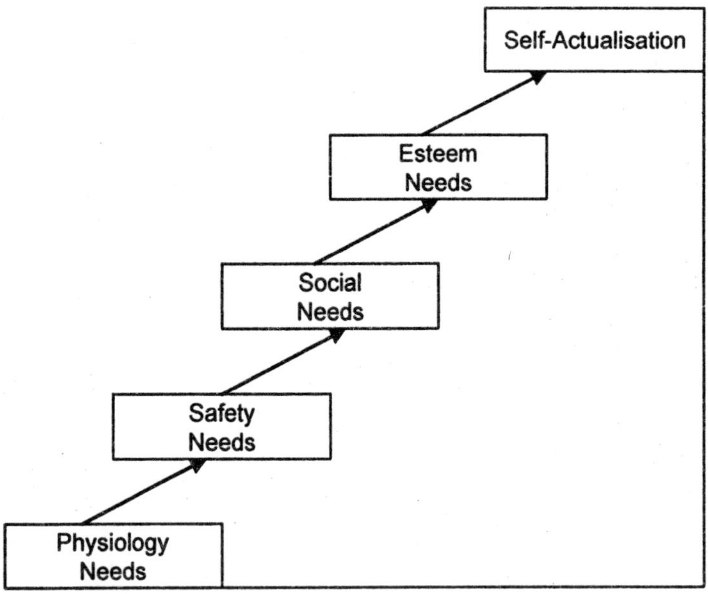


*(a) Physiological Needs*

Physiological needs refer to the basic requirements of human beings, e.g., food, clothings, shelter. These needs are also termed as biological needs since these are concerned with maintenance of the body.

*(b) Safety Needs*

These needs seek an assurance of the physiological needs in future as the future is uncertain and there can be natural calamities or hazards. These needs may include security of job, pension for old age, insurance for accidents and death, compensation for retrenchment, etc.

EXHIBIT 11.1

## Using Need Activation as a Motivational Tool

| *Activated Needs* | *Observable Behaviours* | Do's | *Possible Motivation Action Don'ts* |
|---|---|---|---|
| Physiology | An obvious physical needs deprivation | Provide physical needs | Don't create physical deprivations |
| Safety | Fear<br>Insecurity<br>Seeking protection<br>Financially insecure<br>Work to rule attitude<br>Responsibility avoidance | Reassure<br>Be supportive<br>Be protective<br>Share responsibility<br>Reduce responsibility | Don't create physical Deprivation<br>Don't' put pressure<br>Don't Destabilize<br>Don't violate rules<br>Don't expect initiative |
| Social | People orientation<br>Active in social work<br>Display needs for others<br>Seeks good relation-ships<br>Concern for group harmony<br>Acceptance of group norms<br>Concern for people welfare | Allow sociolising<br>Encourage social work<br>Place in harmonious group<br>Allow greater interaction<br>Give social responsi-bility<br>Use for inter-group liaison<br>Place in group with norms | Don't isolate<br>Don't curb socialising<br>Don't negate social role<br>Don't use for control tasks |
| Self-Esteem | More formability<br>Concern for status<br>Concern for position<br>Desire for authority<br>Desire for prominence<br>Desire to be respected<br>Desire for recognition<br>Desire for status symbols<br>Close to people of status | Give authority<br>Give prominence<br>Give recognition<br>Give public respect<br>Allow share in power<br>Improve designations<br>Provide Status symbols<br>Use loss of face as threat | Don't underestimate ego<br>Don't publicize failure<br>Don't give too much power<br>Don't reprimand in public<br>Don't give very hard talks<br>Don't set unachievable goals |
| Self-Actualize | High Creativity<br>High productivity<br>Independent thinking<br>Respect for compe-tence<br>Disregard of authority<br>High personal standards<br>Great need for autonomy<br>Disregard of other needs<br>Disregard of conven-tions<br>Lack of time con-sciousness | Give autonomy<br>Ask for advice<br>Use loose controls<br>Allow self-discipline<br>Give challenging work<br>Give accurate feedback<br>Use peer group pressures<br>Give flexible work hours<br>Place under competent boss | Don't threaten<br>Use authority<br>Don't give easy tasks<br>Don't impose organisation norms<br>Don't curb initiatives<br>Don't be too rigid on rule<br>Don't challenge competence<br>Don't place with medicores |

*Source*: *Pakistan Management Review*, Second Quarter, 1989.

*(c) Social Needs*

Social needs include man's desire to love and be loved. Maslow calls these 'the love and affection and belongingness needs'. It is suggested that organisations should encourage the formation of constructive informal groups, constructive informal groups should either be eliminated or discouraged.

*(d) Esteem Needs*

Esteem needs relate to one's self-esteem such as self-respect, self-confidence, status, recognition, prestige, etc. The organisation can help the subordinates in their development through the recognition of their good work.

*(e) Self-Actualization Need*

It refers to man's desire for excellence in his chosen field by maximizing his potential. Very few individuals try to achieve these needs. Only such individuals who aspire to fulfil their self-actualization needs can bring about creativity, innovation and development in the structure and functioning of the organisation. The administration must provide congenial and creative environment for them as they are the builders of the organisation. Such individuals may appear to be hostile but they can really contribute to generate social change and modernization.

(i) Human needs are of varied and diversified nature.

(ii) There is a definite hierarchy of the occurrence of these needs, i.e., these move in ascending order. If a particular set of needs, is fairly well satisfied, a man tries to satisfy the higher set of needs.

(iii) The first three can be termed as the needs of 'lower order' while the next two can be classified as 'higher order needs'.

(iv) A satisfied need ceases to be powerful motivator of human behaviour.

Generally speaking, an activated need is associated with a particular set of Observable Behaviours, which can easily be identified by the District Health Officer/Medical Officer. Once the manager has determined which need is dominating a subordinate's phenomenal fields, he can easily evolve a strategy as to how to best satisfy that need and motivate the individual. From the motivational point of View, a clear set of Do's and Don'ts are associated with each activated need. Managers would do well to attempt motivation of individuals by using methodologies complementary to the psychological states, which are created within the individual by the dominant need. A general set of Observable Behaviour and Do's and Don'ts associated with each of the five needs is reproduced. (Exhibit 11.1)

**5. X and Y Theory of Douglas McGregor**

McGregor categorized the traditional motivational assumptions as theory X, a string of self-consistent notions about human nature. First, the theory X assumes that the ordinary man is selfish, lazy and stimulated by only economic rewards. Secondly, the average man is not interested in work unless goaded by the superior. Thirdly, the Individual and organisational goals are contradictory and tend to clash with each other. Fourthly, the average man is devoid of self-discipline and self-control. Finally, he tend to submit himself to the control and direction of others and avoids responsibility.

McGregor, however, points out that man's motivation is far too complex and varied to be explained away wholly by the aforementioned assumptions. In line with other thinkers of social psychology school McGregor describes his alternative model of motivation as theory Y. The assumption of theory Y may be stated as:

1. The average man is not really against doing work.
2. The ordinary man can show self-control and self-direction depending upon the involvement in the work he is doing.
3. The average man craves for self-actualization and it is the responsibility of the management to provide genuine conditions for satisfying his creative abilities and yearnings.
4. The ordinary man under suitable conditions would willingly shoulder responsibility.
5. The average man is capable of making significant contributions to the solution of many administrative problems, but his potentialities are not fully utilized.

After discussing these techniques, let us discuss the various motivators, which can cause positive responses in the medical and health personnel, working in different organisations. The exact nature and extent of these motivators would depend upon the internal and external factors prevailing in a given organisation. We mention here some of the important motivators, which can promote efficiency.

## PARTICIPATION

Participation is an individual's mental and emotional involvement in a group situation that encourages him to contribute to group goals and to share responsibility with them.

We should encourage health personnel participation in the achievement of health goals. An employee's participation would build his morale and ultimately his efficiency. An ILO document mentions that the individual worker "is not just a cog in the very big wheel, but that his personal effort is essential for the achievement of the overall production plan."[2]

The research theory in social organisational psychology has also suggested that participation in group decision-making enhances satisfaction among members and removes tensions. Michael R. Cooper and Michael T. Wood have shown that satisfaction was greater where participation was complete than where it was partial.[3]

There is a need to practise 'Management by Objectives' to ensure fruitful participation. 'Management by Objectives' shifts the focus to goals, to the purpose of the activity rather than the activity itself. It is a process whereby the supervisor and subordinates in an organisation jointly identify its common goals and ensure performance. The manager must encourage the development of such concepts among the employees. The District Health Officer can encourage the participation of all staff members at district and lower levels to ensure that they participate freely and frankly.

## POSITIVE REINFORCEMENT

It means sublimating the energies of the health workers in a desired direction through some environmental and intrinsic reinforcements. This technique was successfully applied by a Harvard Psychologist, B.F. Skinner.

## TERMS OF EMPLOYMENT

The importance of pay or compensation is very great for every health employee. The standard of living and the social prestige of an employee depends to a great extent on the pay he draws. A man chooses his career on the basis of pay, which he expects to receive. Manson Haire remarks, "Pay in one form or another is certainly one of the mainsprings of motivation in our society."[4] Thus, an adequate and sound salary structure, together with other working conditions, is the *sine qua non* for the organisational efficiency and effectiveness. Otherwise, as the Administrative Reforms Commission aptly observes, it has been "one of the major factor for strikes, agitation, inter-service tensions and rivalries, indifferent attitude to work, poor performance, frustration and low morale of the employees."

However, we must be clear that no compensation plan can satisfy all the health employees. The true efficiency in an organisation can be promoted only through dedication and loyalty of its staff members. The managers must motivate the employees through non-financial incentives as financial incentives have little scope in developing countries like India. In the last resort, the quality of the public depends more on the loyalty, the faith and the sense of mission, which staff members bring in the organisation, than on the money expended on them.

## EFFECTIVE ORGANISATIONAL CLIMATE

It is of significance to stress that organisation is not merely a structure; in fact, it embraces a structure as well as the health and medical personnel who man and run it in order to realize goals of health for all. We must always strive through administrative improvements and reforms to remove the irritants, which creep into the organisations. to ensure an effective organisational climate. We may ensure the following:

(a) Clear definition of objectives.
(b) Systematic grouping of related activities.
(c) Maximum delegation of authority.
(d) Minimum layering.
(e) Clear demarcation of line and staff functions.
(f) Correct span of control.
(g) Unity of command.
(h) Proper conditions of work.
(i) Provision for easier communications.

## BUILDING MORALE

In order to make the organisation effective, we have to discard the outdated mechanistic theory of organisation and in its place shall have to adopt a dynamic and creative social theory of public management based upon human morale. The British Civil Service has been praised for its efficient service. Lord Hewart calls it the best Civil Service in the World. W.G. Wells praises the tradition of honour and devotion to duty that animated, the Civil Service in England. What is the secret of the success? Obviously, it is "the tradition of honesty and devotion to duty", i.e. the high morale built up by the services themselves. According to Dr. L.D. White, morale reflects a socio-psychological situation, a state of mind in which men and women voluntarily seek to develop and apply their full powers to the task upon which they are engaged. by the reason of intellectual or moral satisfaction which they derive from their own self-realization, their achievement in their chosen field, and their pride in the service."[5] It is a self-stimulating incentive created within the minds and hearts of the workers. A whole some morale stimulates loyalty. Generates cooperation and encourages team work. All these are essential for the achievement of efficient medical and health services.

### Job Enlargement and Enrichment

A climate of creativity must be developed and maintained by management. Maier and Hyes say that the optimal climate for creativity, is whatever human conditions is optimal for individual freedom and self-expression in social setting. It is the duty of the officers of such units to make the employees feel that their work and their association with a given organisation represent a vehicle which will accelerate the achievement of personal as well as the achievement of goals of the organisation. It means to make the jobs interesting, challenging and meaningful. Koontz and O'Donnell have suggested the following to ensure job enrichment:

(a) giving workers more latitude in deciding about such things as work methods, sequence, and place or by letting them make decisions about accepting or rejecting materials;
(b) encouraging participation of subordinates and interaction between workers;
(c) giving workers a feeling of personal responsibility for their tasks;
(d) taking steps to make sure that people can see how their tasks contribute to a finished product and the welfare of the enterprise;
(e) giving people feedback on their job performance preferably before their supervisors get in; and
(f) involving workers in analysis and change of physical aspects of the work environment such as layout of office or plan, temperature, lighting and cleanliness.

Beside job enrichment, we must inculcate pride in the job among the staff members of an organisation, i.e., doing job with their best ability to achieve excellence in their own fields. The Advertising Council of America once started a campaign which stated: "Are you doing the work you would be proud to sign with your own autograph?" It applied to all persons irrespective of the office they occupy in government. The pursuit of excellence would depend on development of this identity.

## CONCLUSION

The success or failure of an organisation depends, to a great extent, upon the administrative capability, morale and motivation of its top leadership, i.e. state health department and district health officers. The top echelons should facilitate the accomplishment of desired objectives with the least friction and the most satisfaction to those for whom the task is done and those engaged in the health system. In this connection, the leader must understand the nature of social psychology and the methods of motivating the groups and enhancing the morale to achieve organisational efficiency.

Leaders in medical and health system must be the persons with vision, initiative and desire to achieve the operational goals with dedication and preserverance. The greatest efficiency and productivity will flow from the efforts of those who find satisfaction in their work and conditions of service, who sense an awareness of their usefulness of their function who feel encouraged to move ahead and to meet new challenges, who perceive their working environment as one in which high standards of performance are maintained and rewarded and not one in which indolence and incompetence can be ignored or even protected and rewarded. Motivation can do miracles as a motivated worker can achieve more than an expert with no motivation. District health officer; must, therefore, devote considerate time and effort in planning for and achieving high levels of motivation and morale. In such a situation, we would achieve goal congruence, i.e., identity between the individual goals and the organisational goals.

Living together is a beginning.
Keeping together is progress.
Working together success.

## Notes and References

1. H. Finer, Theory and Practice of Modern Government, p. 106.
2. ILO, International Labour Conference, 33rd Session, Provisional Records, p 34.
3. R. Micheal Cooper and Wood T. Micheal, "Member Participation and Commitment in Group Decision-making on Influence Satisfaction and Decision Riskness", *Journal of Applied Psychology,* Vol. 59, No. 2, April 1974.
4. Mason Haire, *et. al.*, "Psychological Research on Pay: An Overview", in *Personnel Administration,* Paul Pigors and Charles, A. Myers, New York. 1969, p. 491.
5. Encyclopedia of Social Sciences, Vol. I, p. 466, Dr. L.D. White, "Article on Administration."

12

CHAPTER

# Time Management

Time is not thought of as a resource. However, it is the most important and crucial factor as time is inelastic and non-renewable. An event cannot take place unless there is a time for it. Time and tide wait for none. We may keep in mind that time is neutral, i.e. it is neither good nor bad by itself. Therefore, to blame the time for any inaptitude for failure will be quite unfair.

Thus, if all the services make the best use of time, we can accelerate the process of development and help the people of the country suffering from abject poverty, ill-health, literacy, unemployment, in leading a good standard of life. In developed countries, the most precious resource is time and that is why they are developed, but in developing countries, time is unconsciously and consciously wasted in useless activities, resulting in underdevelopment and backwardness. Time has a value like currency and like the financial management, it can be organized to get more with less. Time once lost is lost forever. Therefore, we should not waste even a single second.

A study carried out by World Health Organisation revealed that the time utilization by doctors in Primary Health Centre for patient care is only 21 per cent. It is even less in case of preventive health care as most of the time is wasted in travelling. Besides, the medical personnel in rural areas, either absent themselves or come late and go early. Thus devoting very less time to productive work.

Let us support this with some examples:

(i) Many studies have found that nurses devote only 33 per cent of their time on nursing activities while rest of the time is used for non-nursing duties.

(ii) Multipurpose workers devote only 30 per cent of their time for health activities.

(iii) PHC doctors devote only 25 per cent time for patient care.
(iv) Doctors at district level waste 60 per cent of their time in travelling and unwanted meetings.

The statement that "Time is money" sums up the significance of time management. Though most people in Government, Public Enterprises, Private Sector and health sector understand the implications of time management, but in actual practice, we find that time is wasted and its importance is undermined. Most of the executives and workers; in administration complain that they are too busy, but still they while away a lot of their time in unnecessary activities. All other resources can be increased whenever required, but not time, as it is inelastic and therefore, we must make the best use of time. Just to illustrate the importance of time, many studies conducted revealed that persons in administration hardly devote 30 to 40 per cent of their time for the activities they have been primarily engaged for. It means that if proper use is made of time, we can provide services with the existing infrastructure two to three times more and thus the process of development can be accelerated.

Thus, if all the employees make the best use of time, we can accelerate the process of development and help the people of the country suffering from abject poverty, ill-health, illiteracy, unemployment, in leading a good standard of life. In developed countries, the most precious resource is time and that is why they are developed, but in developing countries, time is unconsciously and consciously wasted in useless activities, resulting in underdevelopment or backwardness.

Nation must be committed to utilise even a fraction of second for accelerating the tempo of development to usher in socio-economic democracy, as enshrined in the preamble of the Indian constitution. How to go about it? How to ensure optimization of time? How to make the best use of time? The answers to these questions are very simple, i.e., time management at all levels.

If our country can manage time, we can achieve in a year the work of a decade and thus can move fast towards modernization and development and can say with pride that India occupies a prominent place, as in the past, in the community of Nations.

We have already discussed a number of Techniques like PERTI CPM, Method Study. Work measurement, etc. which can help in managing time, but no technique of time management can compel us to move as time demands. Thus, the ultimate success of time management depends upon the people engaged in the pursuit of socio-economic development and leading the country. If all of us understand the value of time, then there would be no place for strikes, lock outs, work-stoppage, bandhs, dharnas, etc. All these activities are anti-nation and anti-development. In developed countries like Japan, Time is utilised profitably and they don't waste time in any way. If the persons in Government or Industry have to register a protest, they do simply by wearing black badges or present memoranda but not by stoppage of work.

The aim of time management is not to turn workers into machines, who work without interruptions or breaks, nor is it to develop rigid routines. Rather, the aim is to organise and arrange the use of time so that time pressures and overcrowded schedules and wastage are reduced, and that staff can have adequate rest periods without lowering work output.

If forced to work under continuous pressure, people devise means of escape, such as by taking few days off for illness or slowing down their pace and becoming inefficient. These ways of relieving pressure may be observed among staff in an average overcrowded department. It has been repeatedly shown in industry that regular breaks increase work efficiency and work output.

## TIME MANAGEMENT TECHNIQUES (See Chart 12.1)

Laurenr Jaung and Susank Jones in their book, "Time Management for Executives" (Charlo Scriknero Songs, New York, 1981) have said that the happiest people are busy people. But, there are two kinds of busy "harried or disorganised busy and calm effective busy. You can improve your effectiveness quotient and become an enlightened consumer of time if you master the basic lime-management skill." It is very difficult to enlist all the techniques of time-management as these are many and range from simple common sense approach to sophisticated techniques of PERT/CPM, OR, Method Study, Work Measurement, etc. We discuss here some important techniques.

### 1. Assessment of Time Use for Activities that are not Related to Work

In this technique, in columns across a sheet of paper, write down all the activities that are not related to work and that might take place during the course of a working day (e.g. relaxing in staff room or canteen, personal telephone calls, going out to shop, reading a newspaper, tea or coffee breaks, arriving late, leaving early, interruptions by other staff).

Give copies of the papers to staff members who have volunteered to take part in this exercise. Ask them to record the number of minutes spent on each activity not related to work over a period of one or more days. Collect the records and add up the minutes spent on non-working activities each day by each staff member. Request all staff members, who have agreed to record their non-work activities, to meet together to discuss the results or some team of outside experts may be deputed to collect this data. Give the group—the totals from above without revealing the identity of the staff members who provided the data.

Discuss the following questions with the groups:

(a) Is the amount of time spent in non-working activities reasonable, too much, or not enough?
(b) Would it be better to have recognized time breaks (e.g., 30 minutes for tea, shopping, reading the newspaper, or chatting) rather than having many unofficial breaks ?

CHART 12.1

**Time Management**

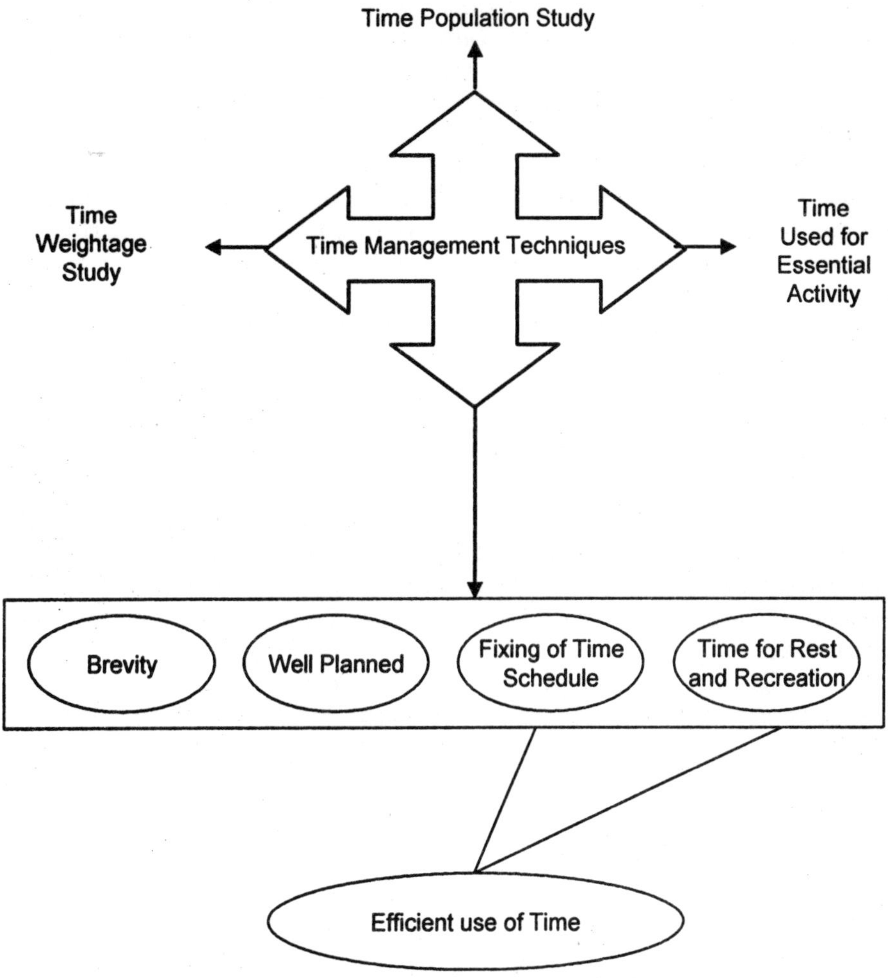


(c) Would recognized or official breaks, be introduced at different times so that the work did not stop?

List the recommendations decided by the group for each of these questions and implement them.

**2. Assessment of Time use for Activities that can be done at Lower Levels**

Most of the senior persons in the organisation perform the work which can be done at lower levels or that does not require the competence of the level where it is being done. If such work is delegated to the lower level, the time spent by the busy people at the higher level can be saved. This would also be economical since the salary scales are higher at upper levels. Let us understand this with the help of a Case Study from Thailand, reported in Public Health Development and Administration by Dr. K. Klinoubol (New Delhi, Deep & Deep, 1989, pp. 336-44). This study was conducted under the guidance of the author.

Acceptance of female sterilization in Thailand has increased considerably, but because of the shortage of doctors, especially in rural areas, long delays occurring before surgery are common. Women are discharged from hospital within 24 to 48 hours of delivery and although many wish to have post-partum sterilization, they often find it inconvenient to return to hospital for tubal ligation. Besides, it is very costly.

The Thai Ministry of Public Health decided to introduce the performance of post-partum tubal ligation by trained nurse-midwives, since this could alleviate the shortage of doctors and so reduce waiting time and free doctors for more skilled tasks. This reduces costs as well.

In 1979, a pilot study was conducted by the Ministry of Public Health in which five nurse-midwives with operating room experience were trained to perform post-partum tubal ligation by a mini laboratory incision under local anaesthesia. The performance of the trained nurse-midwives was compared with that of doctors in a controlled, radxomized clinical trial. The results suggested that trained nurse-midwives can safely perform the procedure.[1]

In the subsequent study, an expanded field trial of the nurse training programme was carried out by the Ministry of Public Health to evaluate the replicability of the training programme in provincial settings.[2] The results of the field trial of the nurse-training programme are similar to those of the pilot study, and further demonstrate that trained nurse-midwives with operating-room experience can safely perform post-partum tubal ligation under local anaesthesia in provincial settings. The nurse-midwives gained both surgical experience and self-confidence in a relatively short period. The average operating time of the nurse after 12 months (15 minutes) was nearly that of the doctors in the previous study (12 minutes).

The acceptability of the service as perceived by the patients was clearly impressive. The attitudes of doctors toward the use of trained nurse-midwives in their hospitals to perform tubal ligation were very positive. As a result of this study, it has been suggested to the Ministry of Public Health that an expanded programme be planned and implemented. Secondly, it is suggested that as medical procedures become accepted and routine, doctors should delegate these tasks to nursing and other personnel.[3] Delegation does not undermine the professional role; it enhances it. The more the doctor delegates the more time he has available for those tasks he cannot delegate and the more his work becomes confined to problems that staff with less training have failed to solve. In addition, more of his time can be devoted to supervising the work he has delegated and to providing continuing education to all engaged locally in activities to improve health.

But delegation is also a matter of economics. The ratio between the remuneration of the doctor and the average worker tends to be much higher in developing countries than in the more developed countries. Auxiliaries can also be trained at much lower cost than can higher grades of professional staff. Thus, it is much more important to ensure that the doctor's time is used only for tasks that require his skill and knowledge. The same is true of other highly trained health professionals—dentists, pharmacists, health inspector, and sanitary engineer and many others. There is a strong case for every highly trained professional grade to be matched by a corresponding auxiliary grade. Furthermore, as their training is shorter, auxiliary staff can be working in the field much earlier than more highly trained personnel.

To quote Allan Rosenfield: "I firmly believe that personnel other than physicians can and should be trained in the techniques of vasectomy, post-partum and tubal ligation, provision of injectable normal contraceptives and where legally and culturally acceptable, the carrying out of menstrual regulation or early first trimester abortion procedures.[4] Sydney F. Loves in his book, "Mastery and Management of Time" (Prentice Hall, USA, 1978) has rightly said that one must prune the trees of his activities so that one may not get lost on the branches. "Not every task requires a high quality level. Time can be gained from one to apply to another."

### 3. Time Proportion Study to Give Weightage to Priority Areas

The Health executives should plan their work according to the priority, so that more attention can be paid to such work. Here the Health executive may analyse the activities done during the day and the time devoted on each activity. The writer has done this exercise on many executives. The analysis of the results of such exercise suggest that the executives spend more time on activities that are less significant and spend less time on activities—that are very important. It means that the executives never devote time in proportion to the importance of the activity, resulting in many wrong decisions, affecting the performance of the organisation. For example, the tertiary health care institutions are created to do research, which can help in policy-making and planning in different areas. However, it is seen that they are engaged in routine activities of patient care. An opening of a department of a subject like Public Administration, Sociology, etc. in a University and a College is done with different objectives: that is why staffing at two levels is entirely different. The University Department is supposed to engage itself in Research, Consultancy and teaching, while a college department is mostly meant for teaching. A careful analysis of practices would indicate that both are engaged merely in teaching and that is why we generally hear that the Universities have become white elephant for the State exchequer. Administrative Reforms Commission examined the problem of administration and observed that in most cases, the top administration only okays the proposal initiated at lower levels. This means that the high level administration finds no time to think of real issues meant for them, like Organisational Development, Management of Change, Conflict Management, etc.

Because of the non-existence of referral system, patients rush directly to tertiary and secondary health care institutions, resulting in high cost and making specialists attend to the work that could be done at lower levels. Hence, there is a need of developing time schedule so that important activities are not missed and due weightage may be given to them.

**4. Time-Proportion Study on Meetings**

In today's administration, top level executives/experts attend a number of meetings, which are not well planned and well focused, resulting in the wastage of time of executives/experts. Whenever one goes to the District health office or State health directorate, one will find that most of the key people are busy in one meeting or the other. The analysis of the agenda and outcome of the meetings would indicate that there is too much wastage of time and that is why the key officials find no time to listen to the grievances of the people and develop a climate of understanding. Let me quote here the study conducted in the context of International Administration by the author (International Administration by Dr. S.L. Goel, New Delhi, Sterling, 1977, pp. 153-54).

The technical staff of the SEARO has to spend a lot of time in attending meetings of other regional agencies for liaison purposes. Besides, they have to prepare a large number of documents to exchange information with other regional organisations. These activities have been increasing over the years, largely because the increasing number of organisations tend to complicate the process of co-ordination. This was also pointed out by the UN Secretary-General who wrote: I detect a sense of concern in many quarters at the growth in the number of bodies and programmes which have been established primarily for co-ordination purpose or in which co-ordination activities play an important and increasing role, in the time and the documentation required to service them, and in the complexities and even the duplications which they involve."[5]

It is strange that even in hospitals, most of the time of the key experts is spent on meeting like Sub-Committees and it is very difficult to meet them and discuss important issues. The key experts get no time for important discussions, as they are exhausted in meetings dealing with matters of relatively lesser importance. It is, therefore, suggested that the time on these meetings may be reduced to be utilized on areas of greater significance.

**5. Time Study to Solve the Problems and Not Symptoms**

Most executives don't find time to deal with a case thoroughly from all angles, but rather deal with the symptoms. In this way, the issue lingers on and continues in this way for long, resulting in wastage of time and resources, not only of the management, but also of the beneficiaries as well as creating bitterness between the two. It has been seen that the cases which could be dealt with in a week's time continue for years.

An analysis of decided cases by various courts in the country would show that the key officials in the administration initiate action, against the employees on disciplinary grounds without due application of mind. This results in the wastage of resources and time of the administration in attending court cases. All these litigations can be avoided if the key personnel attend to these matters in a thorough manner. Key officials, by attending to real problems, can save a lot of time in the long-run and make the administration efficient and responsible.

**6. Well Planned Time Table for Field Visits**

Many of the key personnel at state and district health offices have to control a wide-network of offices. A pan of this job can be carried out through telephone, or by getting periodic response from the field offices. But, there is a need of personal discussion among the headquarter and the field staff, which involves the use of time for travelling and discussion. The officials plan their visit in such a way that they waste most of the time in travelling and less in discussion. It is suggested that field/headquarter visits must be well planned, so that the discussion can be pertinent and all the issues discussed in detail, to avoid meetings off and on. The headquarter personnel must carry with them a well prepared schedule to guide them in the field, while the field people must also come prepared with all the information to clarify the vague points.

**7. Fixing of Time Schedule to Devote Time to Work**

In most of the offices, the time for the visitors, is fixed, so that they may not be thronging the offices throughout the day and waste the time of the personnel. At the Scheduled time, people visit the offices but do not come back satisfied. It is suggested that the Personal Assistants, before sending any person to visit the officials, must listen to him to keep their file ready, so that action can be taken immediately and the person concerned may not visit again and again. A lot of time, as already mentioned, of the officials is wasted when the same people for the same work, visit the offices again and again. A brief training to staff and especially the Personal Assistants can help in quick disposal of public cases and thus avoiding their recurrent visits.

**8. Providing Regular Time for Rest and Recreation to Avoid Fatigue**

Executives are human beings and thus cannot work beyond their capacity. It is, therefore, suggested that they may observe regular rest periods to feel fresh. However, these rest periods may not be done at will but must be already notified to avoid difficulty to the staff and the people, until and unless there are compelling reasons for it.

### 9. Brevity

Besides, the executives must learn to be brief and to the point and discourage relatives/friends to visit them in offices. Telephonic discussions must also be brief.

### Case Study No. I

Time utilization by health manpower, and their productivity, is expected to be influenced *inter alia* by their attitudes to the job, especially their perceptions of the objectives to be pursued; organisational inadequacies and other constraints; job-related tensions and job satisfaction, etc. An attempt was made to ascertain these factors through research studies by Dr. Rajneesh Goel, in Karnataka in 1998.

*Objectives*—To find out the utilisation time of multi-purpose workers—male and female for the promotion of Primary Health Care as well as to find out the weightage given to different health activities out of the utilised time. The emphasis of the study is to locate the factors which consume time on non-productive activities and also to find the weightage given *vis-a-vis* the priority of the Primary Health Care.

*Research Methodology*—He prepared activity schedules both for male and female workers as per their job description and made arrangements to fill the form continuously for four days for each worker, 5 males and 5 females, one for each worker (male for male and female for female) were briefed about observation technique and filling the forms for five days for each worker. This was done in March 1998 from 9 AM to 5 PM. Continuous observation was made from the time they started the work till completion during the day except the lunch break. It is presumed that workers should devote 8 hours leaving aside 1 hour for lunch break.

The Study suggests the following pattern of time utilisation:

| *Sl. No.* | *Activity* | *Time spent by Male workers* | *Time spent by Female workers* |
|---|---|---|---|
| 1. | Movements | 3 hrs | 3 hrs |
| 2. | Personal Work | 1 hrs | 1½ hrs |
| 3. | Late arrivals and early departure | 1 hrs | 1½ hrs |
| | Total | 5 hrs | 5 hrs |

It is presumed that workers should devote 8 hours leaving aside 1 hour for lunch break. An analysis of above record indicates that multipurpose workers, both male and female, spend 62.5 percent of their time in unproductive activities, i.e. only 37.5 percent of the time is used productively. It may be added that out of utilized time, 50 percent is spent on record keeping to maintain their image and reputation on paper. This record is not accurate, causing complications for policy-makers and planners.

*Inferences*

We draw the following inferences from this study: .

(a) We may provide vehicle facility to the workers to reduce time spent in visiting different places.
(b) We may reduce time spent on record keeping by systematizing records management. We may even think of providing computers to ensure the supply of right information with less time consumption with ready made software.
(c) There is a need to ensure quality supervision by PHC Staff, especially Health Assistants, to ensure punctuality.
(d) There is a need for training to make the workers responsive and dedicated.
(e) There is a need to provide residential accommodation to workers with all facilities in the village to encourage them to stay near the sub-centre and improve rapport with the people.
(f) People may be motivated to move to the sub-centre rather than waiting for the workers' visit at their door-steps, after initial meetings.
(g) Advance schedule for a month and its wide circulation can optimise time resource utilisation.

After clubbing various activities carried out during utilised time, he has exhibited them in Tables 12.1 and 12.2, the weightage given by 5 male and 5 female workers for different health activities.

An analysis of the time utilization by service components showed that most of their service time was devoted to family planning activities (percent of service time devoted ranged from 33-49%) followed by MCH services (22-27%), and immunization (5-15%). (See Tables 12.1 and 12.2).

Thus all MPWS (male and female) were found to devote most of their service time on family planning activities. This could well be attributed to the government's emphasis on target achievement in the family planning programme. Since these workers are given a set target to achieve family planning, they are forced to spend more time on this activity, and thus neglect other important activities. However, the target approach has been abolished and its impact is yet to be felt.

The main purpose of the scheme was to devote more time on health education, nutrition, inter-sectoral co-ordination, people's participation, which could not be attended to. There is a need to impart training to these workers to make them realise their true role. Only such understanding on their part can change health scene of rural India, otherwise, it would prove to be another institution with liabilities. The main function of MPW is to make people participate in Primary Health Care activities and get most of the functions performed by them. Besides, they never devoted much time for Inter-Sectoral Co-ordination, an essential Component of Primary Health Care.

TABLE 12.1

**Percent of Time Utilization for various activities (MPW—Male)**

| Sl. No. | Activity/Service | Percent of time utilized Health worker No. | | | | |
|---|---|---|---|---|---|---|
| 1. | Malaria eradication | 27.01 | 22.6 | 32.1 | 23.6 | 32.2 |
| 2. | Control of communicable diseases | 2.1 | 11.1 | 12.6 | 11.6 | 12.5 |
| 3. | Environmental sanitation | 1.1 | 4.4 | 1.2 | 3.4 | 2.2 |
| 4. | Immunization | 2.8 | 6.2 | 4.6 | 32.0 | 3.6 |
| 5. | Family Planning | 41.8 | 31.6 | 31.7 | 2 | 31.8 |
| 6. | MCH Services | 3.1 | 4.6 | 0.2 | 2.6 | 0.1 |
| 7. | Vital Statistics collection | 3.3 | 3.7 | 3.6 | 4.6 | 3.6 |
| 8. | Nutrition | 5.1 | 7.7 | 2.1 | 5.4 | 2.1 |
| 9. | Primary Medical Care | 3.3 | 3.3 | 4.8 | 1.2 | 4.8 |
| 10. | Team Activity | 2.1 | 1.8 | 1.4 | 7.0 | 1.4 |
| 11. | Record Maintenance | 7.7 | 3.0 | 5.0 | .. | 5.0 |
| 12. | Work at PHC | .. | .. | .. | | .. |
| 13. | Interaction with community health volunteers/Dais | 0.6 | .. | 0.7 | 2.0 | .7 |
| | TOTAL | 100.0 | 100.0 | 100.0 | 100.0 | 100.0 |

TABLE 12.2

**Percent of Time Utilization for various activities (MPW—Female )**

| S. No. | Activity/Service | Percent of time utilized Health worker No. | | | | |
|---|---|---|---|---|---|---|
| 1. | MCH | 26.9 | 22.4 | 23.5 | 21.6 | 24.7 |
| 2. | Family Planning | 48.5 | 34.8 | 42.3 | 49.3 | 33.2 |
| 3. | Nutrition | 2.1 | 6.0 | .1 | .7 | 11.7 |
| 4. | Immunization | 5.4 | 16.2 | 15.4 | 5.5 | 9.8 |
| 5. | Vital statistics Collection | 2.8 | 3.8 | .2 | 2.3 | 5.0 |
| 6. | Control of communicable diseases | 5.9 | 6.0 | 5.0 | 7.2 | 6.2 |
| 7. | Primary Medical Care | 4.6 | 3.7 | 7.3 | 8.3 | 4.3 |
| 8. | Team Activity | 3.6 | 5.8 | .. | 2.5 | 2.8 |
| 9. | Record Maintenance | .. | .8 | .. | 2.0 | 2.1 |
| 10. | Preparation (for immunization) | .. | .4 | .. | .. | .. |
| 11. | Interaction with CHV/Dais | .. | .. | .. | .. | .5 |
| 12. | Cleaning | .. | .. | .. | .. | .3 |
| 13. | Group Meetings | .2 | .1 | .. | .. | .. |
| | TOTAL | 100.0 | 100.0 | 100.0 | 100.0 | 100.0 |

We present here the results of some studies conducted earlier on time utilization in the same area.

**Case Study No. 2**

A study of PHC staff Time Utilization pattern was undertaken in a PHC in Uttar Pradesh by S.K. Satpathy et al. (1998). This study included only technical staff (excluded drivers, sweepers, etc.) and the technique followed was a non-participant observation of the staff for several days. From this study, it was found that the non-productive time of such staff was as high as 62%, services time accounted for 27% and travel accounted for 11%.

**Case Study No. 3**

A study on cost analysis of PHCs by M. Kataria and D.P. Srivastava (NIHFW, 1986) included the analysis of allocation of service time at PHC and sub-centre levels. The method used was observation (for field work) and work sampling (at PHC). Besides these two techniques, Delphi technique was also used for supplementing the information collected through the observations. Three districts from two states (M.P. and U.P.) were selected; one PHC per district was selected. Thus 3 PHCs from each state were selected and 12 sub-centres (2 from each selected PHC) were selected. The major findings of the study were:

- 50% of the activity time was spent on travelling and unproductive activities;
- Of the other 50% of productive time, 115th was devoted to 'Direct Services', the major activity being family planning followed by MCH services (by female workers) and control of communicable diseases (by male worker); and
- At PHC, direct services accounted for 47% (UP) and 49% (MP); supportive services accounted for 8% (UP) and 11% (MP); time spent on travel was 22% (UP) and 20% (MP). Thus only 55-60% of total activity time was spent productively

**Case Study No. 4**

Johns Hopkins University conducted studies (1965-68) and came to the following conclusions:

- Only 1/6 of the total health centre effort went into direct service in Punjab, compared to 1/4 in Mysore. Further, in Punjab, supporting activities (33.3%) consumed more than twice as much time than service efforts (15.5%).
- More time was devoted in Punjab to the maintenance of records and preparation of reports than to the provision of services (16.3%), whereas in Mysore a mere 1/3 of the activity time was devoted to records and reports.

## CONCLUSION

Time management would not only be beneficial to the health experts and executives but would also provide more opportunities to the people to share their ideas and views and thus we would be able to lay the solid foundations of People's Participation development and modernisation.

Prabhat Kumar in his article, "A Responsive and Effective Government" rightly suggests that "we forget that time is our most valuable recourse, the only one that is absolutely non-renewable. No one has the right to waste it, every one should control his own time. It can be given but never should be taken away by another. Unfortunately, lateness is the rule in Government and waiting is a national past time."[6]

The Management requires a high degree of self-discipline. The habit of entertaining casual visitors during office hours must be shunned ruthlessly. Designate a prime time, may be an hour or so, during the working hours, which is strictly your own time and distractions should never by permitted to interfere. It is the man who should manage time and not the other way round.

The development and modernization of developing countries can be accelerated by an efficient Public Health Administration. It has been observed that Personnel in Administration are not utilising their time for the assigned job. They are wasting a lot of time in unnecessary trivial activities which are non-productive. We must manage our time purposefully to build Modern India, otherwise we would remain an under-developed country as time and tide waits for none. Health Services can be increased 3-4 times with existing personnel, provided these personnel devote their time to their duties efficiently The failure of the Primary health care in India is the failure of health personnel who never took interest in it and devoted full time for the essential activities,

It is high time for the Union and State Governments to get the time utilisation study conducted for different categories of personnel, so that remedial action can be taken for optimisation of health services.

### Notes and References

1. N. Dustisin, *et. al.*, "Post-partum-tubal ligation by nurse-midwives and doctors in Thailand." The Lancet I, No. 8169.22, March 1980, pp. 638-39
2. N. Dustisin, *et. al.*, cited in Note 2.
3. WHO Poverty Development and Health Policy, PHP, 69, Geneva, 1978, p. 103.
4. Allan Rosenfield, The Ethics of Supervising Family Planning in Developing Nations, Hasting Centre Report, February 1977, pp 25-29.
5. 23rd Annual Report of the Secretary-General to the Central Assembly (1968), paras 80 and 82 (A/720/Add.1).
6. Prabhat Kumar, "A Responsive and Effective Government, in *Management in Government*, January-March, 2000, p. 3.

13

CHAPTER

# Human Resource Development (HRD)

> "HRD in brief is transformation of Potential Human Resources into Kinetic Human Resources for optimization of the potential capacity of employees. It has been rightly said in a study of the Capacity of United Nations Development System that "Human rather than capital is the key to development. Development is not a mechanical process. It is a human enterprise and its success will depend ultimately on the skill, quality and motivation of the persons associated with it."
>
> —*Prof. Iris Claude*

In Ancient Literature HRD is synonymous with total personality development—physical, mental, spiritual and ethical. HRD aims at assimilation of ideas pertaining to life building, man-making and character building. In western countries, emphasis is given only on artificial inducements through various doses of incentives while in Ancient Sanskrit Literature, emphasis is laid on good qualities among Human Beings. Dr. K.M. Munshi rightly says that mere imparting of information is not HRD but it is the building of character. The modern mind has confounded knowledge or achievement with personality. This confusion has been the direful springs of woes unnumbered. In India, it has turned the University graduate into a waste paper basket for odd bits of information. Unshaped in character, dwarfed in personality and devoid of that faith, which alone convert knowledge into power. HRD in ancient literature is to achieve perfection and ethical values while a western countries, the emphasis is on making profits. Ancient Literature lays emphasis on nation-building and does not limit its scope merely to be development of a particular organisation in which one is working. Hence, the scope of HRD in Ancient Sanskrit Literature is more broad based and qualitative in nature as compared to the existing concept of HRD in management literature.

Broadly speaking, HRD is one of the important Human Resource Management (HRM) functions and it includes the areas of individual development, career development and organisational development. The remaining human resource areas like employee-employer relations, human resource planning, recruitment and selection, organisation/job design, etc. come under the purview of HRM. The first area of HRD, i.e. individual development is taken care of by the training and development function, the second area of career development needs both training as well as some organisational interventions like career development-oriented policies and structures and the third area of organisational development is purely an organisational intervention which tries to focus on ensuring healthy inter and intra-unit development relationships and helping groups and organisations to initiate and manage change.[1]

It is recognised everywhere that human resources in an organisation are an essential prerequisite for growth or development, especially in health institutions, where personnel constitute the main resource. It has been rightly said in "A study of the Capacity of United Nations Development System" that the "Human rather than capital is the key to development." Development is not a mechanical process. It is a human enterprise and its success will depend ultimately on the skill, quality and motivation of the persons associated with it. It is therefore, by increasing the efficiency, integrity and the intelligence of its personnel that an organisation will give itself the real means for advancing towards efficiency. The constant improvement of the efficiency of an employee is as much the responsibility of the employee himself as it is of the organisation.

Improved efficiency resulting in higher productivity is of mutual advantage to both the organisation and the staff. Thus, developing the potential of health manpower requires a Human Resource Development all through the health systems. In this regard, within the district health system, the role of District Health Officer is quite crucial and important. In fact the staff working below him spend their major time in the organisation or in the field within the community. The Health Department should make efforts to develop the system in the health system that focuses on HRD approach and ensures that staff working in the health system enjoy their work, feel proud and happy and are committed, competent and loyal to work as a team.

## NATURE AND SCOPE OF HRD

HRD in brief is change of Potential Human Resources into Kinetic Human Resources, that is Optimisation of the potential capacity of employees.

HRD is an effort to develop capabilities and competence among health personnel, as well as to create an organisational environment conducive to the employees, development A.D. Moddies has observed that "Good organisation building has to create around it a bracing atmosphere,

CHART 13.1

**HRD**

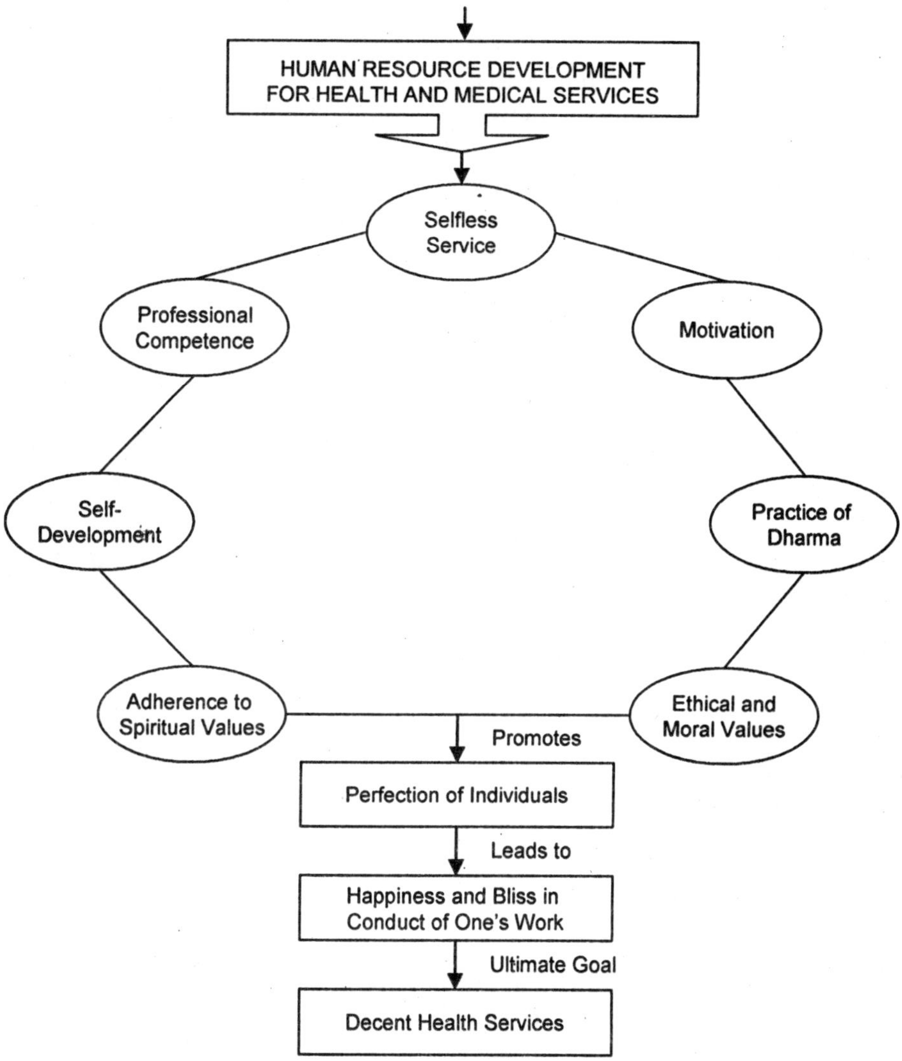


a prideful tradition of integrity, excellence and fellowship. Human beings breathe this ethos around them almost unconsciously and these traditions make for that ethos."[2]

We can thus say that HRD implies a total revolution involving human and organisational issues. Let us now discuss some of the definitions. According to Ishwar Dayal, three things are important in HRD:

"(a) Ways to better adjust the individual to his job and the environment.

(b) The greatest involvement of the employee in various aspects of his work.
(c) The greatest concern for enhancing the capabilities of the Individual."[3]

We may thus define HRD as a process of the development of employees through training, performance appraisal. Potential development, exercise, communication policies, job enrichment programmes, etc., and building of an organisational climate, which may encourage openness, risk-taking, role clarity, awareness of employee's responsibility, increased communication, improvement of personnel policies, management styles, etc. so that employees may be effective in translating their potential energy into kinetic energy and the organisation may be benefited in terms of better image, higher productivity, better utilization of resources, etc. HRD in a way involve total management and for HRD to be effective, we have to introduce changes in management at all levels.

Current Status of HRD in Health System in India—HRD has not caught the imagination of policy-makers and planners of health system. Health systems are suffering in different States, mostly on account of personnel problems. Medical personnel have lost their faith in health care, rather they are busy in exploiting the people through many malpractices. It is high time that we introduce HRD to inject professional growth, dynamism, dedication, commitment and loyalty among health personnel, who are all considered semi-Gods by ailing humanity. This would be able to promote prestige and reputation of health and medical profession.

The current literature on human resource development maintains that HRD is an art and a science as it is very difficult to predict human behaviour. Human beings change from time to time. However, in Ancient Sanskrit Literature, HRD is a science as it lays down definite principles based on thousand years of research which if acted upon can lead to the development of human beings and realize cherished goals. Majority of them do not follow these principles and hanker after petty things causing a low quality profile and deviating from cherished goal. Therefore, it is essential for those who are engaged in teaching and studying HRD principles to possess all these qualities (knowledge) and then implement them. This would a great service to the family, organisation and society at large-international brotherhood. There will not be a divide between developed and developing countries as all of them would be following Dharma leading to peace and development on this earth. When we pray for the welfare of others, all our petty and selfish feelings will go away and our intellect will expand. There are many such prayers in the Vedas and the Puranas, such as:

"May all be happy,
may all be free from disease,
may all realize what is good,
may none be subject to misery."

It has now been proved, country after country that an honest, professionally sound, contended bureaucracy is a critical element of any program. It is thus of utmost importance that the best brains in the country are attracted to the public services. They should not only be motivated to enter the services but also serve in a professional and dedicated manner. This necessitates a careful handling of all the major parameters from their induction to retention. (Central Fifth Pay Commission).

In the present day world, we find an increasing relevance of the statement made by Dr. Radhakrishnan, when he observed that the mind that invented the atom bomb was more powerful than the bomb itself. Every letter can be made into a mantra. Every root has a medicinal value. Every person has some competence and making him realize his potential is HR manager's challenge. Unfortunately, the yojakas, the visionaries, the leaders, the organizers or managers who can make these things happen, are rare. Can we, at the end of our efforts, come up with techniques/methods by which such managers can be multiplied so that their positive impact can help to create the right human capital to meet the challenge of the emerging future.

## ESSENTIALS OF INDUCTING HRD IN HEALTH SYSTEM

(a) An urge and desire on the part of the state health department and district health offices to find better methods of personnel development.

(b) Requisite skill, attitudes and ability in the persons engaged in HRD.

(c) Proper rapport between the HRD team/Deptt. and the key personnel in the health organisations at all levels.

(d) Removal of hurdles and irritants from the organisation affecting efficiency of the employees.

(e) Involvement of the Personnel of the Organisation to get a lot of unwritten information for understanding the dynamics of the organisation for developing an HRD Programme.

(f) The need for suggesting the introduction of only such indigenous methods which can be implemented by the HRD section without much cost and resistance. Besides, the need for technical consideration may also be kept in mind.

(g) Use EDP to keep continuous track of every employee and use performance appraisal, training, etc.. to ensure/change in the desired direction.

(h) Members of HRD team should possess pleasant personality, common sense, imagination, enthusiasm, objectivity and the sense of humour required to induce change towards HRD, as it has been rightly said that it is easier to change the mountains that to change the minds of the people.

CHART 13.2

**HRD**

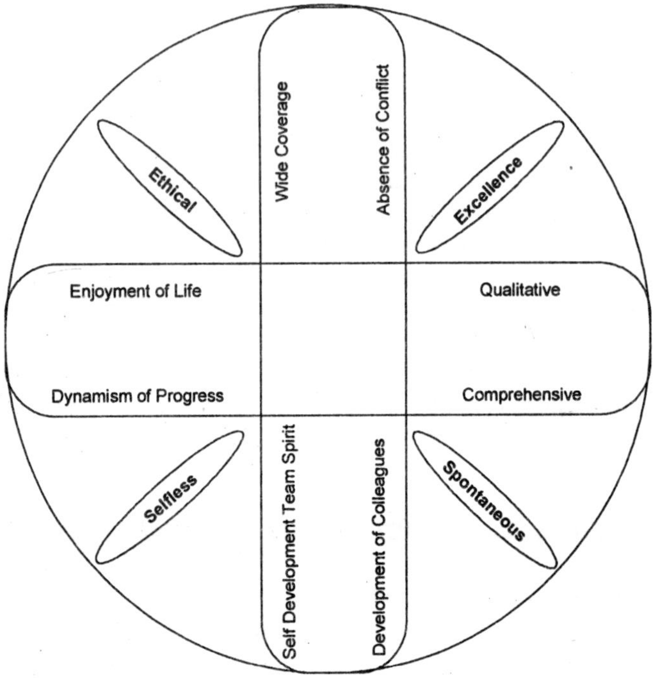


(i) The HRD section must be ready to face resistance to their ideas and dispel these with facts, patience and consideration. The aim should be to develop acceptance through co-operation.

(j) The HRD section must make all the employees in the organisation understand the implications of new methods through seminars, lectures, role playing or any other method to thwart the potential fears amongst the employees of the proposed changes.

(k) HRD to be successful, needs revolution in the total concept of management and not merely sporadic and piece-meal attempts.

(l) The HRD team/section must possess technical competence in HRD, missionary, zeal, the capacity to motivate and communicate with the employees, cultural adaptability, the capacity to organize and manage, the capacity to inspire confidence in employees, and finally patience and dignity.

The above mentioned essentials, when understood and implemented, would help employees to contribute professionally and enthusiastically to the performance of their respective tasks in terms of the objectives, policies and targets of the organisation, as well as to promote a spirit of team work among them. In this way HRD would develop both in theory and practice and this in turn would lead to efficiency and economy in management.

## OBJECTIVES OF HRD IN HEALTH SYSTEM

(a) Revision of the basic concepts, underlying the present personnel policy.
(b) Modernization of clinical and administrative practices.
(c) Introduction of a career development system.
(d) Reform of recruitment methods.
(e) Help the personnel to overcome their weakness and further improve their strengths and thus enable them to improve their performance and that of the health department.
(f) Generate adequate feedback and guidance from the reporting officers or supervisors of the employee.
(g) Contribute to the growth and development of the employee through helping him in realistic goal setting.
(h) Provide input to: (i) a system of rewards comprising salary increments, appreciation, additional responsibilities, promotions, etc., and (ii) better salary conditions.
(i) Help in creating a desirable culture and traditions in the health institution.
(j) Help in identifying employees for the purpose of motivating, training and developing them.
(k) Generation of significant, relevant, free and valid information about employees.

## IMPLEMENTATION OF HRD

Having discussed the definition and significance, let us also discuss the implementation of HRD. It involves all the aspects of management but we will concentrate only on the important ones.

### 1. Commitment

HRD can come into practice only when personnel in an organisation, both at the top and lower levels, have understood the implications of HRD and desire its introduction for better performance. Such understanding would result in commitment. No organisation can develop until and unless the personnel working in the organisation are committed to achieve its ideal. The future of the public services is in the hands of its members, who must strive for creativity, academic excellence, and the pursuit of excellence of service in their professional activities. Faith in the top administrators about their work would generate sufficient energy to get the co-operation of the entire staff in an organisation, as faith is contagious. Staff members would try to make use of the management techniques to promote efficiency in such congenial environment. In this way, we would be able to create a climate of creativity and optimum performance. Such a situation would generate a chain effect.

**2. Specific Action Plan and Strategy**

There is a need to develop a time bound plan to implement the proposed changes within the time frame. We may use here techniques like PERTICPM. There is a need to design the strategy in terms of goals and objectives.

**3. Building Morale and Motivation among the Members of an Organisation**

The most important task of an organisation must be to give abundant and constant evidence of its belief that personnel in an organisation are the key to development. This requires proper motivation of the employees. Motivation is of utmost importance as in constitutes the base for management functions of planning and organising. The personnel must devote considerable time and effort in planning for and achieving high levels of motivation and morale.

**4. Counselling and Mentoring**

The main purpose of counselling and monitoring is to help the employees scientifically to realize their potential-their strengths and weaknesses. It also helps an employee in sharing and discussing his, tensions, conflicts, concerns and problems. The management may devote time to educating the employees and this should continue permanently through the process of:

1. Training;
2. Administrative Reforms;
3. Interpersonal Relations;
4. Recruitment;
5. Performance Appraisal;
6. Career Development; and
7. Manpower Planning

Besides, HRD must develop team-work which would raise the morale and efficiency of the personnel.

> "Team work requires, among other things, that the members have an image of their own team-mates, which coincides as precisely as possible with reality. In addition, each member must have a self-image which adjusts to reality as much as possible and thus coincides with the image the other members have of him."

The critical role of the State in the delivery of public goods and services can be realized only through an efficient, effective and responsive administration delivering quality public service. Measures for administrative reforms have, therefore, acquired urgency as the framework for an effective administration capable of quality service needs to be sensitively achieved. High quality and effective public services are a vital part of a modern state as people are entitled to expect that services which are often central to their lives, should be responsive, sensitive to their needs, easy to use, flexible and efficient.

We are now on the threshold of the twenty-first century. In the new millennium, above all, the government would need to re-invent itself to become citizen-centric and citizen-friendly.

It would need to limit its role to core functions such as security, law and order, social services, creation of infrastructure and macro-economic management. Greater delegation and decentralization of authority and responsibilities would need to be introduced at all levels, combination of Citizens' Charters and the Right to Information would ensure greater accountability in the administrative systems. The process of consultation with the participation of citizen; in decision-making would gradually become more pronounced in order to ensure accountability. At the same time, good citizenry would also need to be emphasized for all round development of the society. Besides enjoying their rights, the citizens would need to behave responsibility and perform their duties to state clearly defined ethical standards would also need to be adopted by the civil servants as well as politicians. In order to achieve all this, innovative use of information technology would be critical.

Transparency and peoples' participation in regulatory and developmental administration is very crucial not only in bridging the gap between the administration and the public but also in nation-building by way of reducing the corruption and complaints against the system. Further it helps the people to understand the limitation of the administration at different levels.

The Human Resource Development in Ancient Sanskrit Literature is to teach the human beings especially those in strategic positions that enjoyment of life consists in achievement and not material possessions through corrupt practices. So, only Ancient Sanskrit Literature through HRD can create positive attitude by which people in Health Administration at top level enjoy work and service to people and not indulge in corruption.

## Notes and References

1. UN: A Study of the Capacity of the UN Development System, Vol. I, Geneva, 1969.
2. A.D. Moddie, The Bureaucratic Culture and Modernity, Asia Publishing House, New York, pp. 106-14.
3. Ishwar Dayal, HRD in Practice: Some Experience and some Reflections, in *Indian Journal of Social Works*, Vol. LII, No. 4, Oct., 1991, p. 485.

14

CHAPTER

# Organisational Development

"Organisation Development is a re-orientation of man's thinkings and behaviour towards his Work Organisations. It applies the scientific methods and its underlying values of open investigation and experimentation to individual and work group behaviours as they are directed towards the solution of work problems. It views both man and change optimistically. It applies a humanistic value system to work behaviours. It assumes people have the capability and motivation to grow through learning how to improve their own work climate, work processes and their resulting products."

—*Hyman K. Randal*

There have been continuous efforts on the part of successive Governments to mould the health organisations to make them more responsive to the health needs of the people and to make them more efficient. Ironically, these reforms have failed to inject necessary changes in health organisational structures and processes. Organisational development is an important instrument to resolve these organisational issues so that these can provide efficient health services.

Organisation Development (popularly known as OD) is a systematic and educative approach to improve the organisation efficiency and effectiveness. It is a dynamic and continuous process to ensure insulation of organisation from being static to dynamic in health delivery.

Organisation Development is a new and dynamic approach, based on behavioural science knowledge to introduce planned change in the total health organisation, with the objective of improving its health and effectiveness. It is based primarily on the action-research model, in which health data is gathered, feedback to relevant teams, leading to joint diagnosis and action planning. The unit of change is not only individual, but mainly the teams and their relationships with other inter-dependent teams. Planned interventions are made in the process system, structure and goals of organisation. OD effort has to be related to the mission of the organisation and it must be oriented to bring about change in the culture and other relevant aspects of the total organisation to ensure health facilities. OD work is based on system theory, is a long-range effort, and is successful only when the top management in the area of health is committed to it. To ensure success of OD interventions, it is necessary that there is an ongoing monitoring and review of plans and outputs of health services.

The objectives of a typical health organisation development programme are:

(i) to increase the level of the trust and support among health personal and groups throughout the health organisation;
(ii) to create an open, problem-solving climate throughout the health organisation—where problems are confronted and differences are clarified, both within group and between groups in contrast to "sweeping problems under the rug";
(iii) to increase the level of personal enthusiasm and satisfaction in the organisation;
(iv) to attain better collaboration and cooperation between inter-department health persons and/or groups;
(v) to increase the openness of communication laterally, vertically and diagonally;
(vi) to increase the level of self and group responsibility in planning and achievement of goals through optimum resource utilization; and
(vii) a shift in values so that human factors and feelings of health personnel come to be considered as legitimate.[1]

OD is defined as a "complex educational strategy which aims to bring about a better fit between the human beings who work in and expect things from organisations and the busy unrelenting environment with its insistence on adapting to changing times."[2]

Warren Bennis has called organisation development "a complex educational strategy intended to change the beliefs, attitudes, values and structure of organisations so that they can better adapt to new technologies, markets, and challenges, and the dizzying rate of change itself."[3] Richard Bechhard provides the following definition, "Organisation development is an effort: (1) planned, (2) organisation-wide, (3) managed from the top, (4) to increase organisation effectiveness and health through, and (5) planned interventions in the organisations processes using behavioural-science knowledge.[4] Paul Lawrence and Jay Lorsch describe organisation development as a complex application of diagnoses and prescriptions based on behavioural-science knowledge, which facilitates changes that "will lead to either a better fit between the organisation and the demands of its environment and/or to a better fit between the organisation and the needs of individual contributors. For example . . . if a particular change enables specific units to conduct transactions with their part of the environment more effectively, it is in the direction of developing the organisation . . . If a particular change results in individuals being more highly motivated to contribute to organisational purposes, it is also in the direction of organisation development."[5] What do applied behavioural scientists do in organisation development programmes? Lawrence and Lorsch emphasize the use of behavioural-science concepts and methods for gathering data and making diagnoses. "How differentiated is the organisation? Where are problems occurring in achieving integration?[6] How are members managing conflict? Where are the sources of individual satisfaction and dissatisfaction? Where do member feel the individual contribution contract is inadequate?"6 Beckhard discusses four kinds of activities in organisation development: "(1) working with teams on team development, (2) working on planning and goal-setting processes for individuals, teams and larger systems, and (3) working on educational activities for upgrading the knowledge, skills, and abilities of key personnel at all levels."[7]

Hyman K. Randall has defined this concept as "Organisation Development is a reorientation of man's thinkings and behaviour toward his Work Organisations. It applies the scientific method and its underlying values of open investigation and experimentation to individual and work group behaviours as they directed toward the solution of work problem. It views both man and change optimistically. It applies a humanistic value system to work behaviours. It assumes people have the capability and motivation to grow through learning how to improve their work climate, work processes and their resulting products."

Alexander Winn defines the concept as a normative, re-education strategy intended to affect systems of beliefs, values, and attitudes within the organisation, so that it can adapt better to the accelerated rate of change in technology, in our industrial environment and society in general. It also includes formal organisational restructuring, which is frequently initiated, facilitated and reinforced by the normative and behavioural changes.

OD depends upon the purely internal initiative of the employees of health organisation. The present emphasis in administration is only on structural changes, but structural changes without personnel dedication and capabilities would be of no avail. It is high time that we must introduce OD in all our health institutions toward off the bureaucratic attitudes which result in low output and stagnation. We have the other techniques to achieve this objective, e.g. Management by Objectives, Participative Management. We must try to integrate all these techniques for optimizing the efficiency of health personnel in an organisation.[8]

The most important task of Personnel Department must be to give abundant evidence of its belief that personnel in an organisation are key to development. This requires proper motivation of the health employees.

Motivation is of utmost importance as it constitutes the base for the health management functions of planning and organizing. It has been noticed that the performance of the personnel either as individuals or members of a group is less as compared to their capabilities in terms of skills, abilities, and capacities. Finer, for example, states that demonstrated performance generally never exceeds more than fifty per cent of the individuals ability to perform.[9] Most individuals tend to balance their efforts around an assessment of relative costs (time and energy) and benefits.[10] A climate of creativity must be developed and maintained by management. Maiser and Hayes say that "the optimal climate for creativity . . . is whatever human conditions optimal for individual freedom and self-expression in social setting.[11] It is the duty of the officers of such units to make the health employees feel that their work and their association with a given organisation represent a vehicle which will accelerate the achievement of personal goals as well as achievement of goals of the organisation.

Henry B. Schacht, commenting on the changing trend in Organisational design and the use of human resources, has stressed that health managers must learn to handle both the underprivileged and the bright young people, especially those who were calling for change. He states:[12]

> "What this means is shorter, flatter Organisations; it means responsive management; it means a true willingness to allow people to participate in setting their own destiny; it means that militaristically-oriented hierarchy that has characterized societies and most business enterprises is a thing of the past, and the quicker we recognize it the better . . . all organisations will have to think of their key assets in terms of people and knowledge. People can be the most flexible of all assets; knowledge is the one thing that will give us insight into change and the consequences of change."

The success of this technique depends upon its proper implementation by the top health executive. He has to use the information generated for the good of the organisation. The emphasis in all O.D. programmes is on changing the attitudes, values and beliefs of health employees, so that the health employees themselves can visualize and implement organisational changes to promote efficiency.

## GOALS OF OD

The goal of OD is to ensure dynamic health organisation to accommodate existing and potential problems so that the health organisation remains action-oriented. The health personnel working in these organisations would feel satisfied and are encouraged to make use of creative ideas with dedications. The OD builds trust and confidence among health employees and there is no dichotomy between organisational goals and individual's goals. OD promotes both individual and organisational efficiency.

Organisation Development is one of the few recent educational programmes on all aspects of health organisation as well as managerial responsibility. It has the potential to create an institution capable enough of coping with turbulent future. Probably the organisational sciences owe their rescue from classical malaise to especially the OD movement. The goals of OD is to make every health employee in an organisation to work with full capacity and get satisfaction in giving best health delivery services.[13]

Keeping in mind the role played by the Private Sector in delivering health care services to the masses, their potential can be used for the improvement of health care delivery systems.

Scope in organisation development:

1. Capacity building through the HRD programme.
2. Re-organising the department.
3. Formation of a Public Health Act.
4. Strengthening of a Strategic Planning Cell.
5. Drafting of medical manual.
6. Providing schemes of incentives to encourage for further improvement.
7. Formation of State Level Health Care Accreditation and Regulatory Authority.

These above when well planned and effectively implemented would set the wheel in motion for achieving a result-based approach.

The strategies for Organisation Development would—

1. Bringing about an 'attitudinal change' in the personnel delivering health care services.
2. A behavioural change communication would strengthen the integrity of the Human Resource Development in the health organisations.
3. Development in the skill and knowledge of the people through trainings, workshops, meetings, group discussions, tele-conferencing study tours and visits, etc.
4. Recognising marked achievement and rewarding would encourage and uplift the enthusiasm of the health care personnel.
5. Counselling for recruitment and transfer along with timely eligible promotions would facilitate people to give their best services for health care.
6. Refurbishing method of accountability of services rendered would drive the organisation towards a result-oriented approach.

A well studied change in The Cadre and Recruitment Rules would be effective to achieve the target, objective and the goal of the Department. Similarly the drafting of Public Health Laws and Rules would stream-line the department. A comprehensive Public would keep the department in a disciplined and systematic form, taking into account, the involvement of private sector the concept of Public Private Partnership (PPP) has evolved, to deliver better health care services. Similarly, Health Insurance would remove the insecure feeling in the population specially vulnerable and economically backward group of people.

### Strengths of OD

1. It borrows freely from the proven procedures for improving functioning of individuals, groups and organisations.
2. Adoption of action research model, and a change strategy that focuses on the culture of work teams and the organisation make OD more powerful and relevant than most change strategies.[14]

### Weaknesses of OD

1. Its over preoccupation with human and social dynamics of an organisation, to the detriment of attending to the task, technical and structural aspects, and their interdependencies;
2. Conceptual foundation underlying OD strategies have limitations, as most of their models were built on collaborative approach rather than on power, coercion and competition; and
3. OD has no quick remedies, and no shortcuts to total organisational improvement.[15]

## OD IN INDIA

Problems of OD in India in Health Organisations:

(a) Top health management in theory accepts the sharing of authority and goal formulation by all health personnel in the Organisation, but in practice, they hesitate and want to remain supreme and above the subordinates who feel neglected and do not devote much attention.

(b) The Organisational climate in India is not suitable for OD interventions. Political, Social, Economic, Cultural, environment encompassing Organisations do not allow the introduction of OD.

(c) Health Organisation Structure in India is designed on formal relationships and unproductive lines and hence, in such a situation, OD interventions cannot be a success. Health employees feel alienated.

(d) In India, most of the health organisations are managed on adhoc basis rather than having long-term objectives. Under such situations, OD interventions become difficult. There is lethargy among health professionals.

What is required is to create genuine Organisational Climate, wherein techniques like OD can bear fruits and health delivery can become a success and health resources optimized.

## OD INTERVENTIONS

A large number of OD interventions are used to promote (see Charts 14.1, 14.2 and 14.3) organisational efficiency. French and Bell identified twelve interventions: (1) diagnostic, (2) team-building, (3) inter-group activities, (4) survey-feedback methods, (5) education and training programmes, (6) techno-structural activities, (7) process consultation, (8) the management grid, (9) mediation and negotiation activities, (10) coaching and counseling, (11) career planning, and (12) planning and goal setting activities. On the other hand, Warren Bennis classified intervention into nine categories, according to the purpose of OD. These focus on, (1) discrepancies, (2) theory, (3) procedures, (4) relationships, (5) experimentation, (6) dilemmas, (7) perspectives, (8) structures, and (9) cultural problems.

The exact intervention is applied to solve a definite problem or a combination of interventions are applied to remove organisational irritant or irritants. It is very difficult to discuss all of them here. We may examine here only the widely used techniques in the area of health management.

1. Sensitivity Training.
2. Team Building.
3. Grid Training.
4. Survey Feedback.
5. System 4 Management.

### 1. Sensitivity Training

It is a method of changing behaviour of the health personnel in the organisation, relying on unstructured group interaction to smoothen inter-personal relationships. In this process, the actual technique employed is termed as T-group. 'Sensitivity' in this context means sensitivity to self and self-other relationships. In this training, 10-12 persons are involved, who are assisted by a professional behavioural scientist, who acts as a catalyst. It provides a free atmosphere, which breaks through the barrier of intellectualization and verbalization. It emphasizes "open your eyes, look at yourself, see how you look to others. The decide that changes if any, you want to make and in which direction you want to do." Thus the health organisation emphasis of T-group is on self-improvement based on the analysis of one's behaviour *vis-à-vis* the other members of the organisation to ensure individual and organisational goal achievement.

Leyland Bradford, Jack-R. Gille and Kemeth benne have mentioned the following objectives of Sensitivity Training:

CHART 14.1

**Different Types of OD Interventions are shown in the following table**

| *Target Group* | *Types/Technique of Intervention* |
|---|---|
| Intervention designed to improve the effectiveness of Individuals (Health Employees) | Life and career planning activities; Role analysis, technique coaching and counseling; T-Group (Sensitivity training); Education and training to increase skills, knowledge in the areas of technical tasks needs—relationship skills, process skills, decision-making, problem-solving, planning, goal-setting skills, Grind OD Phase I. |
| Interventions designed to improve the effectiveness of health Dyads/Triads | Process consultation; Third Party peace-making Grid OD Phases 1, 2. |
| Interventions designed to improve the effectiveness of health TEAMS and GROUPS. | Team building—Task directed—Process directed Family T-group Survey, feedback process consultation, Role analysis techniques,"Start Up" team-building activities. Education in decision-making, Problem-solving, planning, goal-setting in group settings. |
| Interventions designed to improve the effectiveness of health Inter-Group Relations. | Inter-group activities—Process directed—Task directed: Organisational mirroring (three or more groups), Techno-structural interventions, Process consultation. Third party peace-making at group level. Grid OD Phase 3. Survey feed-back. |
| Interventions designed to improve the effectiveness of the Total Organisation. | Techno-structural activities, confrontation meetings, Strategic planning activities. Grid OD Phases 4, 5, 6. Survey feedback. |

*Source*: Wendell French and Cecil Bell, Jr. Organisation Development (Englewood Cliffs, N.J. Prentice Hall Inc., 1973), p. 107. (Adopted)

(a) To make health trainees sensitive to emotional reactions and expressions in themselves and others.
(b) The health participants sharpen their ability to perceive and to learn the implications of their actions in the process of drawing their attention to their own or other's feelings.
(c) To stimulate and develop personal value and goals which are commensurate to social goals and scientific methods of personal decision-making.

CHART 14.2

**Techniques of OD**

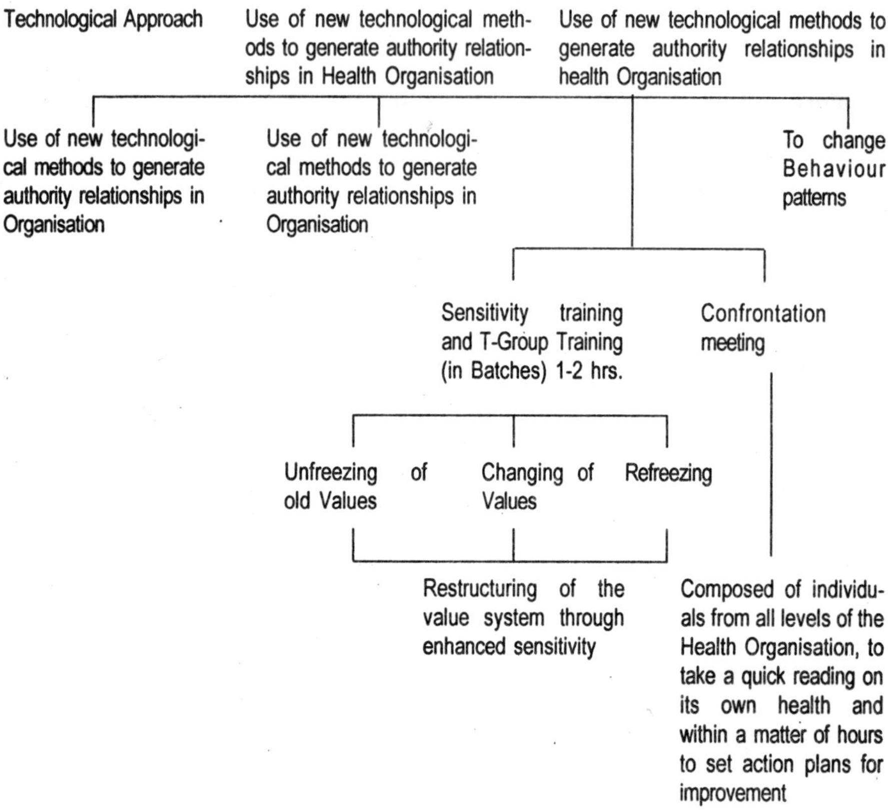


(d) To develop a scientific attitude to tackling future situations among head of its employees.
(e) To help achieving behavioural effectiveness in transactions in environments obtained around the health participants.

The application of this technique has demonstrated both positive and negative results. The negative results are mostly based on the wrong introduction of this technique and improper handling. Rober J. House suggests that there is a need of careful selection of health participants, so that the members do not suffer from the symptoms of emotional instability, low tolerance and anxiety and psychiatric case histories. Dunnette and Campbell rightly conclude, "Laboratory education has not been shown to bring about any essentially negative results on objective measures, individuals who have been trained by laboratory education measures are more likely to be seen as changing their job behaviour than are individuals in similar job setting who have not been trained.[16]

CHART 14.3

| *Climate setting* | *Information collection* | *Information Sharing* | *Priority setting and group action* | *Organisation action Planning* | *Immediate Follow-up* | *Progress review* |
|---|---|---|---|---|---|---|
| ↓ | ↓ | ↓ | ↓ | ↓ | ↓ | ↓ |
| The top health executive communi-cates to the entire management group, its objective and his concern for and interest in open discussion and problem facing. (45 mts. to 1 hrs.) | Entire health group is divided into small heteroge-neous units consisting of 7 to 8 members. Each unit is advised to choose a reporter to present its findings at a general information sharing the monitor of health unit session to be con-ducted an hour after (1 hrs.) | Information collected is shared among all the health persons after getting the report of each group cyclostyled. | Priorities are set in each functional area of head (1 hrs.) | Separate functional plans are integrated into total organisational Plan (2 hrs.) | Preparing a follow up healthy action and reporting it to all its members (1-3 hrs.) | Follow-up (2 hrs.) |

*Note:* The steps given in this Chart need to be followed with meticulous care, otherwise it can have a negative effect. Before introducing these steps, leaders must be trained in the art and science of OD.

## 2. Team Building

The emphasis in team building is on improving the effectiveness and efficiency of the group and not of the individuals alone, as is the case in T-group. It is a set of techniques by which health personnel in an organisational group diagnose as to how they work together and plan the needed changes that will improve their performance and ultimately organisational health efficiency.

Health Personnel have to work in a team. Team building is very important whether it is OPD, ward or operation theatre. Team work among health personnel can be used for promoting Organiational Development.

Organisations produce very little solely from individual effort. According to Margulies and Raia,[17] "Most effective team action is not easy to achieve in which Tom, Dick and Harry are trained independently or separately..."

The research in the utility of this technique has clearly indicated that properly planned Team Building Approach has positive impact and influence. Michael Beer concluded pervasive OD technology available to the change agent. Its design provides data for diagnosis and unfreezing, incorporates experimental learning, and provides the means for refreezing new behaviour. Furthermore, the process of team development is likely to change organisational inputs (needs, values and skills) and a wide variety of group (cohesiveness, communication, planning). Through problems identification, it can also effect immediate change in organisational output.[18]

Arthur C. Bech (Jr.) and Ellis D. Hillmar have rightly mentioned the following ingredients for developing team approach:

(a) *High Expectations*—Always expect a lot from people. They will not disappoint you very often.
(b) *Respect for the individual*—Ask for his ideas and use them when they are better or as good as yours. If you do not use his ideas, tell him why. Requesting his help is a high compliment.
(c) *Honest Relationships*—Play it straight. Scott Myers said, "when in doubt, be honest."
(d) *Freedom to Act*—Within the framework and limitations set-up in objectives mutually agreed upon between boss and subordinate, give the employees freedom to achieve results.
(e) *Team Orientation*—Through objective-setting or problem-solving sessions develop teamwork and commitment to objectives and solutions.

In this way health employees of an organisation would promote efficient and effective health care delivery system.

### 3. Grid Training

Grid training combines the training to ensure the change in behaviours in both task-oriented and people-oriented styles. Grid Training based on the Managerial Grid developed by Robert Blake and Jane S. Mouton of the University of Taxes.[19] It is comprehensive approach and try to achieve the Managerial Grid (9-9) in which the health leader has high concern for production as well as for his people. The Grid is the framework of 81 squares on which styles of behaviour can be plotted. On the X-axis is plotted the "concern for production" and Y-axis the "concern for people."

There is a set of underlying values in relation to the nature of man and his work in the organisation which according to Margulies and Raia are as follows:

(i) Providing opportunities for people to function as human beings rather than as resources in the productive process;

(ii) Providing opportunities for each organisation member, as well as for the organisation itself, to develop to his full potential;
(iii) Seeking to increase the effectiveness of the organisation in terms of all its goals;
(iv) Attempting to create an environment in which it is possible to find exciting and challenging work;
(v) Providing opportunities for people in organisations to influence the way in which they relate to work, the organisation and the environment; and
(vi) Treating each human being as a person with a complex set of needs, all of which are important in his work and in his life.

The specific objectives[20] of a grid organisation development programme are to:

(i) Study the organisation as an interacting system and apply techniques of analysis in diagnosing its problems;
(ii) Understand the importance and rationale of systematic change in contrast to change by evolution and revolution; and
(iii) Evaluate the style of leadership and technique of participation most likely to produce high-quality results.

**Phase of Grid Training**

It is conducted in two parts, involving six overlapping phases which are discussed below. Part I concentrates on individuals and single work groups, Part-II laboratory-Seminar Training—Here the health managers are assured about their level of leadership individually, so that base line survey is available.

*Phase 1*

Managers selected are then acquainted with the desirability of achieving 9, 9 style of leadership. They are told about the potentialities of this style.

*Phase 2*

*Team Development*: Health Managers are given training in human relations as to how to build a team in the organisation. The managers would be made familiar with the process of group dynamics and how to foster team work, team culture, team traditions, team spirit and thus change the human beings to make them to move together.

**Part II: Organisation Development**

*Phase 3: Inter-group Development*

In this phase, the emphasis is on training in inter-group relationship. The light is thrown on the causes of the emergence of inter-group conflict and the ways of promoting harmony are developed. The conditions of mutual cooperation are analysed to ensure goal congruency.

*Phase 4: Organisation Goal-setting*

An ideal model for the health organisation is developed with all its aspects—structure, goals rewards system, management practices, etc. The model so developed is shared among lower level functionaries to achieve their cooperation and commitment.

*Phase 5: Goal Attainment*

In this phase health participants discuss the implementation of organisational goals. Here the achievement of goals is discussed in detail with the possible obstacles.

*Phase 6: Evaluation*

After a year or so, the pros and cons of Grid training are evaluated. All efforts are made to continue the practice yielding positive results and to identify the weak areas to be tackled.

Grid has been adopted in many organisations with partial success. Experts are critical of the basic assumption of 9, 9 Grid approach. Critics like Bernardin and Alvares expressed that a 9, 9 orientation applied to the organisation as a whole will foster a new kind of corporate Darwinism. Inspite of its criticism, it is considered to be an effective and efficient tool for organisation change.

**4. Survey Feedback**

The main purpose of survey feedback is to asssist and equip the organisation in diagnosing problems and developing action plans for problem-solving. Besides, it encourages the members of the organisation to remove the impediments in the way of smooth relationship. This technique includes a package of four distinct steps:

(i) *Collection of Data*: Either through the specially designed questionnaire or adopting standard questionnaire, the information is collected from the personnel in an organisation on various aspects like leadership style, process of decision-making, delegation, decentralization, etc. The data is processed in an intelligible form.

(ii) *Sharing the information*: The data collected and processed in clear words is presented to all the members of the organisation to solicit their views and discussion among the members under the guidance of OD specialist. The purpose is to acquaint the members about the existing health of the organisation with special reference to its positive and negative indicators.

(iii) *Designing an Action Plan*: Participants in view of the existing health of the organisation suggest some action plan to remove the negative indicators and promote the positive one so that the organisation is rejuvenated to sound health. The Action Plan must be definite and specific.

(iv) *Follow-up*: At regular intervals of time, this exercise may be repeated to ascertain the progress made and to change the action when needed.

The Institute for Social Research of the Michigan University has come to the conclusion that the "available data seems to indicate that survey feedback can be an effective approach towards meeting organisational goals and individual needs." However, we may keep in mind that top management must be willing to use the information it gathers and the participants do not feel deceived, manipulated or misrepresented.

(v) *System Four Management*: Rensis Likert has developed this scheme of OD. He devised a four-level model of organisation effectiveness incorporating the basic categories of task-orientation and people orientation. Likert feels that personnel are the precious assets and therefore must be treated and managed carefully. Likert classifies management philosophies into four convenient systems.

An analysis of the Chart 14.4. indicates that the system one believes in exploitative and authoritative approach, in which the leader acts as a dictator. In this approach, authority is centralised at the top and the subordinates are asked merely to obey under the threats of punishment. In system two, the leader is benevolent and autocratic. He allows the people to express themselves, but by and large, he behaves like a dictator. These managers have "Condescending Confidence" in employees. The system three refers to consultative management, wherein managers have substantial, but not complete confidence in employees abilities. The leader invites suggestions and ideas, shows his willingness to listen to his subordinates and may consider their views. He may, however keep control over decisions. In system four, the manager runs the administration with the full consent and co-operation of the employees. Decision-making is highly decentralised and the subordinates are delegated authority to a great extent.

Likert's conclusion is that most efficient organisations have system 4 characteristics and therefore organisations should move to system 4. Since the employees feel belongingness to the organisation in system 4, it can yield positive results. W. Heesler mentions a number of other methods besides above. These are:

1. Sole enrichment/job enlargement.
2. Seminars.
3. Mechanisation/Automation.
4. Confrontation/Meetings.
5. Lectures.
6. Career Planning.

CHART 14.4

| *Organisational Variable* | *System-1 Exploitative* | *System-1 Benevolent* | *System-1 Consultative* | *System-1 Participative* |
|---|---|---|---|---|
| 1. Extent to which superiors have confidence and trust in subordinates | Have no trust and confidence in subordinate | Have conde-scending confidence and trsut such as master has to servant | Substantial but not complete confidence and trust, still wishes to keep control of discussions | Complete confidence and trust in all matters |
| 2. Extent to which superiors behave so that subordinates feel free to discuss important things about their jobs with their immediate superiors | Subordinates do not feel free at all to discuss things about the job with their superior | Subordinates do not feel very free to discuss things about the job with their superiors | Subordinates feel rather free to discuss things about the job with their superiors | Subordinate feel completely free to discuss things about the job with their superiors |
| 3. Extent to which immediate superiors in solving job problems generally tries to get subordinates idea and makes constructive use of them. | Seldom gets ideas and options of subordinates in solving job problems | Sometimes gets ideas and opinions of subordinates in solving job problems | Usually gets ideas and opinions and usually tries to make constructive use of them. | Always gets ideas and opinions and always tries to make constructive use of them. |

## CONCLUSION

Which method is more useful and when it may be used needs probing. The analysis of answers would indicate that the use of technique would depend upon the nature or the situation and the maturity of the top management. The top management must find sufficient time to plan Organisational Development. In India, the Machinery of Public Administration and Management has failed to live upto the expectations of the people and have not been able to optimise resources because the top management in India never find time for OD, rather remain busy with petty things, which can be done by other people. Most of the organisations in India have become dead woods and unproductive. In order to vitalise and rejuvenate them, we must plan OD to give fresh life to Indian administration and management. All the top administrators in India should be given training in Organisation Building and Development, so that they can make use of this training in maintaining the Organisational health, through consistent and persistent efforts. This would require the restructuring of the administrative apparatus, so that the top managers are really managers and not managers by virtue of merely sitting at the top. The managers must create the desired climate where the achievements of results become the main concern—both quantitatively and qualitatively.

## Notes and References


1. S.K. Bhatia and Nirmal Singh, Principles and Techniques of Personnel Management/Human Resource Management, Deep & Deep, New Delhi, (2nd Ed., 2000), p. 106.
2. Wendell, L. French and Cecil, H. Bell, "Definition and History of Organisation, Developments: Some Comments", Organisational Behaviour: A Book of Reading. ed., Keith Davis, Reading No. 38, McGraw-Hill Book Co., New York, 1977, pp. 247-55.
3. Warren G. Bennis: Organisation Development: Its Nature, Origins and Prospects (Reading Mass, Addison-Wesley Publishing Co., 1969).
4. Richard Bechkard: Organisation Development: Strategies and Models (Reading. Mass, Addison-Wesley Publishing Co., 1969.
5. Paul R. Lawrence and Jay W. Lorsch: Developing Organisations: Diagnosis and Action (Reading, Mass, Addison-Wesley Publishing Co., 1969).
6. *Ibid.*
7. Bechard, *op. cit.*, p. 35.
8. Hyman K. Randhall, A Practical Approach to Organisation Development through MBO, Ed. by Back and Hillmach, Wesley, 1972, p. 4.
9. H. Finer: Theory and Practice of Modern Government, p. 106.
10. Eli Ginzberg: "Perspective on Work Motivation", *Personnel,* Vol. 31, No. (July), 1959, pp. 48-49.
11. Maier Bennis, Organisation Development: Its Nature, Origins and Prospectus, Reading: Mass, Addison-Wesley, 1969.
12. Henry B. Sachacht, Business Horizens, August, 1970, pp. 29-34.
13. R. Anuradha, Organisation Development as a Theme of Seventies and Eighties, in *IJPA,* Oct.-Dec., 1988, p. 985.
14. *Ibid.*
15. *Ibid.*
16. Marvin D. Dunnette and John P. Campbell, "Laboratory Education: Impact on People and Organisation", *Industrial Relations,* October, 1969, p. 23.
17. N. Margulies and Raia, A.P., "Organisation Development: Values, Process and Technology", New York: McGraw Hill, 1972, p. 363.
18. Michael Beer, "The Technology of Organisation Development", Marvin D. Dunnette, *et. al.,* Handbook of Industrial and Organisational Psychology, Chicago, Rand McNally 1979, p. 960.
19. Robert R. Blake and Jane S. Mounton, "The Managerial Grid", Houston, Gulf Publishing Company, 1964, and Blake and Mouton, "Building a Dynamic Corporation through Grid Organisation Development", Reading, Mass, Addison-Wesley, Inc., 1969.
20. Brochure From Scientific Methods, Inc., Austin, Texas, (Also see Andrew Perspective, Prentice Hall, Inc., Englewood Cliffs, N.J., New York, 1984, pp. 459-61).

15

CHAPTER

# Management of the Employees Health

"Happiness, Happiness, Happiness
It may of different origin on this earth
But the happiness of being healthy
Is the real happiness."

*—Author*

Health is becoming top priority for Indians.[1] Good health, and not career or money as many may imagine, appears to be the most important thing in the life of consumers in the Asia/Pacific region, including India. This was revealed in the latest Asian Ideals Survey from Master Card International, which studied the values and attitudes of consumers in the region. The consumers rated health (45 percent), family and friends (22 percent), and happiness (19 percent) as most important. Wealth occupies only the fourth slot with an unexpectedly small percentage (5 percent) among the most important things in life. An equally small percentage (5 percent) indicated that career and religion were the top priorities in their lives. In India, consumers rated health (32 percent), happiness (24 percent) and career (16 percent) as the three most important things in life. These were followed by family and friends (15 percent), wealth (9 percent) and religion (5 percent).

Various techniques of management may therefore not help in achieving organisational development, unless the persons working in the organisation are healthy. In his address to 31st Session of WHO Regional Committee for South-East Asia held at Ulan Botor, Mongolia (22-28 Aug. 1978), Dr. Nyam-Osor, Minister of Public Health, Mongolia read a passage from a poem by Dashdorji in Natragdorj, which glorifies "Health". It is being reproduced below.[2]

Health is man's greatest possession, for it lays a solid foundation for his happiness. Charaka, the renowned Ayurvedic physician is known to

CHART 15.1

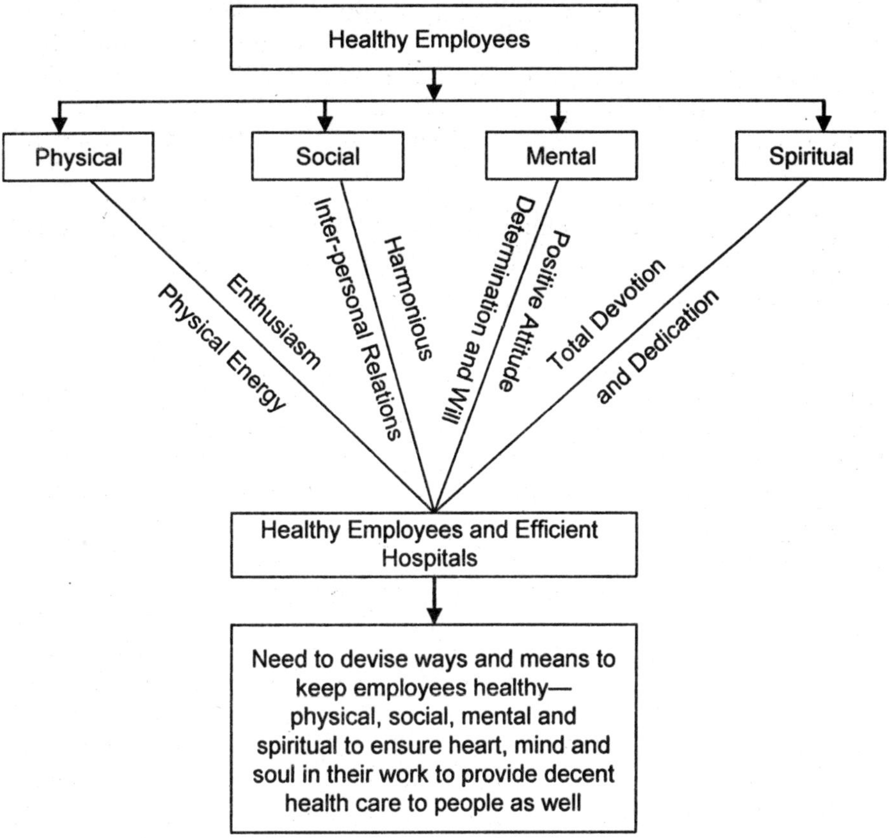


have said: "Health was vital for ethical, artistic, material and spiritual development of man." To quote Herophilas, C. 300 B.S.

> When health is absent
> Wisdom cannot reveal itself
> "Art cannot manifest
> Strength cannot fight,
> Wealth becomes useless
> And Intelligence cannot be applied."

Buddha has said that of all the gains, the gains of health are the highest and the best. Health is not only basic to leading a happy life for an individual, but it is also necessary for all productive activities in the society. Who could deny the fact that if a soldier is not keeping good health, he cannot be expected to defend the frontiers of his country, even when he is provided with the latest sophisticated weapons? Similarly, who would deny that an unhealthy farmer with the best possible technological know-how would not succeed in producing the best that can expected of him? Obviously, what is true of an unhealthy soldier or an unhealthy farmer is also true of other categories of workers. Thus, no industry or office can expect the optimum output, if it does not employ healthy workers or does not make and provide adequate facilities for proper maintenance of their health. Undoubtedly, professional efficiency, good health and productivity are inter-related.

Good health can promote high labour morale and productivity, i.e., a healthy worker can work full-time and has a greater productivity potential. According to Benjamin, in countries 'where health conditions are worst, relatively simple and low cost health programmes can produce dramatic lessening of the disability of the labour force."[3]

Good health effects intelligence. Improper nutrition and lack of mother-care can cause parental retardation and other mental problems. A study carried out by Correa and Cummins in Contribution of Nutrition to "Economic Growth" covering 18 countries reveals that in 9 countries of Latin America, there was an increase in the gross national product with improving nutritional standards, whereas the contribution of nutrition was zero in the economically developed countries. The poorer the country, the greater the role of improved nutrition in its development.[4]

Good health is a basic right and produces 'civic consciousness.' We should not look at health only as a means of economic development. What is more important is to view economic growth as contributing to the betterment of the health of people. It must be recognised that health is a basic human right. Thanis Kraivixien, former Prime Minister of Thailand, rightly said in his inaugural address to the 30th WHO Regional Committee for South-East Asia, held at Bangkok, Thailand (2-8 August, 1977); "Any society should consider that a high quality of life, and I dare say happiness of the people, which can only be obtained through a sufficient level of health, is not only a basic prerequisite to development but should be the basic objective of any development effort."[5]

Better health is generally associated with better capability and leadership. In a study by ILO on qualitative difference in the labour force, health was found to be the factor most clearly related to difference in economic growth.[6] According to Myrdal: "The required personal qualities are certainly multiple and probably have a synergistic action. However, there can be no doubt that health plays an essential part."[7]

Better health induces positive attitudes, conducive to economic growth and modernisation. The individuals become better citizens as they hope for future betterment and work hard to make the future more pleasant and enjoyable. Improved health may drive people to increase productivity and reduce family size.[8] The people with good health are generally enthusiastic and try to achieve higher and higher goals in life.

The employees working in health organisations whether public or private must be healthy as they are to:

(i) Treat the patients who can be affected if the health of health employees is not well.
(ii) Patients can follow the examples of good health from healthy employees.
(iii) Medical personnel in good health can work with enthusiasm and treat the patient efficiently.
(iv) Medical personnel in good health would be regular and they would not be on leave.

In view of the above, we have included this chapter "Management of the Health of Employees" equally apply to Health and Medical Employees.

## MEANING OF HEALTH

Health is viewed differently by different people all over the world. The World Health Organisation defined health as "a state of complete physical, mental, and social well-being and not merely an absence of disease or infirmity." Thus, good health is a synthesis of physical, mental and social well-being. As stated in the First Five Year Plan, "Health is a positive state of well-being in which harmonious development of mental and physical capacities of the individuals lead to the enjoyment of a rich and full life. It implies adjustment of the individual to his total environment—physical and social."[9]

Some people even define it as a condition under which an individual is able to mobilize all his resources—intellectual, emotional and physical for optimum living. Thus, health is not static; on the contrary, it fluctuates on a scale which ranges between optimum health as defined by WHO to complete lack of health.

S.C. Seal, in his presidential address, defined health as: "flexible state of body and mind which may be described in terms of a range within which a person may sway from the condition wherein he is at the peak of enjoyment of physical, mental and emotional experiences, having regard to environment, age, sex and other biological characteristics due to the operation of internal or external stimuli and can regain that position without outside aid."[10]

"Health" has found an important place in the Constitution of all States and the UN agencies. Of the 30 Articles of the Universal Declaration of Human Rights, Art. 25 is particularly concerned with the right to health. Everyone has the right to a standard of living adequate for the health and well-being of himself and his family, including food, clothing, housing and medical care and necessary services and the right to security in the event of unemployment, sickness, disability, widowhood, old age or other lack of the livelihood, in circumstances beyond his control. Motherhood and childhood are entitled to special care and assistance. All children whether born out of wedlock or otherwise shall enjoy the same social protection. The preamble of the WHO Constitution also states that the enjoyment of the highest attainable standard of health is a fundamental right of every human being and that governments are responsible for the health of their people and can fulfil that responsibility by taking appropriate health and social welfare measures. Let us now discuss the responsibility of employers to keep the health of the employees fit from all angles.

## PROMOTION OF PHYSICAL HEALTH

A physically fit individual has the ability to function at the optimum level of efficiency in its daily activities. He maintains his cardiovascular, nervous and endocrine systems working in perfect order. He is able to do hard work for a long duration of time without undue fatigue. Therefore, if the employees are physically fit and free from diseases, they can concentrate on their work and absenteeism can be minimised. It has been seen in most of the organisations that staff members are not enthusiastic and active in their work because of poor physical health.

Consciousness is the most essential aspect of human personality. The neuro-physiological, muscular, glandular, and digestive systems must be in very healthy condition so that they carry on their perceptual and intellectual activities very efficiently. Body is the instrument through which human mind functions. Physical fitness is, therefore, absolutely necessary for intellectual alertness and ascent of consciousness from lower to higher planes.

What can be done to prevent the deterioration of physical and mental health? We suggest here the following important responsibilities of an organisation to promote the physical fitness of its employees.

### (a) Providing Health Facilities

It is the prime responsibility of all organisations to provide health facilities nearer to their work place. There is a provision for it in many organisations like Central Government Health Scheme (CGHS) for Central Government employees. However, these facilities have failed to provide decent health services, because of their negative attitude restricting it to curative functions. Thus besides clinical services, the following other services should be provided as well, e.g.

(i) Health Education to the employees and their family so that they are made health conscious and less and less dependent on medicine. It has been rightly said that prevention is better than cure.

(ii) Doctors and other staff should visit the employees in their work place and discuss with them the seasonal health problems, which can forewarn the employees to take necessary precaution.

(iii) The environs of health facilities should be hygienic, so that employees can feel safe and may not get infected.

(iv) Equipment and drugs should be of standard quality and sufficient checks on corrupt practices should be exercised.

**(b) Cleanliness**

Cleanliness is the most important factor in keeping the employees healthy and aesthetic.

Cleanliness has a soothing impact on the minds of the employees. Waste Bins should be so designed that they cannot leak and can be maintained in sanitary conditions. A visit to most of the offices, even in a beautiful city like Chandigarh, would reveal a horrible state of affairs. The rooms must be free of insects, rats, rodents, etc. Besides, the arrangement of articles must be done aesthetically. The chairs, tables and other furniture should be well kept so that its impact on the employees and clients is pleasing.

**(c)** Essential facilities like drinking water, good lavoratories, lighting ventilation, heating and cooling, stationery, etc. should be provided to the staff members. All these would enhance the working efficiency. We find in many offices that there is inadequate arrangements for lighting and drinking water. They move away from the working place resulting in wastage of precious time. These appear to be small but are of immense value in terms of their impact.

**(d)** Good management takes care of arranging the space where the staff works. There are no complex rules about space arrangements. It is a common-sense approach. Thus, a layout which provides comfort and convenience is very important for doing work satisfactorily.

**(e)** Tobacco dependence has been classified as a behavioural disorder in the WHO International Classification of diseases. Tobacco smoking is responsible for blood cancer, lung cancer, coronary heart diseases, stroke and chronic bronchitis. Hence, smoking should be banned as even passive smoking is identified as a major cause of morbidity.

## MENTAL HEALTH

There is very close relationship between mental equanimity, peace and happiness of an individual and his physical health and efficiency. A mentally tense, anxious and sick person has a tendency to develop various symptoms of organic disorders. Thus, other conditions remaining equal a normally serene and cheerful person may be expected to have various pathological symptoms in his body.[11]

Consciousness shrinks in a mentally abnormal person, and his shrunken consciousness finds expression through his pathological organic disorders. The consciousness of a diseased person has a trend towards continuous contraction. The domain of consciousness of a mentally and organically sick person becomes narrow, clouded and depressed. The ancient Indian seers used the conception of 'mental equanimity' instead of the concept of 'mental health'. Sri Aurobindo used the concept of mental serenity in the same sense as the concept of 'mental equanimity' of ancient Indian seers. The concept of 'mental equanimity' is more satisfactory than the concept of mental health because the former alone can produce spiritual development in an individual.[12]

Mind is the most powerful part of the human system. It is a Super Computer. Staff members in the organisation don't realise its potential or devise ways and means to harness this most important source. Organisations can achieve excellence provided they know the secret of tapping human mind. We generally notice that most of the employees are not mentally positive as one or the other problem concerning their employment continuously bogs them down. Many of them become mental wretches and a liability on the organisation. The Organisations instead of solving their problems, cause further deterioration. 25 percent of employees in every organisation are a liability and the other 75 percent are not contributing as per their potential.

Employers should try to create positive mental attitudes among the employees. Positive mental attitude is a state of mind that reflects the strength of employee's belief in what they do. It generates inner and voluntary emotions which enhances motivation, resulting in positive thoughts. Positive thinking is the key to development and is result-oriented.

Ethical behaviour in the public service is considered as a blend of moral qualities and mental attitudes. The requisite moral qualities include not only the willingness to serve the public but also the willingness to behave competently, efficiently, honestly, responsibly, objectively, fairly, and accountably. Mental attitudes include awareness of moral dilemmas inherent in policies and conflicting claims on the substantive and procedural aspects of policy, a sympathy for divergent views held not only by some members of the public but also by professional colleagues and a sensitivity to paradoxes of rules that may lead to frustrating and unkind actions. Thus, an appropriate blend of moral qualities and mental attitudes become an essential ingredient for moral government and administration. Such a mixture strengthens the basis of legitimate and effective government which is founded on public trust and confidence.

We get a moral government by creating those conditions within which a moral government can operate. This is done by making it possible for officials to acquire the necessary traits and by practicing the same. An exemplary public servant, is not simply the one who obeys and behaves within the confines of law but is also one who strives for a moral government. Such is the duty of those who wish to be involved in the difficult and complex world of government. This is the essence and basis of a moral State.[13]

Public life is in a desperate state today, with vice-regal regalia dominating it with its fierce ferocity and crushing criminality, sounding the death-knell of ethics, morality, and value-system. There is a dire need to save it. Public men, at whatever station of life they function must be 'men' for the public; leaders must lead; and, most importantly, politicians must stop 'politicking'. Public opinion—which is often branded as meaning neither public nor opinion—must be built up against acceptance and tolerance of unethical behaviour and action by anybody, howsoever high and mighty he may be. Crisis of confidence—which admittedly is a function of culture—must be restored in public life; otherwise, the ancient civilisation that we boast of, will be no more; there will remain no public, no life, worth living, without ethics.[14]

The ancient Indian philosophers laid stress on mental equanimity for the general well-being of individuals. The mind of an ordinary person is usually very restless. Myriads of desires produce upheavals in the mind of an individual. Over and above this, the mind of an ordinary person is afflicted by several tensions.

The ancient Indian philosophers maintained that if the mind of an individual usually remains in a disturbed state, he is very likely to develop pathological symptoms. An individual with pathological mental symptoms quite often develop certain pathological organic symptoms because there is very close relationship between the body and the mind of an individual. The mind of an individual becomes free from anxiety and miseries, if there is peace in his mind.[15]

Let us mention the methods to maintain the mental health of the employees.

**1. Ensuring all Facilities to Employees in Time, to Avoid Tensions and Diversion of Mind**

Most of the employees in an organisation waste about 25 percent to 50 percent of their time in getting their due benefits, e.g. arrears of salary, leave salary, duty leave, sanction for various allowances, due to the unsympathetic attitude of establishment sections/employers. Such situations create frustration, indolence and indifference, leading to lack of interest and enthusiasm. Thus, there should be a specialised cell responsible for timely disposal of cases. The progress should be regularly reviewed by the head of department. These are simple acts but can promote greater efficiency, if acted upon.

**2. Prompt Decision-making Concerning the Cases of the Employees**

Many differences crop up between administration and employees on account of issues arising out of their daily work. For example, a wrong promotion can cause mental tension and the employee loose all interest in his work. In such situations, employees approach the court of law with vengeance. They give up their loyalty to the organisation and even most efficient employees can become dead wood or hardliners. Their minds become deranged and they start behaving negatively. It is therefore, suggested that the administration should be prompt and judicious so that employees are relieved of their mental agony. Even if the decision does not favour them, still they would feel satisfied with timely and fair decision.

**3. Ensuring Transparency in Administration to Develop Confidence and Commitment among Employees**

Personnel in administration at top level are secretive and some times use their discretion wrongfully to oblige those who are otherwise ineligible.

Such instances demoralise those who work hard with all sincerity. For example, a Vice-Chancellor appointed 23 persons during last days of his tenure, causing heart bum and jealousy down the line. In the absence of explicit criteria and indicators, there is lack of transparency in operations. Genuine efforts to make the system transparent would develop commitment among employees and—they would work to their full mental capabilities and capacities.

**4. Encouragement to Honest and Hardworking Employees to Create Mental Happiness**

Most of the persons who achieve excellence and self-actualization are ignored or not given enough recognition. They develop a negative attitude as they feel that there is no purpose in, what they're doing. As a result, they slip into the category of mediocres and below averages. It is thus the duty of the employers to encourage honest and hardworking employees through various means, e.g. sending a letter of appreciation, getting the news published in the paper, getting the item noted in the governing body and so on. This would accelerate the development of the organisation and may stimulate even the dead woods. Psychologists have proved the motivational value of non-monetary factors, as mentioned above. Such motivation to self-actualise would lead to mental happiness.

Lawyers, Doctors, Company Secretaries, Chartered Accountants, Engineers and Scientists, not to speak of the talented bureaucrats, are all slowly selling their souls for a mess of pottage. Even the leaders in the professions have let us down.[16]

In such other areas of governance, as professional services, like teaching, medical, legal, accountancy and engineering, ethics is perhaps the ultimate principle which can keep them on the right track. No amount of laws and rules, and threats of punishment can proverbially bring the horse to water but cannot force it to drink. Unless the experts and professionals are guided by a sense of accountability and ethics, it is almost impossible to receive good service from these people. As Harold Laski pointed out, political-legal rights must have a moral basis. Men must earn to subordinate their self-interest to the common welfare. This is the only definition of morality.[17] As Swami Vivekananda said: "That which is selfish is immoral, and that which is unselfish is moral." Unless this kind of moral basis of government could be created, it would be impossible to build up a democratic, social-welfare state.

**5. Locating Shirkers and Providing Counselling to them**

There are many employees who lose interest in work and become a liability. Their existence dampens the enthusiasm of good workers. Their lethargy becomes contagious and we discover in the long-run that indiscipline spreads, causing short fall in output and poor quality of services. The employers should follow the proverb "Nip the Evil in the Bud." The employers should not ignore them but should try to sublimate their mental energies in a purposeful direction. This may require counselling in the initial stages. However, if it does not work, such employees may be dealt with sternly by conducting disciplinary proceedings and awarding minor/major penalties. In this way, the mental health of the Organisation would be protected.

### 6. Inculcation of Ethical Values

The ethical degradation and moral decline within the bureaucracy in Bangladesh is almost similar, if not worse, to that in other developing countries: They don't believe that they are serving anyone else but themselves and exploit their positions for personal gain. They generally arrive at work late and leave early. They take extra long lunch recesses. They steal public property. They accept bribes for the performance of duties that are contractually part of their responsibilities. When they do work they work very slowly... They stymie the public by losing the files; through excessive review of the issue at hand or by simply pretending that they have not heard of the matter before. For all of this, they acknowledge now wrong doing, for they do not believe that what they are doing is wrong.[18]

This situation is rampant in third World countries and calls for defining morality in governance. Morality signifies pursuit of ethical conduct and performance of duties assigned in such a manner that the declared purpose is realised. In the Greek tradition, it implied the development of the latent capabilities of an individual for the full flowering of his/her personality to deliver public good. To this end, there was rigorous training and preparation for the holders of public office so that the aims of public office were served. Dharma, in the Indian tradition, commands morality in terms of righteous conduct. As propagated by Emperor Ashok, it further implied inculcation and practice of virtue in the performance of assigned duties. To an extent, the normative morality would subjugate personal interests to community interests and particular aims to general aims of the society. Mahatma Gandhi has raised Dharma to a higher pedestal, signifying a quality through which we know "our duty in human life and our relation with other selves." Thus, ethics in public life is important to understand our place in society and the duties we owe to the society by virtue of what society gives us.[19] Employees should be given regular inputs in different forms in order to inculcate ethical values in work situation.

### 7. Stimulating Leadership to Create Qualities of Head and Heart among Employees and Removing Mental Tensions/Fears

Employees look for standards from the top. As is the king, so are the subjects. Leaders should possess mental agility which they can percolate among employees. Thus, the organisation should be careful in selecting their top personnel as they are rare birds.

We must remember that it is the top men in each department who set the tone of the administration. It is they who set the example for those under them to emulate. When the acts of those at the top become tainted, when their reputation becomes shady, they will not be able to enforce high standards of integrity in those below them. It is, therefore, imperative that men at the top should personify the highest standards of personal integrity, probity and rectitude. As Sir Iyor Jennings observed, the most elementary qualification demanded of a minister is honesty and incorruptibility. It is, in addition, necessary not only that he should possess this qualification but also that he should appear to possess it.

Dr. Narendra N. Wig, WHO consultant in his article "Mental Health and Work" in *The Tribune*, dated Sept. 27, 2000 has made the following observations: "It is important that the place of work should be made conducive to mental health" Unfortunately, very little attention is being paid to this aspect in our offices and factories. In view of the rising cost of mental illness because of stress at work, it is high time the senior management in offices and industry paid attention to this aspect. The following are some of the suggestions for de-stressing the modern workplace:

1. Modify the pressure placed on the working people by creating a healthy environment and sound management policies and practices.
2. Keep the mental health of the workers as an integral part of the business agenda and regularly briefing the senior management about it.
3. Improve interpersonal communication at all levels.
4. Provide recreational facilities for workers.
5. Arrange regular sessions to teach workers how to reduce stress by techniques like yoga, relaxation exercises, etc.
6. Organise professional help by counsellors and such other persons for the vulnerable members of the staff at an early stage.[20]

## SOCIAL HEALTH

Another dimension of health is social health, i.e. how an individual can have healthy relations with persons with whom he comes in contact. We find that there are many persons who sit in isolation and they get socially marginalised. Such persons get sick as socialising with others is essential aspect of human nature. Aristotle has rightly spelt out that man is a social animal in an organisation, the colleagues with whom one is working should be friendly and one could share with them about his personal and official problems. One should have good relationships with superiors and subordinates. Social health is a buffer stock to avoid physical and mental breakdowns. Let us examine as to what the employers can do to provide a decent social environment and social health to his employees.

I.M. Somi in his article, "Spreading Sunshine with a Smile" in *The Tribune*, dated August 20, 2000 rightly exhorts to set out with the intention of cheering others when they are depressed, and lifting their depression with a witty remark. It is the sharing of a gift that gives its value. This is equally true to spreading sunshine in other's life. Make a daily reflection and you will find your attitude gradually changing in practice. The benefit, in health and happiness, that such a change of attitude can bring is well worth the effort required to achieve it. The following measures may be initiated to secure social health of the employees:

**(a) Provision of Good Staff Clubs with All Amenities of Indoor and Outdoor Games**

Organisations should provide for staff clubs wherein employees with their family can come and relax through games and get together. The most important part is that clubs provide outlet to feelings and emotions. One can make groups of his likings through various permutations and combinations. This informal relationship can generate the bonds of friendship, love, and affection and these feelings can be transferred to work situations.

**(b) Arranging Meeting in Office Time to involve the Employees**

Top managers must arrange informal meetings for discussion on personal problems affecting work situation with employees to create in them the feeling of belongingness. This would also make them feel important as well as tap their potential energy. However, these meetings must be well arranged ensuring participation of one and all.

**(c) Free Access to Seniors**

An employee should be encouraged to see his seniors whenever there is any difficulty or problem. He should come prepared with details and tell in advance as to the purpose of his meeting so that the seniors are receptive. Such arrangements can remove a large number of tensions and unnecessary references.

**(d) Arranging Cultural Programmes during Festivals or other Occasions**

Organisations should encourage informal get together during some festivals and occasions so that employees can get relaxed and feel charged.

**(e) Arranging Tours**

Tours to nearby hill stations and scenic places can refresh the minds of the employees and accelerate the rate of social interaction. We can understand our colleagues better when we interact in an informal atmosphere. Relationships developed in this way are lasting and permanent and can be mutually supportive at the times of personal distress.

## SPIRITUAL HEALTH

In sum, individuals can have perfect health only when they are able to ascend from the lower to the higher states of consciousness, and remain perfectly poised in the higher plane of consciousness for a considerable duration of time. Perfect health is a comprehensive concept which includes mental equanimity, physical fitness and spiritual development of an individual. The most crucial problem with which mankind is faced at present is the problem of health in its comprehensive sense. Health in its comprehensive sense means perfect physical fitness, mental serenity and vivid comprehension of the higher planes of consciousness in an individual. Healing means restoration of an individual to his normal state of physical efficiency, mental equanimity and clear comprehension of the higher planes of consciousness.

Health has its base in spiritual powers. Organisation can arrange different lectures on spirituality which can keep the health of the employees in good shape as well move them to positive actions. J.L. Gupta in his article, "Power of Prayer" in *The Daily Tribune*, dated August 31,2000 stated that, "Today, we care for what we eat, but not for what is eating us. We worry about what we wear, not what is wearing us out. We build houses and furnish them at considerable cost to make them comfortable. Then we look for the fastest cars to get away from our homes. We get every place air-conditioned so that we do not sweat-at work or on the road of life. Then we spend more—we buy a treadmill or join a gym, even to go to a health club—all to be able to sweat out."

Such indeed is the dichotomy in our lifestyle. In the new millennium. we are moving fast, at a rather rapid pace, but we are not aware of the direction. We are rudderless. No wonder, we have problems of body and mind. All tension and lot of stress. There is not a moment of peace and rest. No time to stand and stare. Resultantly, the medicos claim a substantial share of our earnings, regularly.

Shirish Joshi rightly stresses the need of spiritual health. To quote that the notion that religious faith can promote physical well-being is not new. Most of us have heard of cases in which someone, seemingly by sheer faith and will, has miraculously recovered from a terminal illness or survived far longer than doctors thought possible. What is new is that such rewards of religion are becoming the subject of study by scientists.[21]

A large study found that religious folks had lower blood pressure, less depression and anxiety, stronger immune system and generally spent less money on medicines than people who not believe in the existence of God and were less involved in religious activities in temples. Scientists cannot prove that God heals, but they can now prove that belief in God has a beneficial effect. There is little doubt that healthy religious faith and practices can help people get better.

As a result of many studies, which say that prayer can help people feel better and live longer, many medical schools in the USA are offering courses in spirituality, religion and health.

Man without divine knowledge wanders in darkness. He is like a tree without fruit, flower without fragrance, a stream without water. Such a life is absolutely barren and worthless. Yoga can help us achieve all aspects of our perfect health. Yoga is a system of physical, mental and spiritual training. It starts with the purifications of body and ends with the unfoldment of the spirit.

## CONCLUSION

S.K. Kiran Kumar and K.A. Geetha have rightly summed up: Holistic approach to health represents a re-visioning of the human endeavour to restore order in the organismic functioning, that has occurred in the past several centuries within the medical profession. The holistic health movement is the reflection of the growing dissatisfaction among the professional as well as lay people about the capacity of modern medicine in delivering the health care. A shortcoming of modern medicine is its failure to recognize the inactive nature of the different aspects of human existence viz., physical, psychological, social and spiritual in the etiology of illnesses and in the maintenance of health and well-being.

Since modern medicine is itself a development within the framework of science, many have argued that the change needs to be brought about in the very framework. Thus, holistic health movement is viewed as a by-product and manifestation of the contemporary thrust on the revision of the scientific framework. One can find this trend in the works of behavioural, natural and social scientists which are contributing for a major change in the world view. It involves a fundamental shift in cognition leading to radical alternations in the belief and assumptions about the nature of the universe, about the human nature, about organism-environment interaction, and about the nature of consciousness. The newly emerging world view is described as holistic paradigm (Krippner, 1991).

In the final analysis, the physical, social, mental and spiritual balance is the most desirable for holistic health. Unless a person is physically fit and active; he cannot perform at his best level. On the other hand, it is the mind which accounts for 80 percent of physical and social problems. These are called psychosomatic diseases. Lastly, it is the spirit which ultimately directs the mind and through it to the body. The employers should devise ways and means to ensure synergy of the physical, social, mental and spiritual capabilities, which would release the infinite potential powers of the employees and generate efficiency and happiness in the organisation.

### NOTES AND REFERENCES

1. *The Economic Times*, dated 20 August, 2001.
2. World Health Organisation, South East Asia Regional Office, South East Asia, Regional Committee, 31, p. 59.

3. B. Benjamin, "Social and Economic Factors Affecting Mortality" in Confluence: Surveys of Research in the Social Services, Vol. V, (Hague, Mauton and Co.), 1965.
4. H. Correa and G. Cummins (1970): "Contribution of Nutrition to Economic Growth", *American Journal Clin., Nutr.* 23, 560-63 in World Health Papers, 49, p. 47.
5. WHO, SEARO: SEA/RC 30, p. 64.
6. Galenson and C. Pyatt, "The Quality of Labour and Economic Development in Certain Countries, Geneva, ILO, p. 1964.
7. G. Myrdal, Asian Drama—An Inquiry into the Poverty of Nations, New York, Pantheon, 1968.
8. M. Perlman, "On Health, Population, Change, and Economic Development, in M. Perlman and other (eds.) Spatial, Regional and Population Economics, Essays in Honour of Edgar M. Hoover (New York and Breach, (1972), pp. 293-300
9. Govt. of India, First Five Year Plan, p. 488
10. S.C. Seal, (1963), Presidential Address, 50th Science Congress, Delhi.
11. WHO, Public Health Papers, No. 49, 1973, p. 9
12. A.K. Sinha, Science and Tantra Yoga, 1993, p. 91.
13. O.P. Dwivedi, Reflections on Moral Government and Public Service as a Vocation, in *IJPA*, July to Sept., 1995, p. 297.
14 O.S. Dwivedi, "Conclusion: A Comparative Analysis of Ethics, Public and the Public Services", James S. Bowman and F.A. Elliston (eds.), Ethics, Government and Public Policy, New York, Greenwood Press, 1988, p. 318.
15. Bata K. Ethics, Maladies and Remedies, in *IJPA*, July-Sept., 1995, p. 461.
16. A.K. Sinha, *op. cit.*, pp. 70-71.
17. Justice V.R. Krishna Iyer, Ethical Entropy in Public Life, in *IJPA*, July-Sept. 1995, p. 350.
18. Ashok Mukkopadhyay, Ethics in Governance, in *IJPA*, July-Sept., 1995, p. 399.
19. Mohammad Mohabat Khan, Politics of Administrative Reform, the Case of Bangladesh, New Delhi, Ashish, 1999.
20. Kamla Prasad, Pursuit of Public Government in *IJPA*, July-Sept., 1995, p. 430.
21. *The Sunday Tribune*, Shirish Joshi, August 19, 2000.

# 16
CHAPTER

# *Management Techniques for Inculcating Aesthetic Sense among Medical Personnel*

"The employee spend the productive time of the day in working for the organisation to earn their livelihood. However, most employees consider official work as a drudgery to be avoided and postpone on one pretext or the other and this makes their life dull, insensitive and non-creative. In contrast, if the employee take pleasure in discharging their duties, they can remain active, healthy and efficient. Life should thus remain always joyful. Employment provide extra opportunity to meet and share views with colleagues as well as with the beneficiaries. The quality of job content and the situational context are equally important for gaining the job satisfaction while much has been written about the working in government, enough attention has not been paid to the ambience/environmental factors which are so critical for ensuring the desired output."

*—Author*

The medical and health employees spend the productive time of the day in working for the health organisation to earn their livelihood. However, most employees consider medical work as a drudgery to be avoided and postponed on one pretext or the other and this makes their life dull, insensitive and narrative. In contrast, if the employees take pleasure in discharging their duties, they can remain active, healthy and efficient. Life would thus remain always joyful. Employment provides extra opportunity to meet and share views with colleagues as well as with the beneficiaries. The quality of job content and the situational context are equally important for planning job satisfaction. While much has been written about the working in government, enough attention has not been paid to the ambience/environmental factors which are so critical for

CHART 16.1

**Healthy Aesthetic Sense**

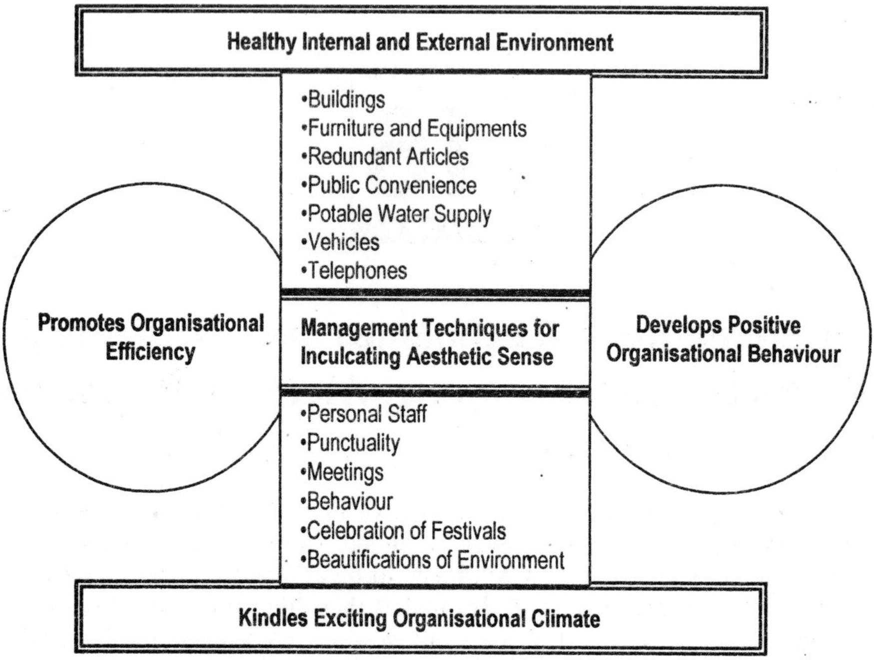


ensuring the desired outputs. It is commonly seen and felt that the employees do not seem to be bothered about the place they are working, its surroundings and the general atmosphere. A visit to most health organisations would reveal the following:

(i) The outlay of the hospitals is dull, shabby and disorderly. Various pieces of furniture do not match, and are so positioned that it appears to be lying scattered and uncared for.

(ii) The bath rooms are stinking, making it unbearable and unusable. Besides, drinking water of good quality is not available, which leads to many diseases.

(iii) Disorderly parking of vehicles outside the health organisation premises causes inconvenience to visitors and the whole place books like an unorganized market area.

(iv) The medical personnel come to the office at their own time, disregarding all norms of punctuality, depicting an attitude of apathy and indifference.

(v) Building maintenance is poor and it appears that employees have no concern with the surroundings. Most of the walls and floors have been spoilt by spitting, throwing refuse, painting and pasting posters/slogans, etc.

(vi) We find many useless articles, equipments, papers, etc. scattered all over, causing repulsion for any visitor. There is no display of aesthetic sense in decorating the building and its exteriors with plants, flowers, etc.

(vii) Most of the health employees are always busy in one meeting or the other, leaving very little time for substantive office work or even interaction with the public.

(viii) We find that most health employees start quarreling with the patients on one pretext or the other, assuming themselves to be the owners of the organisation rather than being public servants/facilitators.

(ix) We often find employees talking on a telephone for long, thus wasting office time and reducing efficiency.

(x) The senior officers draw more and more peons and clerical staff to their personal establishments in keeping with their 'status' and 'prestige'. This deprives the office of its productive hands leading to decrease in overall efficiency.

(xi) There are no occasions for intellectual discussions, lectures, symposia, etc. wherein the employees can open up and suggest ways of improving the office outlook, work culture and administrative practices.

(xii) Holidays are observed on important days without having even adequate knowledge about them and the necessity felt for celebrating them.

The question is how to manage all these inputs? How to make the quality services available? Although above issues are considered to be peripheral and incidental yet these are actually the pre-requisites for building an efficient organisation. For example, a good office layout helps in the following: These are considered to be unimportant but otherwise, these are the pre-requisites on which to build efficient health organisation and hospitals.

1. Proper utilization of office space.
2. Effective work flow.
3. Speedy communication.
4. Better use of office equipments.
5. Proper supervision.
6. Necessary comfort and reduced fatigue.
7. High morale of the personnel.
8. Improved overall efficiency of the health and hospital organisations.

Keeping the above benefits in mind the Department of Administrative reforms has sponsored a scheme for office modernization by subsidizing

75% of the costs in order to promote office environment conductive to work. However, obtaining good office accommodation and luxurious furnishings may not be sufficient unless it is kept clean and tidy, free from bad odour, and infection. Let us discuss some of the areas of management to develop aesthetic sense among the medical employees in an health organisation and to promote happiness and efficiency among the staff.

## A. HEALTH AND HOSPITAL BUILDINGS MANAGEMENT

Buildings should be well maintained to keep the minds of medical employees happy as well as to create good image in the minds of the visitors. Most of the government buildings especially in the fields are in dilapidated conditions. PWD, an organisation created at the union and state levels to maintain and upkeep of these buildings has failed to discharge its duties because of corrupt practices as well as shortage of staff and finances. What can be done to maintain buildings?

(i) Each health and hospital building should be placed under the control of a caretaker, and even if more than one office exists in that building, the responsibility of maintaining that building should be with a single person. The care-taker must examine the building at regular intervals and note all the problems being faced.

(ii) A committee should be constituted and empowered to effect the required changes.

(iii) White washing and painting of walls and doors respectively should be done at and when required instead of fixed intervals. Maintenance contracts would be awarded accordingly.

(iv) Safety of the buildings should be regularly examined and those found unfit for occupation should either be demolished or reclaimed in order to prevent danger to the life and property.

(v) Adequate lighting and fan arrangements may be made as per the need of each room/seating patterns rather than sticking to uniform standards of space.

(vi) Leakages in buildings may be checked in time so as to avoid permanent damages.

(vii) Modifications/alterations may be made only under the advice of architects having innovative ideas for efficient and active use of space.

## B. MANAGEMENT OF FURNITURE AND EQUIPMENT

Furniture is essential to provide comforts and working atmosphere to employees. Furniture costs money and hence must be used carefully and maintained properly. We can take the following steps to make the furniture serve our purpose:

(i) Proper assessment of the needs of all rooms/employees may be done before ordering new equipment. It has been seen that because of lack of coordination furniture at one place is lying surplus while at another place it is in demand causing artificial scarcity. Sometimes the stores are still full of old furniture which can be made of good quality with minor repairs and polishing while the orders are placed for buying fresh furniture.

(ii) Peons employed for the upkeep of furniture need be trained in the upkeep of furniture through regular dusting, spraying to avoid rusting, and keeping them in good conditions.

(iii) Furniture should be neatly arranged to provide aesthetic outlook and look presentable.

(iv) Every year/every single article of furniture should be physically counted and examined for repairs and polish or condemnation, etc.

(v) Furniture, which is unserviceable and beyond repairs, needs to be condemned rather than piling them up in stores and wasting precious spaces.

(vi) The staff should be convinced about the importance of cleaning, inspecting and keeping equipment in good order; of reporting defects immediately; and of returning equipment to its correct place after use.

(vii) There is no easy way to convince the staff of the need to clean equipment and to keep it in good condition. The best way is for the supervisor to set a good example by ensuring that equipments are cared for kept in a good condition (dirty or damp equipment deteriorates more rapidly than when it is kept clean and dry).

(viii) An inspection check-list and inspection schedule should be drawn up and duties decentralized among responsible employees irrespective of their technical charges. These officials should help in detecting discrepancies and taking remedial action.

Thus, good management take care of the management of equipments by:

- instructing and motivating staff to feel responsible for the equipment they use,
- ordering supplies when needed,
- storing them safely, and
- controlling their use.

The salient advantages of such a system would be:

(a) Reduction in idle time and continuous availability of equipment.
(b) Increased life of the equipment.
(c) Continued service.
(d) Less operational costs.
(e) Satisfactory quality of services.
(f) Safety of operation.

## C. MANAGEMENT OF REDUNDANT ARTICLES

Health Hospital institutions are full of redundant articles and no one takes pains to write them off. These articles on one hand present an ugly look and on the other hand block the space, especially in metropolitan cities, where the value of space is quite prohibitive. In addition, these can spread diseases. Thus articles/papers/equipments which have become useless need to be discarded as early as possible. How can we go about it? We suggest a few measures as follows:

(i) There should be stock taking in every section, once a quarter to identify of what is relevant and what is not. This exercise would help in disposing of unwanted articles.
(ii) The auctioning of discarded items should be decentralized for field offices. The depreciated value rather than book value should be the criteria for evaluating the auction bids.
(iii) Removal of redundant articles should thus be a continuous process.
(iv) There may be many articles like fans, tube lights, heaters, boilers, etc. which have become outdated or inefficient. These need to be discarded on regular intervals and substituted by efficient models.

## D. MAINTENANCE OF PUBLIC CONVENIENCES

Bath rooms and toilets in health and hospitals premises are the most essential infrastructural component for health employees as well as patients. They should be kept clean, as cleanliness is next to godliness. Many of the diseases are the product of insanitary conditions prevailing in many offices besides causing physical discomfort and inconvenience to the users. We suggest here the following actions to keep them clean:

(i) Sweepers engaged for cleaning bath rooms may be given training by pinpointing the importance of cleanliness in the upkeep of bath rooms.
(ii) Necessary materials like phenyl, cleansing agents, etc. may be supplied regularly.
(iii) Some persons may be appointed to supervise the upkeep of bath rooms regularly and maintaining a record of the action taken.

(iv) Bath rooms may be constructed away from working places so that the stink does not adversely affect the working of employees and patients.

(v) Employees and patients may be requested to keep the bath rooms clean.

(vi) Sufficient water arrangements may be made.

(vii) Privatisation of cleanliness of bath rooms can be tried.

## E. SUPPLY OF POTABLE WATER

Water is the basic requirement of every human being. Most of the employees and patients get health problems and infections because of poor quality of water. They cannot afford bottled water available at a high cost. The organisation should attend to management of supply of good water for all employees and patients. The following can be done in this direction:

(i) Water storage should be done in clean tanks. Besides tanks should be washed on Saturdays/Sundays when offices are closed. Besides insecticides like potassium permagnate may be used once a month to keep the water infection free. Tanks which have become too dirty should be discarded.

(ii) Employees and patients should be requested not to waste the precious resource, i.e. water. Taps may not be kept open.

(iii) Plastic jugs and glasses used for taking water in the rooms are mostly dirty. They need be regularly cleaned and well maintained.

(iv) Contract for mineral water at cheap rates may be tried if feasible.

(v) Water testing may be got done through laboratories once in six months to assess its quality.

A study carried out by Dr. Rajneesh Goel for his unpublished doctoral research "Analysis of Primary Health Care Administration in Karnataka" indicates that at sub-centre, Primary Health Centres (PHCs) and Community Health Centres (CHCs) the buildings are neither sufficient to accommodate all activities, nor well maintained. Buildings are not regularly white washed, broken glasses not removed, repairs not done, making it impossible for Primary Health Care functionaries to carry out their activities in a dignified manner.

The analysis of sub-centre, Primary Health Centre, CHC indicate that lavatory facilities are in a very bad shape resulting in foul smell in the area, making it difficult to sit both for the health staff and the patients. Urinating near Health Centres can result in serious infections. It is suggested that lavatory services may be provided adequately and well maintained either by its own staff or through the contractual system.

The above study also found that both the health personnel as well as the patients were unhappy and even annoyed over the quantity and quality of furniture provided. Even simple examination tables, beds in the wards, trolleys were non-functional. Most of the chairs were broken. It is suggested that health department must ensure the availability of good quality at health centres to make them functional.

There is no proper handling and upkeep of equipment, resulting in low performance. Most of the persons handling these equipments are not trained and need to be trained.

Preventive maintenance is systematic maintenance procedure, wherein the condition of the equipment is constantly watched through a systematic inspection programme and preventive action taken to reduce the incidence of breakdown.

## F. MANAGEMENT OF VEHICLES

This is an age of vehicles as most of the employees and patients use cars/scooters/vans to come to hospitals. Parking of these vehicles has become a big challenge and even nuisance. We suggest the following to manage vehicles:

- (i) Parking zones may be earmarked separately for cycles, scooters and cars so that there may be clear-cut demarcation.
- (ii) Vehicles of the staff who are to park for the whole day should be done separately from visitors as their movement would be limited.
- (iii) Parking rules may be framed and in case of violation, huge fines may be imposed as a deterrent.
- (iv) Persons may be engaged to guide the vehicle owners. His salary can be paid from the collections made from vehicle owners.

The old vehicles are a liability to the organisation since they generally consume more money on repairs and maintenance as well as on fuel. They tend to be highly uneconomical and much less efficient in operations. Future these old vehicles create a number of budgetary imbalances in utilisation of funds. In this context, condemnation of old vehicles in a phased manner following the principle of "eight years of age" or "1.60 lakh km. run" should be done. Besides age of vehicle and kilometers run, the Department may also consider the operational factors like fuel consumption, maintenance costs, etc. for condemnation. The present practice of scrapping/condemning the vehicles is not very much conducive to the quick disposal of the condemned vehicles and to its efficiency. It is a pity to see large number of vehicles getting rusted without either making them useful or condemn them. There is a need to form a joint committee of Transport Department representative alongwith the financial and administrative representatives to arrive at a logical decision.

## G. MANAGEMENT OF TELEPHONES

Telephones have been installed to facilitate the communication and save the time of employees in seeking information, clarification, etc. However, we notice that telephones are used for personal purposes and that too for unnecessary activities wasting time and money. We can enforce discipline by introducing following measures:

(i) Private calls may be allowed only in emergencies. These may be entered into the register indicating the number, purpose, etc. Modern EPABXs have the call tracking facilities to monitor the frequently called numbers. The users would have to justify the official purpose of the calls if needed.
(ii) The need for frequent use of telephones for seeking information/ clarification may be studied in depth to point out the lacunae in the existing MIS. Telephone should be used only when necessary.
(iii) Telephone should not become a distraction for non-users sharing the room. Hence, its location needs to be worked out accordingly.
(iv) Pay phones with private enclosures should be provided in office premises to encourage officials to make their private calls outside the office room.
(v) Recent studies have pointed out that 30-40% of the time, senior executives tend to spend over phone. Half the time, things could have been attended at subordinate levels. Automated exchanges could be used screening the incoming calls and ensuring that the call goes to the right person. This could save the time of the client as well as officials, if planned properly.

We can save a lot of expenditure by maintaining a discipline well as save time for productive work.

## H. MANAGING PERSONAL STAFF

It has become fashion to engage a large number of personal staff who misuse the name of officers on whose behalf they talk and work. In this connection we should do the following:

(i) Personal staff should be minimum to avoid unnecessary rush and confusion.
(ii) Training may be given to personal staff of their duties and responsibilities.
(iii) Activities of personal staff should be checked so that they may not misuse the powers of the officers.
(iv) Personal staff should act as a filter and funnel for the officers.
(v) Personal staff should be polite.

## I. PUNCTUALITY

Punctuality which was cherished by all has become a casualty causing great problems. It is good for better time management. We give here abstracts of a study conducted for health services by Dr. Rajneesh Goel for his doctoral work "Analysis of Primary Health Care Administration" in Karnataka from Panjab University Chandigarh (unpublished) in 2000 in support of the above contentions.[1]

The opinion survey indicated that there is lot of indiscipline among functionaries of the PHC. Doctors and Paramedical Staff remain absent without leave. Besides 100 percent respondents said that they come late and go early, thus making themselves available only for a short period. Murali Manohar and Kameshwarn pointed out that the medicos do not like to serve in the rural areas because of their urban culture and background. Former Prime Minister Atal Bihari Vajpayee strongly emphasised that, "The people want to see action, and not to hear words of promise repeated again and again." How to ensure punctuality? We suggest some techniques to ensure punctuality:

(i) Head of Deptt. should show seriousness about this issue by calling for all employees to be punctual as a preventive and educational measure.
(ii) Induction training may be given to all employees to be punctual as preventive and educational measure.
(iii) Late arrivals should lead to deduction of half day casual leave and 3 consecutive defaults invite censure and adverse entry in SRs & CRs.
(iv) Punching of cards to mark attendance can be introduced.
(v) Habitually non-punctual employees may be served warning/censures/stoppage of increment and even suspension including termination.
(vi) Extra-benefits in the form of deputation for training, other assignments, etc. may be refused to those who are not punctual.
(vii) Strict monitoring may be done to prohibit late coming.

The Administration Reforms Commission (ARC) has rightly stated that, "the healthy functioning of the administration depends not only on the competence of its personnel, but also on the maintenance of a high standard of personal conduct and the observance of discipline. It is, therefore, essential that there should be a clearly enumerated code to correct official behaviour and a provision for the punishment of those who deviate therefrom. There would, of course, also be provision for punishing slackness and inefficiency."[2]

Punctuality enforcement is not a difficult task provided the culture of non-punctuality is discouraged. Employees are being paid for devoting time and time is money. How can we pay them if they are not producing. The Indian Administration is suffering a lot on this count.

Government of India and state Governments must give top priority to this issue as we find that because of non-punctuality of doctors, teachers, administrative staff, people suffer a great agony in waiting for them. The government must be harsh and no leniency should be exhibited to persons who are not punctual. This is the first and foremost requirement of any administrative success and responsive administration.

## J. MANAGEMENT OF MEETINGS

Meetings have become essential to sort out many issues and problems. Meetings are generally held without much forethought and preparation, resulting in wastage of resources.

Serving of tea/coffee and refreshments has become a major preoccupation. Sarcastically, people interpret 'Committee' meeting as 'come for tea' meeting. Besides, huge expenditure is incurred by government in running departmental canteens to cater to a chain of meetings. Some officials even abuse this as a pretext for not being available in their OPD ward to the patients, etc. Most often the meetings indicate the starting time and are open ended. This jeopardizes the working schedule of most participants. Besides, most meetings are *adhoc* and do not give sufficient notice to the members. This often causes clash of activities and priorities. Officials have to give greater priority to the superiors' meetings than to the commitments of the clients/citizens. What can be done to reduce the number of meetings? How can we make them useful? Let us mention some action points.

(i) Agenda should be well prepared in advance with clear-cut spelling out the details of the points.
(ii) Members may be given sufficient time to go through the agenda in order to participate/contribute meaningfully.
(iii) All the members should be encouraged to participate in a business-like manner.
(iv) Minutes of meetings should be recorded faithfully.
(v) Decisions arrived at may be communicated quickly.
(vi) Meeting should be held only when there are some real issues otherwise formalities could be completed by circulation of material among the members.
(vii) Intranets should be used to display the meeting schedules to make the process transparent.
(viii) Serving of tea/coffee should be avoided when the duration is less than an hour.

The Ministry of Personnel, Public Grievances and Pensions (Department of Administrative Reforms and Public Grievances) in its report. Initiatives and best practices of Government of India for effective and responsive administration suggested the following:

(i) A meetingless day on every Wednesday should be observed strictly. The designated officer or his/her immediate subordinate should be accessible on this day and for emergent complaints at stipulated hours on other days.
(ii) The receptionists, security personnel and peons should be given suitable instructions about the meetingless day so as to allow the members of the public to meet officers without prior appointment. This should be enforced also in respect of all the attached offices and public agencies under the supervision of the Ministry/Department.
(iii) The name, designation room number, telephone number, etc. of employees should be displayed prominently at the reception and other convenient places in the office buildings/ministries.

## K. BEHAVIOUR MANAGEMENT

Most of the problems today are the result of rude behaviour of majority of health employees towards patients. Their behaviour has alienated the people from the functioning. Inspite of 73rd and 74th amendment, people still are not been given their due place and recognition in public governance. How to go about it. We may suggest the following remedies:

(i) Training may be imparted in art and science of communication.
(ii) Employees using filthy language should be dealt strictly by imposition of fines or recording the demeanour in the confidential reports.
(iii) A column about behaviour should be incorporated in ACR.
(iv) Employees should be encouraged to be polite, nice and courteous. Superiors should set a personal example by observing same standards while dealing with their bosses as well as subordinates or members of public.
(v) Supervision should be done strictly and if required dialogues of citizens and employees depicting different situations—very negative, negative positive, very positive, be recommended for training purposes. To quote Aristotle, "Anyone can become angry—that is easy. But to be angry with the right person, to the right degree, at the right time, for the right purpose and the right way is not easy."
(vi) A new concept called "Equilibrium Thinking" has been tried out with police trainees both with veterans having thirty years' experience and freshly recruited officer trainees. Several of the trainees reported remarkable breakthroughs in managing anger and other emotions.[3] Equilibrium is produced when positive values or vices are balanced. The positive values need to be affirmed or reinforced and the negative values need to be

denied, weakened and uprooted. Current success literature talks only of the power of positive thinking but mere positive thinking does not generate sufficient power to overcome the challenge of ingrained negative attitudes, habits forces and values. Mere positive thinking does not produce an equilibrium that comes from a habit of self-realisation. The method is quite simple. Continuously hold the words Beat it to Beat it in one's mind. In order to overcome anger, continually issue the following commands to self:

| | | |
|---|---|---|
| 1. | Be calm | Beat anger |
| 2. | Be gentle | Beat stress |
| 3. | Be peaceful | Beat tension |
| 4. | Be patient | Beat Impatience |
| 5. | Be poised | Beat imbalance |
| 6. | Be tactful | Beat tactlessness |
| 7. | Be cheerful | Beat depression |

It takes only about 10 seconds to run the series of commands through one's mind. So even if one repeats the exercise, ten times a day it will take only 100 seconds.

| *Do's* | *Don't's* |
|---|---|
| 1. Make haste, slowly. | Don't merely make haste. |
| 2. List areas of interface. | Don't be unrealistic. |
| 3. Phase out areas for introduction of small steps. | Don't take on more than you can commit. |
| 4. Involve customer and staff in formulating and implementing it. | Don't involve only senior officers in the formulation and implementation. |
| 5. Prepare a Master Plan for formulation and implementation over five years and budget for it. | Don't rush into an overall package for the whole Ministry/Department/ Organisation. |
| 6. Win consumer confidence with small, highly visible measures. | Don't promise more than you can deliver. |
| 7. Remember, citizens' charter is a process. | Don't look upon it as a one-time exercise, with constantly evolving a final outcome. |
| 8. Inform the customer of the proposed commitments. | Don't inform the customer unless you are sure of delivering the service. |
| 9. Use simple language. | Don't use difficult language or jargon. |
| 10. Train your staff. | Don't leave yourself out. |
| 11. Delegate power. | Don't centralise. |
| 12. Set-up system for feedback and independent scrutiny. | Don't continue blindly without regular, periodic reassessment of performance. |

The repetitive reinforcement on a daily and continuous basis will help in internalizing values and overcoming flows and weaknesses. Equilibrium thinking lends itself to the all round development of the human personality and character. Prabhat Kumar, the then Cabinet Secretary of India in his Article, "A Responsive and Effective Government" rightly stresses the need for making the administration sensitive to the citizens' needs.[4] To quote him:

We are now on the threshold of the twenty-first century. In the new millennium, above all, the government would need to re-invent itself to become citizen-centric and citizen-friendly. It would need to limit its role to core functions such as security, law and order, social services, creation of infrastructure and macro-economic management. Greater delegation and decentralisation of authority and responsibilities would need to be introduced at all levels. A combination of Citizens' Charters and the Right to Information would ensure greater accountability in the administrative systems. The process of consultation with the participation of citizens in decision-making would gradually become more pronounced in order to ensure accountability. At the same time, good citizenry would also need to be emphasised for all round development of the society. Besides enjoying their rights, the citizens would need to behave responsibly and perform their duties to the state. Clearly defined ethical standards would also need to be adopted by the civil servants as well as politicians. In order to achieve all this, innovative use of information technology would be critical.

Ministry of Personnel, Public Grievances and Pensions (Department of Administrative Reforms and Public Grievances) has given some tips which need be followed to keep offices in order.[5]

## L. CELEBRATION OF FESTIVALS AND IMPORTANT EVENTS

In order to promote patriotism, national integration and enlightened citizenship, it is essential that the ministry/department/subordinate offices should celebrate festivals and important events for small duration wherein, the following activities can be undertaken:

1. A brief lecture about the purpose of festival/event.
2. Cultural programme.
3. Discussions.
4. Simple tea and snacks.

Such acts would promote the bond of friendship among the medical personnel in the hospitals and help in building a good team. This would also take care of regionalism, caste and narrow loyalties

## M. BEAUTIFICATION OF ENVIRONMENT

Internal and external physical environment should be soothing and stimulating to generate enthusiasm, activity and high spirits. A visit to most of the hospitals reveal that no attention is paid by administration to this aspect.

The internal environment of any hospital essentially consists of the files which act as a medium for transaction of office work. The sections generally are overflowing with files and files and papers which have literally gathered dust for ages. Although there is a regular mechanism of weeding out of the files, most of the material does not get classified into the redundant category e.g. books/publications/printed material/registers. The task of binding the files before sending to record room is to be performed by daftaries. For many reasons, this never gets done. As a result, not only space constraints and congestion arises but smooth functioning of the current work is also hampered. Thus, unless the supervisory authority inspects and regulates the records/files management and sensitizes the staff for the need to keep the office environment spic and span, this situation is likely to perpetuate—

(i) Plants in pots may be kept at various locations. These may be changed according to the season. The weeds should also be regularly removed through contract arrangements.
(ii) Proper spraying may also be done to ensure infection free atmosphere. Some sprays with fragrance may also be used. Spread of rodents, flies, mosquitoes should be checked.
(iii) Proper play cards may be displayed for the guidance of visitors.
(iv) Dustbins and waste paper baskets may be provided to avoid littering and proper disposal of waste material.
(v) Preparation of Tea/Coffee or any other article may be banned in the individual rooms. Tea/Coffee, etc. can be had only in the canteen. Canteen should be equipped with proper exhaust fans to avoid pungent smells.
(vi) Good ideas may be written on the board specially provided for the purpose at the entrance of the building to infuse good thoughts.
(vii) If there is space surrounding the hospitals, it should be well maintained. There should be regular removing of the congress grass and weeds and planting of flowering plants depending upon the season.

The dynamics of hospitals management can thus be summarized in a graphical form given on next page.

The task before the hospitals administration today is to manage the appropriate inputs in such a way that the hospitals strives towards excellence. We can thus conclude that the dynamism in the hospitals cannot be declared by fiat, nor can it be generated artificially imposing systems, procedures, and job demands. The enthusiasm and the aesthetic sense of hospitals employees express about their jobs, about each other and

| Input |  | ORGANISATION |  | Output |
|---|---|---|---|---|
| Beautification of internal and external environment | → | ORGANISATION | → | Feeling of pride and belongingness |
| Health Employees and patients welfare through essential facilities | → |  | → | Sense of well-being and job satisfaction and appreciation by patients |
| Inculcation of values of Punctuality and good behaviour | → |  | → | Responsive, accountable and patients centric administration |
| Efficient conduct of meeting | → |  | → | Proper use of time and money for patients |
| Joint celebration of festival events | → |  | → | Team spirit |
| Input | → |  | → | Output |

about their organisation is a priceless corollary of effective management. Without it, the whole management effort can easily become a kind of drudgery, never moving beyond a mechanical process with little sense of personal involvement. The hospitals employees have a great potential which need be optimised through the development of their attitudes and philosophy through aesthetic development. A well maintained hospital, from within and outside can be a source of delight for medical and health personnel working within and patients visiting the hospitals.

## Notes and References


1. Rajneesh Goel, "An Analysis of Primary Health Care Administration in Karnataka", a Ph.D. thesis from Panjab University, Chandigarh, 2000, (unpublished).
2. Atal Behari Vajpayee, Indian Administration Today, Reading Its Weaknesses, in *IJPA*, Jan.-March, 1999.
3. Partap Philip, Managing Anger, Aggression and Stress, in *Management in Government*, Jan-March 2004, pp. 45-48.
4. Prabhat Kumar, A Responsive and Effective Government, *Management in Government*, January-March, 2004, p. 8.
5. Ministry of Personnel, Public Grievances and Pensions Deptt. of Administration Reforms and Public Grievances, Initiatives and Best Practices of GOI for Effective and Responsive Admn., November 1997, p. 4.

17

CHAPTER

# Selfless Service for Building Health and Medical Organisations on Truth, Beauty and Goodness

"A reasonable degree of excellence in at least one productive skill through which individuals can experiment the truth that work is worship when performed in a spirit of service, and can secure little means of existence with dignity and honour."

—*Swami Vivekananda*

Swami Ranganathananda in his note, "Democratic Administration in the Light of Practical Vedanta" portrays a poor picture of the prevailing value system in India. To quote, *India Today* is at the cross-roads. We are in a curious predicament. The obverse of the coin is bright, the reverse grim. We are heirs to a glorious civilization whose mighty stream has been following uninterruptedly down the millennia, enriching and ennobling all on its path. Sixty years back we have also recovered our political independence from the largest empire the world has seen, and that without firing a single shot-something unique in history. Yet chaos stalks the land. Things are falling apart. Values cherished over the centuries are getting eroded. In a country of rich natural resources the poverty of the masses is abysmal. The haves exploit the have-nots in a hundred ingenious ways. Women and the weaker sections of society reel under injustice and handicaps. Corruption is rampant. Mindless violence maims and destroys the precious lives of the innocent. The sensitive citizen finds himself asking, "Whither India."[1]

The reputation medical profession is going down as most of the medical professionals are exploiting those who are already burdened with sickness and are not working. The main aim of medical profession is to earn money by hook and by crook. In recent years, they have started malpractices of taking out organs from one person and selling at a huge cost to others. Medical personnel today, can do any sort of activity which can bring money to them.

What is the problem? It is selfishness of people especially intellectuals. What is it then that gives peace of mind to a man? The answer is: selflessness. A man is happy to the extent he is selfless. A selfless man is happy because he thinks less of himself and more of others. He wishes to see everybody happy —it is against his nature to wish that he will have something which others do not have. This what is expected from health medical personnel.

A selfish man like the present day medical expert or doctor on the other hand, thinks of himself alone and he is too egotistic which others do not have. A selfish man, on the other hand, thinks of himself alone and he is too egotistic to care for others. He has an exaggerated notion about himself, as if the whole world depends upon him. He wants everything to happen the way he wants and if it does not, he is distressed. A selfless man, however, is modest in his expectations; he knows he has no right to impose his will upon others. And it is never his wish to deprive others in order that he may have more. He is happy with whatever he has in the normal course of things and he is happier if others have what he himself has. It hurts him to see others in pain. He is happy if others are happy, unhappy, if others are unhappy. His goodwill includes everybody irrespective of race or religion. The whole world is his friend, says a Sanskrit proverb. He may be, humble man without any influence at any level, yet if there is any wrong done to anybody anywhere, he feels as if the wrong has been done to him.[2]

Swami Chinmayanand beautifully warns those who want to serve others as it is demanding exercise on the part of individuals. To quote:[3] "Missionary work is subtler than art, more demanding than science, more precise than literature, more adventurous than space-walking. Therefore, we must exhaustively and thoroughly prepare ourselves before we enter out fields of action, to serve others, to lead and guide the seeker. All discordant and undesirable elements in our life must be eliminated. The sovereign remedy for all ailments in us is found nowhere else but just within ourselves. The great secret of true success, of true happiness, then, is this; the man who asks for no return, the perfectly unselfish man, is the most successful. It seems to be a paradox. Do we not know that every man who is unselfish in life gets cheated, gets hurt? Apparently, Yes, "Christ was unselfish, and yet he was crucified." "True, but we know that his unselfishness is the reason, the cause of a great victory—the crowning of millions upon millions of lives with the blessings of true success."

Swami Harshanand says that ask nothing; want nothing in return. Give what you have to give; it will come back to you—but do not think of that now. It will come back multiplied a thousand fold—but the attention must not be on that. Yet have the power to give; give, and there it ends.[4]

Medical personnel can get real happiness to ailing personnel which give him everlasting joy and bliss which is a rare commodity. Money is only the means and not the end.

"Man is born to give not to grab", "grabber pays the penalty in the form of misery"; the giver reaps the reward in the form of joy.

The resources, the bodily effort and the mental disposition becomes multiplied in the man of yajna. Stich a man is never in want, always in affluence. His bounteous mind is the real Kamdhenu. Because of his frame of mind he is ever in prosperity. This is the plan and purpose of cosmos. This medical personnel should always follow the principle of service without anything in return.

When the Creator said that fostered by sacrifice, the gods would surely bestow on man all the desired enjoyments unasked, he meant that, for his own part; man should go on scrupulously performing his duty. If man did not fail in the performance of his duty, there could be no doubt that fostered and nourished by his sacrifice, the gods could ever continue to supply him with all the means of leading a happy and contented life; for the gods were bound to perform their part of duty. Health and medical personnel who perform their duties as Dharma would get everything in life.

The essence of the spirit of service is contained in the following words of Vivekananda:

"This is the gist of all worship—to be pure and to do good to others. He who sees Shiva in the poor, in the weak, and in the diseased, really worships Shiva; and if he sees Shiva only in the image, his worship is but preliminary. He who has served and helped one poor man seeing Shiva in him, without thinking of his caste, or creed, or race, or anything, with him Shiva is more pleased than with the man who sees Him only in the temples. He who wants to serve the father must serve the children first. He who wants to serve Shiva must serve His children and all creatures in the world first."[5] (Chart 17.1) Swami Vivekananda says the great secret of true success, of true happiness, then, is this; the man who asks for no return, the perfectly unselfish man, is the most successful. It seems to a paradox. Do we now know that every man who is unselfish in life gets cheated, gets hurt?"

Apparently, yes, "Christ was unselfish, and yet he was crucified." True, but we know that his unselfishness is the reason, the cause of a great victory—the crowning of millions upon millions of lives with the blessings of true success.

Ask nothing; want nothing in return. Give what you have to give, it will come back to you—but do not think of that now. It will come back multiplied a thousand-fold—but the attention must not be on that. Yet have the power to give; give, and there it ends. Learn that the whole of life is giving, that nature will for. you to give. So, give willingly. Sooner or later you will have to give up. You come into life to accumulate. With clenched hands, you want to take but nature puts a hand on your throat and makes your hands open. Whether you will it or not, you have to give. The moment

CHART 17.1

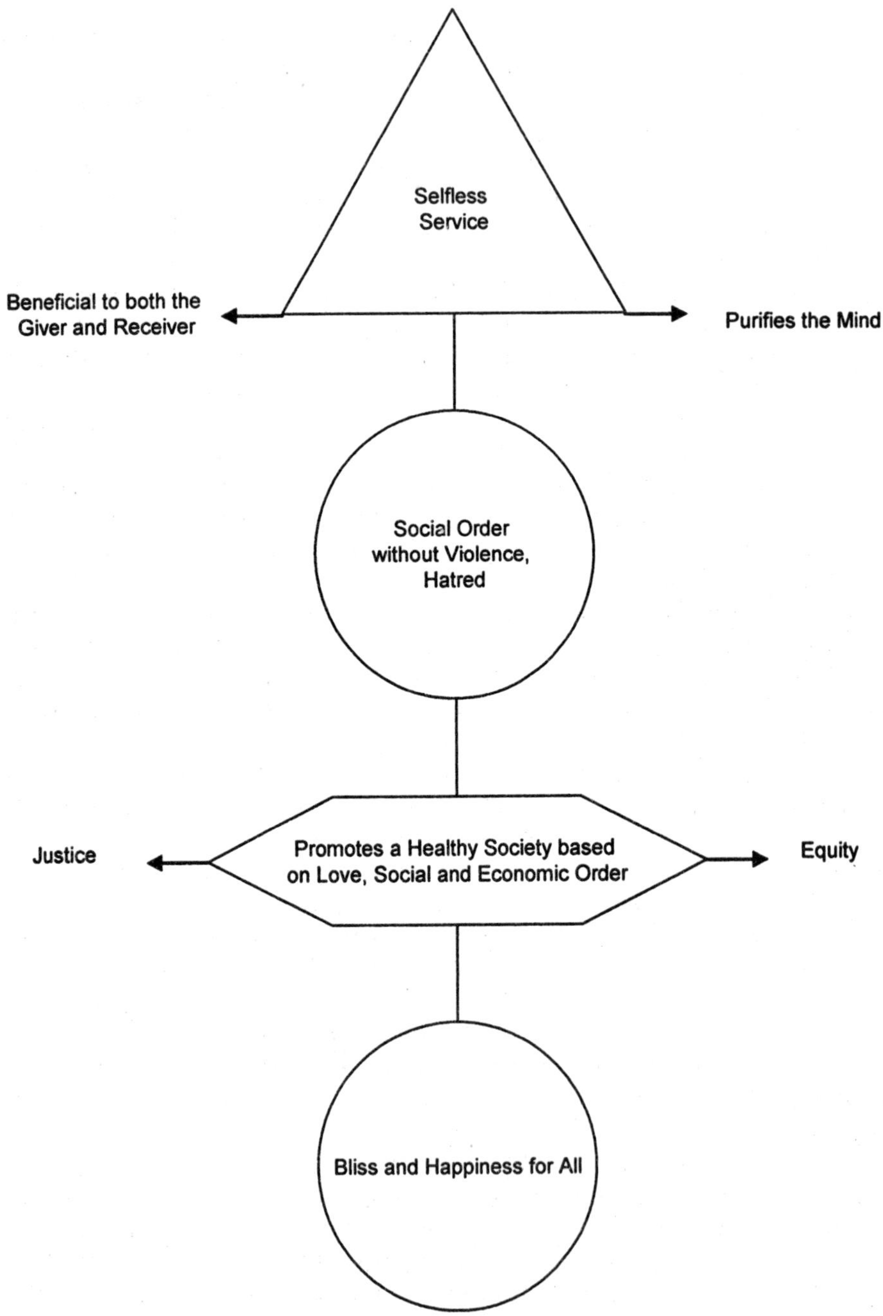
Selfless Service
Beneficial to both the Giver and Receiver
Purifies the Mind
Social Order without Violence, Hatred
Justice
Promotes a Healthy Society based on Love, Social and Economic Order
Equity
Bliss and Happiness for All

CHART 17.2

**Selfless Services**

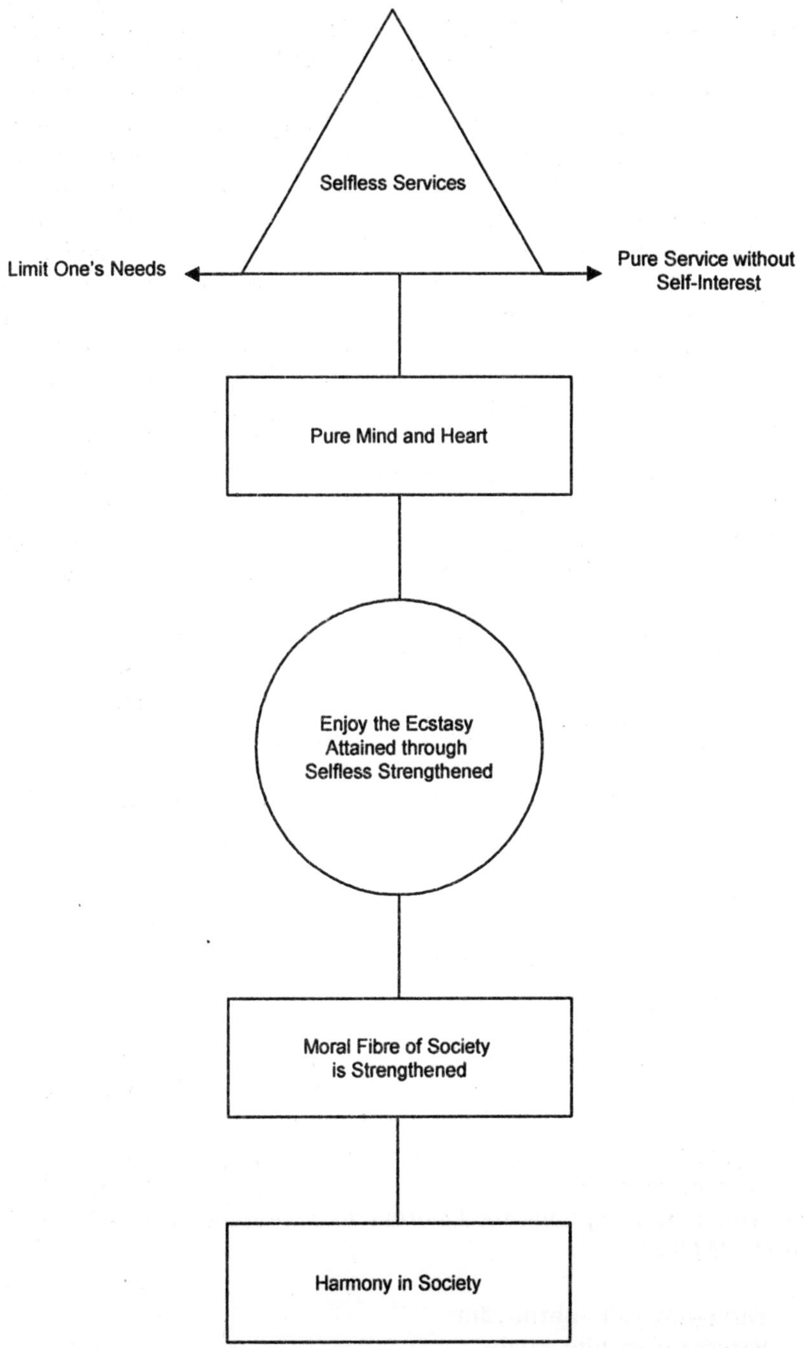

You say, "I will not", the blow comes, you are hurt. None is there but will be compelled, in the long-run to give up everything. And the more one struggles against this law the more miserable one feels. It is because we dare not give because we are not resigned enough to accede to this grand demand of nature, that we are miserable. The forest is gone, but we get heat in return. The sun is taking up water from the ocean, to return it in showers. You are a machine for taking and giving; you take, in order to give. Ask, therefore, nothing in return, but the more you give, the more will come to you. The quicker you can empty the air out of this room, the quicker it will be filled up by the external air; and if you close all the doors and every one, that which is within will remain, but that which is outside will never come in and that which is within will stagnate, degenerate and becomes poisoned. A river is continually emptying itself into the ocean and is continually filling up again. Bar not exit into the ocean. The moment you do that, death sizes you." The health and medical personnel follow the Philosophy of selfless service. This would compensate them through the blessings of those to whom you have served.

This world is not for cowards. Do not try to fly. Look not for success or failure. Join yourself to the perfectly unselfish will and work on. Know that the mind which is born to succeed joins itself to a determined will and preservers. You have the right to work, but do not become so degenerate as to look for results. Work instantly, but see something behind the work.

Even good deeds can find a man in great bondage. Therefore, be not bound by good deeds or by desire for name and fame. Those who know this secret pass beyond this round of birth and death and become immortal.

In the Mahabharat, "there are two beautiful definitions of Dharma; throughout our cultural history, this word was never used to mean a dogma or creed or ethnical religion; we are making this mistake only in the modern period. The first definition is by Sri Krsna, occurring in the Kama Parva (8.49.50):

Oharanat dharma ityahllh
Dh.trmo dharayate prajah;
Yah syat dharana-samYuktah
Sa dharma iti niscayah—

dharma is so called, because it holds the period together in a society, it integrates man with man; that value which has this integrating capacity, that is determined as dharma (by the wise)."

In the Santi Parva of the same Mahabharata, the Pandavas and Sri Krsna and many sages were told by Bhisma the story of a merchant, by name Tuladhara, expounding Dharma to a Brahmana ascetic, by name Jajali (12.254.9):

Sarvesam yah suhrnityam
Sarvesam ca hite ratah;

Karmana manasa vaca
Sadharmam veda jajal —

'That person understands Dharma who is always the friend of all beings, who is engaged in doing what is good for all, through action, thought, and speech. The health and medical personnel must do service to the people as they are meant to do good to suffering humanity. The people will worship them through thought and action. Doctors must feel solace in giving better life to the ailing humanity.[6]

H.H. Jagadguru in his book, "Acharya's call" beautifully suggests that those who want to serve others must limit their needs. To quote,

Bharthari hailed from the Malwa region of neighbouring Madhya Pradesh and lived over thirteen hundred years ago. Says he in his Nitisataka (Verse 64):

Ete satpurusah paraarthghatakah svarthan paritayajya ye
Samanyastu pararthamudyambhrta svarthavirodhena ye;
Te ime manavaraksasah parahitan svarthaya nighnanti ye,
Ye tu ghnanti nirarthakam parahitam t eke na janimahe . . .

"There are some sat-pursas, good people, who engage themselves in the good of others' sacrificing their own self-intesest; the samanyas, the generality of people, on the other hand, are those who engage themselves in the good of others so long as it does not involve the sacrifice of their own self-interest. There are those others, the manava-raksasas, devilish men, who sacrifice the good of others to gain their own selfish ends; but alas, what am I to do say of those who sacrifice the good of others without gaining thereby any good even to themselves or to anyone else." Doctors and paramedical staff should serve the common man without any personal interest. This will provide them extra energy and real happiness.

When USA was passing through a period of despondency and disillusion, Senator Paul Douglas remarked that:

"It is fortunate that there are in government large number of men and women who lead devoted lives of public service. They work extremely hard for far less pay than they could get in private industry. They never sell out the public interest but instead defend it with great difficulties. They do all this moreover, without receiving appreciable praise. They are generally either little known or actually ignored by the public. Sometimes, they are bitterly attacked by interests which are seeking to obtain unfair privileges or which are swayed by unfounded prejudices. These men and women are indeed unsung heroes, who deserve far more recognition than they receive.. Swami Vivekananda has put beautifully the ideals of service, which must be practiced by the medical experts.

"It is a great privilege for all of us to be allowed to do anything for the world; in helping the world we really help ourselves." To quote Enstein, "A hundred times every day I remind myself that my inner and outer life are based on the labours of other men, living and dead, and that I must exert myself in order to give in the same measure as I have received and am still receiving."

Medical profession must follow these examples of selfless service which can bestow upon them bliss and grace of almighty. The future of the medical profession is in the hands of its members who must strive for creativity, academic excellence, and the pursuit of excellence of service in their professional activities. Faith of the top administrators in performance would generate sufficient energy to get the co-operation of the entire staff in an organisation. In this way, we would be able to create a climate of creativity and optimum performance. Such a situation would have its chain effect. "Good organisation building has to create around it a bracing atmosphere, a prideful tradition of integrity, excellence and fellowship. Human beings breathe an ethos around them almost unconsciously, and these traditions make for that ethos."[7]

An attitude of dedication to the goals of an organisation should be an indispensable trait of the top leaders of health and medical profession. This is their primary qualification to operate and function effectively and efficiently to build self-confidence in themselves and in turn in the public. It is not just performing development-linked administrative duties; it is taking action and encouraging people to take action required to bring about structural change and growth in the economy. This needs to be supplemented by the leader's belief in the organisational goals.

Lal Bahadur Shastri National Academy of Administration, Mussorie and Department of Administrative Reforms and Public Grievances, Government of India, New Delhi, in International Workshop on good governance, New Delhi (30.11.2000 to 1.12.2000) stressed the role of values for good Leadership. To quote, "Value must be lived. Chosen well, they won't wear out from overuse. They will become more durable with time. Measure your efforts, and those of your people, by values. Promote those who operate in line with them. Reprimand or fire those who don't. Keep values in mind whenever you make a decision. Remind people often of the values and why they are important. Let them know, in every way you can, that the values are real and must be acknowledged in every organisational practice or policy."

Swami Chinmayananda rightly observes that in order to live and to bring out the maximum happiness from ourselves, to work out the best for ourselves, everyone of us must have a goal in life, a mission, an inspiring ideal; looking up to that ideal and bitching our eyes to it, we must work on in the world outside. Thereby, the work becomes chastened; the work itself become its own reward for the individual and a great joy wells up in his mind, not in terms of what he gets on the first of the month, but what he gives to the society as best as he can, from the place where he is.[8]

Let us explain the role of serving others with the help of medical profession.

Dr. H. Mahler is very critical about the inability of health workers in contemporary society to influence those social and environmental factors which truly determine public health. He states:

"There persist widespread negative attitudes among health professionals towards the health care of the poorest strata in the rural and urban population in the developing countries. Most of these attitudes imply-with a repetitiveness of an old gramophones records caught in a narrow, arrogant, condescending and indifferent groove—that these poor people are too apathetic, too superstitutious, too illiterate to benefit from the health care potentially availability to them. Health professionals and those who train them should be much more radicals in accepting a social responsibility for the health needs of the people in these poor rural-urban communities so that they can act as agents for change."[9]

"Thus, we can say that there is a need to train health administrators and workers in the new art of Public Health Administration so that they can take the benefits of the modern science to the common man and maintain the spirit of Geneva Declaration."[10]

Now being admitted to the profession of Medicine, I solemnly pledge to concentrate my life to the service of humanity. I will give respect and gratitude to my deserving teacher. I will practice medicine with conscience and dignity. The health and life of my patients will be my first consideration. I will hold in confidence all that my patients confides in me. I will maintain the honour and noble traditions of the medical profession. My colleagues will be my brothers. I will not permit considerations of race, religion, nationality, party politics or social standing to intervene between my duty and my patient. I will maintain the utmost respect of human life. Even under threat I will not use my knowledge contrary to the laws of humanity. These promises I make freely and upon my honour. The same feelings has been expressed in the Tokyo Declaration. To quote the preamble to the Declaration of Tokyo:

"It is the privilege of the medical doctor to practice medicine in the service of humanity, to preserve and restore bodily and mental health without distinction as to the persons to comforts and to ease the sufferings of his or her patients."[11]

Prof. J.S. Neki has rightly said in this connection that "to help, to heal, to reconstruct, to comfort-and all along the line' to act with compassion-all these bear testimony to the moral consciousness of the doctor. Whatever the new strains imposed upon medical ethics, this structure will survive and continue to guide doctors in their professional conduct. Legal and judicial obligations they have, of necessity, to fulfil. But these are not genuine ethics. Genuine ethics has to be ingrained into character and does not have to depend upon external controls.[12]

Swami Vivekanand stressed that if you want to find god, serve man, Gandhiji concern for self-less service can be seen when he says, "Recall the face of the poorest and the most helpless man whom you have seen and ask yourself, if the step you contemplate is going to be of any use to him to control over his own life and destiny. Civilization in the real sense of the term consists not in the multiplication, but in deliberate and voluntary reduction of wants. This only promotes real happiness and contentment and increase the capacity to service. True economics is the economics of justice.

Selfless service requires individuals to forget themselves and concentrate on society at large. To quote Swami Chinmayananda.

The life of harmony can be lied by rising above our limited egocentric view of things and happenings, and expanding our mind to accommodate a constant awareness of the totality of the world, the entirety of mankind and the vastness and wholeness of the universal problems. When the total and consummate perception is developed and maintained, man's individual problems sink into insignificance and absurdity, our life of harmony with the ampler scheme of the cosmos brings to our heart an inward peace and poise. When poise is maintained within us, problems and challenges vanish like mist before the rising sun.[13]

Medical profession is a good gift which should be employed to serve the poor, unprivileged and common man. This act would give peace and harmony to them. Swami Jagadatmananda beautifully explains: Another spirit that issues from a firm faith in the divine principle, is the spirit of service. Service may have become a worn out coin today. Selfish and weak men discredit every field they set their feet on. Christ said that we should not judge the quality of a tree by a rotten fruit. We should judge the importance and quality of service on the basis of its steady followers. Service is to be characterized by goodwill and selfless love for all. The spirit of service manifests itself when those who are at the topmost rungs of progress offer a helping hand to those who are on the lower rungs, masked and unsolicited. It expresses itself when advantages or gifts are shared with others or when one joins hands with others in accomplishing a common deed. Selfless love is the light of the divinity latent in every individual. It is manifest when we do good to others without expecting a reward in return. Service doesn't crave for flattery, it doesn't resort to the strategy of blowing its own trumpet, and it doesn't seek publicity or advertisement. Even a bit of work, sincerely done in one's small place, intended to bring about the general welfare, is service. The attitude and bent of mind behind the work are important, not the actual work done. The method of work is important. The intention behind the work is important. Each individual, by cultivating from faith in the divine spirit, and by trying to realize the spirit hidden within him will imbibe the virtues of wishing the good of all, patience, hope, industriousness and the spirit of service. Undoubtedly, these virtues lead to an all round development of the individual and a total development of the society.

If our studies environment, and education instill these qualities in us, our society will rise high. The moment we realize the unlimited energy within us, that very moment will herald the dawn of prosperity for all mankind.[14]

A hundred thousand men and women, fired with zeal of holiness, fortified with eternal faith in the Lord, and nerved to lion's courage by their sympathy for the poor and the fallen and downtrodden, will go over the length and breadth of the land, preaching the gospel of salvation, the gospel of help, the gospel of social raising-up, the gospel of equality. Then only will India awake, when hundreds of large-hearted men and women, giving up all desires of enjoying the luxuries of life, willing and exert themselves to their utmost, for the well-being of the millions of their Countrymen who are gradually sinking lower and lower in the vortex of destitution and ignorance.[15]

Swami Ranganathananda in his book, "Philosophy of Service" published by Advaita Ashrama, Kolkata, in 2003 has right observed that our country can come out of all types of crisis only through the spirit of selfless service. To quote him: Renunciation of the little self with a view to manifesting the higher self and the spirit of service are the twin ideals of India. In the wake of our great national renaissance of the last century, the country did inspire itself with this spirit of renunciation and service and threw bands and bands of dedicated workers in all parts of India for the cause of India's freedom and India's nation-building as a result of their contributions, the country became free and ended its centuries-long stagnation and slavery in 1947. Why we failed to continue in that great mood and temper thereafter is a mystery. It is amazing how our people, emerging from the darkness of their slavery of centuries to the light of freedom, could easily forget the lessons and warnings of their history and cease to be creative.

History is replete with instances of nations bursting with creative energy on emerging from a spell of political slavery. The classical example of this is Athens. When it succeeded, by united and sustained struggle, in defeating its Persian invaders and freeing itself from their brief but deeply galling yoke, Athenian democracy experienced an ecstasy of freedom which issued forth during the next fifty years in an outburst of creative activity in every department of its national life cultural, social, political and artistic—which has brightened not only its own but all subsequent Western history as well. Why did we fail to experience a similar sustained ecstasy of delight on the attainment of freedom, not after centuries of bondage, and why did we allow our creative centuries of bondage, and why did we allow our creative energies to dry up within a few brief years of independence? With the drying up of our creative spirit, we soon slipped back into our erstwhile stagnant ways, into moods of complacency and way of selfishness and self-centeredness. This is the tragedy of our brief post-independence. This is the tragedy of our brief post-independence history. And we have paid the price in shocks of military defeats, economic disasters, political disintegrations, and social upheavals. Whereas every one sought only his or her own happiness, no one is happy today.

Thus, there is a need to promote selfless service among health and medical experts so that they can transform India into a Welfare State. In the words of Swami Ranganathananda, "The subject of the philosophy of service, therefore, is not meant for academic discussion in the dull philosophy courses of our universities; it should stir the minds and hearts of every section of the population. It is thus, that the nation will get the necessary strength to meet the recurring challenges that this age of revolutionary transition will throw at it. If India succeeds in responding to these challenges adequately, he will become a beacon of hope not only to herself but also to the whole of humanity. We have responded successfully to many a challenge to our national existence and integrity in our long history. And we shall face and overcome this challenge as well. With this faith in ourselves and in our national destiny, let us, from this day onwards, enter our respective fields of life and activity with hope and courage"[16]

Mahatma Gandhi nicely observed, "Living the Gandhian life is supremely hard, for it means stripping oneself of all wants. The people at Sewagram and Sabarmati have made their own uneasy compromises with modernity, but what gives their lives meaning and purpose is that they continue along the Gandhian path. In doing so they remind us that there are higher goals than earning a livelihood, and that in serving our fellowmen, we may best serve ourselves."

Health and medical experts would find it rewarding if they engage themselves in selfless service through their expertise.

## Notes and References


1. Swami Ranganathananda, Democratic Administration in the Right of Practical Vedanta, Sri Ramakrishna Math, Mylapore, Chennai, 2003, p. (iii).
2. Swami Lokeswarananda, Practical Spirituality, Sri Ramakrishna Mission, Institute of Culture, Calcutta, 1995, pp. 95-96.
3. Swami Chinmayananda, We Must, *op. cit.*, p. 49.
4. Ram Parshad Gupta, Food For Thought, New Delhi, 1996, pp. 78-23.
5. The Complete Works of Swami Vivekananda, Vol. IV, p. 324.
6. Swami Ranganathananda, *op. cit.*, p. 246.
7. A.D. Moddie, The Brahamic Culture and Modernity, Asia Publishing House, New York, pp. 106-14.
8. Swami Chinmayananda, *Kindle Life, op. cit.*, p. 192.
9. Text of Address by Dr. H. Mahler, to the Thirteenth Session of Regional Committee of South-East Asia.
10. Geneva Declaration.
11. I swear by Apollo by Christian Viedma, *World Health*, July 1979, p. 28.
12. J.S. Niki, Medical Ethics, *World Health*, July 1979.
13. Swami Chinmayananda, *Kindle Life*, pp. 40-41.
14. Swami Jagadatmananda, *Learn to Live*, Vol. 1, pp. 255-56.
15. Swami Jagadatmananda, *Learn to Live*, Vol. 2, p. 8.
16. Swami Ranganathananda, *op. cit.*, p. 251.

**18**

**CHAPTER**

# Techniques to Promote Human Excellence and among Health and Medical Professionals

"Transformation of individuality into personality, thus, is an essential for spiritual growth—for the manifestation of all potentialities lying latent in the man. When this happens excellence naturally comes in its trail . . . Spiritual intelligence is always to be regarded as the supreme guide in all human exercises, because it is this spiritual intelligence that leads to fulfilment of human march, it is this spiritual growth, which enables the man to discharge his obligations to the community in an excellent manner."

— *Prof. Ramaranjan Mukherji*

Health and Medical professionals were highly respected in India. That respect and our surrounding medical profession is slowly dwindling as this profession is being equated like other business activities. Health and Medical professionals are today engaged in money making and that doctor who makes a huge money is equated with excellence which is totally baseless and irrelevant. Such medical professionals are cheats and a slur on the fair name of the profession. Health and medical professionals are basically educated to serve the ailing humanity and lessen the grief in the society. Today, in a hospital only personnel with money can get any facility and get top priority because they can pay money liberally to health and medical personnel. In the present times, the medical profession has bad reputation. This noble profession must achieve excellence which entails a number of qualities. Let us discuss these qualities.

We mention below the prerequisites, which can be developed through right education, to ensure holistic development of people and keep them away from modern influence of materialistic tendencies, that are responsible for stresses and strains and other mental problems We have to remember one thing today The maladies, difficulties and distress which mankind is facing throughout the world, are spiritual in nature That is why medical science has almost failed, that is why psychology has almost failed, that is why technological wealth and prosperity have almost failed that is why most civilized, organized disciplines and political orders have almost failed. Distress is related to the quality of his mind, it is related to the quality of his soul, it is related to the quality of his philosophy.

Dr. M. Lakshmi Kumari in her forward to Yoga in Education, Vol. I by Dr. H.R. Nagendra and Sri T. Mohan Swami Vivekananda Yoga Prakashan states that the aim of all education, undoubtedly, is the attainment of human excellence and perfection, not just in any field of knowledge or activity but life in totality. Education should be the means to fashion excellent characters out of the very ordinary human raw material. This means culturing of the qualities of head and heart in a way congenial to the growth and development of oneself and others around him. In practical life, this has to be translated as qualities of truthfulness, righteous living, purity in personal life, self-confidence, integration of body, mind and intellect, love and compassion towards all living beings and surrender to Almighty. These are steps leading to the unfolding of perfection, already existing in man. Such a truly educated and cultured man alone can meet the challenges, internal and external, in a positive way, converting them into opportunities, thus helping in his ultimate evolution. Pursued further, one's entire thought, behaviour and life itself would come to express the spiritual oneness of the creation and this would be the manifestation also of the divinity inherent in man. A truly educated man, like a true scientist, satisfied with nothing but the one truth, has to be necessarily spiritual as well.

Swami Vivekananda stressed on man-making and character-building through education. To quote him, "Education is not the amount of information that is put into your brain and runs riot there, undigested all your life. We must have life-building, man-making, character-making assimilation of ideals. We want education by which character is formed, strength of mind is increased, the intellect is expanded, by which one can stand on one's feet. What we want is Western science coupled with Vedanta, Brahmacharya as the guiding motto and also Shraddha and faith in one's own life. Education is the panacea for all the ills affecting us individually, socially and nationally.

The education as is obtained today is not at all aimed at character-building. As a result that we find even highly educated men, who have so much of power and service machinery at their command, failing miserably while tackling problems in the right way, in the human way, in the interest of our nation. Highly talented individuals are there in every field, second to none, but devoid of patriotic fervour and personal integrity, the impact they produce is minimal. Today, we are urgently in need of men and women of character, integrity and dedication and of tremendous capacities, happily blending dignity of man with dignity of labour.

In health and medical field, India has top most physicians. Surgeons and experts in other health and medical areas, but they lack integrity, character, mission of service resulting into poor health services.

Concentration of mind, its purity and chastity alone can bring out the amazing qualities and capacities that lie hidden in the health and medical experts. Lack of these has created a crowd of health and medical personnel who is debilitated, inhuman, selfish and indifferent to human values. Swami Vivekananda stresses the value of Shraddha, faith, as one of the most potent factors capable of elevating human life. He wanted this, "Life saving-great, ennobling, grand doctrine" to be taught to our children from their very birth. Where the different streams of consciousness in man, namely, concentration of mind, purity of life, faith in oneself, strength of body and fearlessness of mind are combined together in a single personality, the force of that character becomes invincible. Men of such stature alone can rebuild a shattered society. It is such men that our educational system should create to safely carry over our country through the 21st century. Such values must be practiced by our eminent and professional experts.

Excellence in general discussion is associated with outward manifestation and temporary achievement. However, the real definition of excellence is found in Ancient Sanskrit Literature which is permanent and based on spirituality. In advanced countries, people are following what is written in our scriptures and that is why they are developed materially while people in developing countries are not following their own ideas enshrined in Ancient Sanskrit Literature resulting in backwardness. However, the people in advanced countries concentrate only on material advancement which is causing imbalance in development. What is needed is to imbibe qualities of service to humanity along with material advancement to make this world a real place of enjoyment and bliss.

The medical and health experts must follow the ideas of excellence as were prevalent in ancient India and develop excellent health institutions based on excellent service. Excellence is not theory but must be exhibited by our excellent health care system.

Excellence consequently, is not a figment of imagination incapable of being achieved at any stage; it is a reality capable of being obtained through spiritual growth. And the prescription given by Sanskrit Literature on attainment of Excellence in all spheres is unique and is itself excellent. Human excellence is based on human strength and not human weakness. Swami Vivekananda was a great exponent of this view. Let us elaborate its components.

## I. CHARACTER

"Some say knowledge is power,
others say, the above is not true.
Character is power and wealth" —*Satya Sai Baba*

Excellent character is first and foremost quality of a man of excellence. It is very difficult to remain firm in character. We generally find unsteadfast health and medical personnel in day-to-day life. They are not steadfast. Let us quote an example: We find the wonderful character of Nachiketa in the Katha Upanisad; a boy of eleven years, but with what maturity! At such a tender age he wanted to know the Truth about man. He asked Yama and Lord of death (1.1.20):

'When a man dies there arises a doubt: some say that he exists; some others say that he does not which is right, I should like to know, being taught by you'. Nachiketa's question regarding this profound truth was like a bombshell to Yama: How could he impart this great truth to a mere boy? Instead of answering his question he tried his best to divert the boy mind by offering him tempting alternatives. He offered him plenty of wealth, sense enjoyments, progeny, a kingdom on earth But the boy stood firm he said:

"All these pleasures that you have offered, are transient. O Death, they also wear out the vigour of all the sense organs of mortal man. Moreover, all life, long or short is only little compared to eternal life. Let your chariots, dance and song remain with you only. All good character traits have a common denominator of social courage, usefulness common sense besides self-acceptance and self-confidence. Men of character may not be popular but they are respected and followed. They are true leaders of men and times. They will fight but not quarrel, differ but will not oppose or criticize, will be firm but not rigid, dogmatic, appreciate without flattery, cooperate without surrendering, self-confident but not self-important, cooperate, compromise and reconcile on non-essentials but put up a valiant, relentless fight for basic principles, act and never react. We need our health and medical experts to be men of character to make excellent health and medical institutions which can be second to none."[1]

## 2 USE OF INTELLECT

The man of excellence exercises his mental faculty to discriminate between real and unreal. He gets guidance from authoritative sources like the Ancient Sanskrit literature. Sri Krishna clearly says that even to perform work in the right spirit, one must exercise his intellectual faculty even a little work, done with the spirit of self-sacrifice and dedication, gives a sense of fulfilment. Therefore, intelligent people always choose the path of selfless work using their discriminative faculty. To work and yet to be free from the effects of work requires subtle understanding of the secret of work and such understanding comes from Buddhi. Sri Krishna says in the Bhagavad-Gita (2.39). Being endowed with such intellect you will get rid of the bondage of actions, O partha, Discrimination between the real and the unreal is called 'Viveka'. Buddhi alone has the capacity to determine the real nature of an object. In the path of knowledge, the aspirant- has to realize the Truth by constant reasoning. Sankaracharya emphasizes this view in the Viveka Chaudamani (Verse: 16)

An intelligent and learned man skilled in arguing in favour of the Scriptures is the recipient of the knowledge of the Atman.[2] Health and Medical experts must follow their intellect so that they can achieve excellence in their professions and make the institutions in which they are working excellent.

### 3. POSITIVE ATTITUDE

The person of excellence should develop positive attitude and firm faith in himself and the scriptures This will create respect towards scriptures and such a person would welcome challenges and solve them intelligently.

An health experts with a positive attitude does not like an easy going life. He welcomes challenges, obstacles, difficulties, problems and faces them with great courage. He always likes an adventure in life. Such heroic spirit is a quality needed to become a successful health experts. Such health experts alone can lead the society who has developed a positive intellect Shakaracharya defined this attitude in the Viveka Chudamani (Verse 25). 'The firm conviction that the words of the scriptures and the Guru are true is called shraddha, by which the Real is attained.[3]

### 4. SELFLESSNESS

Health and Medical experts of excellence do not believe in their own welfare and development. They are keen to promote the welfare of all as in their welfare lies his own welfare. In Mahabharata, the Victory of Pandavas was because, the persons on their side were highly skilled, spiritual and desireless while on the other side that is Kauravas were desirous of usurping the territory of legal heirs. Ram Rajya in Ramayana was based on the Character of Ram and his brothers

When we pray for the welfare of others, all our petty and selfish feelings will go away and our intellect will expand. There are many such prayers in the Vedas and the Puranas, such as:

May all be happy, may all be free from disease, may all realize what is good, may none be subject to misery.[4] Patanjali Yoga Sutras, Chapter 2, Sloka 4 says that Ignorance creates all other obstacles. They may exist either in potential or a Vestical form or they may have been temporarily overcome or fully developed Patanjali Yoga Sutras, Chapter 1, Sloka 30 says that sickness, mental laziness, doubt, lack of enthusiasm, sloth, craving for sense pleasure, false perception, despair caused by failure to concentrate and unsteady in concentration, these distractions are the obstacles to knowledge

Mahayana Buddhism makes out that the Buddhas appear on earth for the redemption of mankind, "The exalted one appears in the world for salvation to many people, for joy to many people, out of compassion for the world, as a blessing, as a salvation, as the joy of Gods and men." The excellence therefore is not purely for brightening one's life but it is to help other people in this world to achieve salvation. (Sadharma Pundarika, XV)

Excellence for health and medical personnel cannot be exhibited by merely qualifications and a lot of wealth but depends upon their sincere and dedicated services to patients. The test of excellences is service to patients selflessly.

## 5. PURSUIT OF KNOWLEDGE

A man of excellence is keen to pursue knowledge as knowledge is power A person is great not because of money but because of knowledge. Knowledge alone can remove ignorance. A beautiful verse in Chanakya Niti (XV1147) says 'What distinguishes a man from an animal is his capacity to acquire knowledge. Without knowledge men are equal to animals'. There is a popular saying:

'The King is honoured only in his kingdom whereas a learned person is honoured everywhere'.[5] In this context, it may be of interest to note that without the expert trainers and desirous trainees, there can be no knowledge. Knowledge depends both on the teacher and taught. There is no purifier as great as Knowledge, he who has attained purity of heart through a prolonged practice of Karmayoga automatically sees the light to Truth in the self in course of time.

There is nothing that can replace the special intelligence that a worker has about the workplace. No matter how smart a boss is or how great a leader, he/she will fail miserably in tapping the potential of employees by working against employees instead of with them.

—Ronald Cantmo, former Deputy Commissioner,
New York City Sanitation Department

Excellence demands constant hard work on the part of medical experts. The excellence of health and medical experts is not a one time activity. The Disciplines of medical sciences are growing. There is a need of constant need of gaining knowledge otherwise he may not remain excellence.

## 6. SELF-RESTRAINT

A man of excellence understands that all life is a continuous struggle with temptation and evil which can be avoided by a disciplined life Neither by work, nor through progeny nor through wealth but by renunciation alone is life eternal reached (Mahanarayana Upanisad VIII 14.) Sacrifice of self is the best sacrifice by speculative knowledge, we come nearer to the gates of reality but we cannot approach Truth by means of thought alone. It can be reached only through the perfection of the whole human nature, we must practice the tortures of body, mind and spirit. The control of passions means transmutation into spiritual energy and bliss. This state of poise can be attained only by vigorous practice. Those health and medical experts who have detained a state of mind which spure can do a first rate job and do miracles. They work with deep conception.

## 7. PERFORMANCE OF ONE'S DUTY WITHOUT ATTACHMENT

Therefore, go on efficiently doing your duty without attachment. By doing work without attachment man attains the Supreme, i.e. excellence. Renunciation of attachment implies renunciation of desire as well for it is from attachment that desire springs up (II 62). It is, therefore, that renunciation of the desire for fruit has not been separately mentioned. People who become attached to senses, they cannot achieve excellence. They become slaves of their senses. Health and medical personnel must carry out their duties without any monetary considerations or other benefits. They must work with quality as work in its own reward. Those medical experts who work for selfish motives go down in their own eyes and cannot achieve excellence.

They should work without having any personal interest. The man dwelling on sense objects develops attachment for them, from attachment springs up desire and from desire (unfulfiled) ensues anger. Sri Krishna explains Yoga as balance of mind (Chap II 48) When an action is motivated by desire, anxiety as to whether the desired result is going to be obtained or not will surely disturb the peace of mind of the doer Again, when an action is inspired by self-interest, the doer is likely to lose sight of what is right or what is wrong even when he has chosen to do the right thing undue eagerness for obtaining the result is likely to make him swerve from the path of rectitude, whereas a doer, if he is detached towards the result, is saved from all anxiety There is nothing to divert him from the righteous path This teaching that we ought to discharge our obligations, social or otherwise, with a sense of responsibility, at the same time banishing from our minds all thought of obtaining personal benefit therefrom and in a spirit of dedication to the Lord is what is meant by Karma-Yoga.[6]

By constantly dwelling on objects of enjoyment man develops an intensive form of attachment for them. This awakens in his mind a keen desire to obtained various forms of enjoyment. This is what is meant by attachment giving rise to desire. And when some hindrance appears in the fulfilment of this desire, he develops hatred for the cause of this hindrance, and the hatred is transformed into anger. This is what is meant by desire producing anger. Anger causes stress and poor mental status.

Neither think yourself as actor, because no actor can attempt to do anything. Discharge whatever is your duty, and remain at your ease with having done your part. (Yoga Vasistha Utpatti-Prakarana, Book 3) If you want to secure real happiness, then renounce all. By so renouncing you will secure happiness infinitely greater than what you could have had through your property. You can enjoy more as you will remain stress free.

The essential nature of true penance is not to possess anything. Nothing even a single thing will bring back the delusion of property. Only those who have completely renounced will reach the highest goal of life, Moksha the others still with the delusion get entangled in the net of Samsara with all the mental problems associated with it.

Health and medical experts must remain busy in their profession with total dedication and thus helping the ailing humanity to promote good health without consideration of any monetary or other benefits. This would keep the medical experts in equilibrium otherwise, their mind would remain disturbed.

The object of Gita is to discover a golden mean between the two ideals of action and contemplation, preserving the merits of both Karma-yoga is that golden mean in which the merits of both the ideals are happily integrated. It advocates a life of activity with detachment as guiding spirit and one's spiritual unfoldment as the goal of one's activities. Thus it discards neither ideal but by integrating the spirit of renunciation of the one and the activism of the other, it purifies and elevates man. This fusion of the two ideals in Karma-yoga gives due regard to social welfare on the one hand and the other leads an individual to the fulfilment of his spirit aspirations. Thus the Gita ignores neither the society nor the individual It does not advocate life of inaction but instead recommends a life of intense action in which self is effaced in all aspects[7] (*Ibid.*, pp. 25-26). The first verse of the Isa Upanisad says:

All the changing things and events of this world have to be covered with Isa (God—the Supreme Reality). Live your life in a spirit of non-attachment. Don't crave for possessions which are not yours.[8] The Chandogya Upanisad, for example, prescribes:

All this is Brahman Meditate calmly on Him as the One from whom everything is born by whom everything is maintained and annihilated.[9] Such feelings would develop integrated personalities free from all modern ailments—anxiety, fear, tension, stress, etc.

## 8. HONESTY

Therefore, so long as while performing actions or enjoying their fruit, a participant found to have the feeling of possession and desire with regard to those actions and their fruit or so long as his mind is subject to morbid feelings such as attraction and repulsion, grief, etc. it should be clearly understood that all his actions have not been dedicated to god.

Pt. Jawaharlal Nehru, while addressing the Fourth Annual General Body Meeting Indian Institute of Public Administration, appropriately remarked that: "In a period of dynamic growth, however, we want as civil servants—persons who are not, if I may use the word without any disrespect, merely head clerks but people with minds, people with vision, people with desire to achieve, who have some initiative for doing a job and who can think how to do it. But, the person who is to be completely neutral is a head clerk and no more. He would do his work efficiently as a head clerk, no doubt but nothing more. Can a person be neutral, I ask you, about basic things which we stand for, our state stands for, our plan stands for, e.g. a socialist pattern of society."[10]

The health and medical experts must work with honesty of purpose and sincerity. They should be honest in their duties otherwise patients would have no confidence in him. Honesty, which is the most essential ingredient of excellence. He says that: Honesty is another essential quality like patience. Honesty is a great force. Honesty means integration of the three aspects of personality, thought, speech and deed. For instance, when you give a promise to the workers, honesty demands that you act accordingly or at least make a sincere attempt to act according to the promise. Otherwise it is dishonesty or deceit. A victim of deception does not easily forget the humiliation, or shock that he has felt. It explodes—one day or the other, in some form or the other. If it doesn't explode it remains simmering within. Honesty can win the hearts of men Though one may not be able to fulfil one's promise or keep one's word, if the effort is sincere, it has its value, it will earn respect, it will have a good effect.

The medical experts should dedicate their whole energy upon the task on which they are engaged to optimise the results. This would be beneficial as both medical experts and patients can lead a life of harmony and not conflict.

True, that spiritual illumination shines of itself in a pure heart, and as such, it is not something acquired from without; but to attain this purity of heart means long struggle and constant practice, has also been found, on careful enquiry in the sphere of material knowledge, that those higher truths which have now and then been discovered by great scientific men, have flashed like sudden floods of light in their mental atmosphere, which they had only to catch and formulate. But such truths never appear in the mind of an uncultured and wild savage. All these go to prove that hard Tapasya, or practice of austerities, in the shape of devout contemplation and constant study of a subject, is at the root of all illumination, in its respective spheres.[11]

Men should act according to buddhi or understanding. If we are victims of our impulses, our life is as aimless and devoid of intelligence as that of the animals. If we do not interfere, attachments and aversions will determine our acts. So long as we act in certain ways because we like them and abstain from others because we dislike them, we will be bound by our actions. But if we overcome these impulses and act from a sense of duty, we are not victims of the play of prakrti. The exercise of human freedom is conditioned and not cancelled by the necessities of nature.[12] Health and medical professionals should practice through pure hearts to achieve excellence.

## 9. ACTION ORIENTATION

Mere accumulation of knowledge would be of no use unless put to action. The Yoga of Knowledge and the Yoga of Action both lead to supreme Bliss. Of the two, however the Yoga of Action (being easier to practice) is superior to the Yoga of Knowledge. A person who possesses all other powers but is wanting in the power of action will not be appreciated as a desirable person by the world at large. Dr. Radha Krishna says that there is more happiness in doing one s own work even without excellence than in doing another's duty well. Each one must try to understand his psycho-physical make-up and function in accordance with it. It may not be given to all of us to lay the foundations of systems of metaphysics or clothe lofty thoughts in enduring words. We have not all the same gifts, but what is vital is not whether we are endowed with five talents or .only one but how faithfully we have employed the trust committed to us. We must play our part, manfully, be it great or small. Goodness denotes perfection of quality. However distasteful one's duty may be, one must be faithful to it even unto death.[13]

Whatever result a persons intends to achieve he may succeed in realising it according to his idea provided he pursues his end with a steadfastness of will. In executing an action that is clearly discerned to be the right one, the adequate course must be pursued with the steadfast will without hesitation or procrastination.

Swami Jagadatmanarda in his book, "Learn to Live", Vol. I, rightly says: Instability and indecision mark the state of mind which is not subject to any discipline The energies of an undisciplined mind are scattered in many directions and are wasted. A person with an unsteady mind can not achieve any thing worthwhile. By doing all work big or small, with concentration and methodicity, one gathers the ability to work with efficiency and ease."[14] Thus health and medical professionals must implement their knowledge for the welfare of the society.

## 10. CONTROL OVER SENSES TO AVOID ANY TEMPTATION TO DO WRONG ACTIONS

The Karmayogi, who has fully conquered his mind and mastered his senses, whose heart is pure, and who has identified himself with the Self of all beings, remains untainted, even though performing action. So long as one's mind and senses are not controlled, they naturally run after sense enjoyments; and so long as impurities in the form of likes and dislikes exist in the mind. It is difficult to remain equipoised in success and failure. Hence, until the mind and senses are fully controlled and perfect purity of heart is attained one, cannot be called a real Karmayogi. Medical experts must be Karmoyogi and should not bow before their sensual pleasures.

## 11. LOVE AND AFFECTION FOR PEOPLE TO ACHIEVE PEACE

Happiness on earth and bliss above are certainly the fruits of living the life of love. The changeless abode of the soul is reached by the path of love. Those that are devoid of love are just the skeleton covered with skin. The journey of this world is delightful to one, who after the removal of his errors and dispersion of the cloud of his ignorance, has come to the knowledge of truth.

In Isavasya Upanisad, Sloka 6 it has been advised that the wise man who perceives all beings as not distinct from his own self at all and his own self as the self of everything, he does not by virtue of that perception hate anyone. Love and emotions are a great strength and source of tremendous power. Swami Vivekananda has beautifully put, "If there is a conflict between the intellect and the heart, always follow heart", the above mentioned teaching has to be perfected through constant use to achieve excellence. To quote Swamiji again, "various feelings in the human heart are not wrong in themselves; only they have to be carefully controlled and given a higher direction, until they attain the very highest condition of excellence."[15]

## 12. SPIRIT OF SERVICE

The essence of the spirit of service is contained in the following words of Vivekananda: "This is the gist of all worship—to be pure and to do good to others. He who sees Shiva in the poor, in the weak, and in the diseased, really worships Shiva; and if he sees Shiva only in the image, his worship is but preliminary. He who has served and helped one poor man seeing Shiva in him, without thinking of his caste, or creed, or race, or anything, with him Shiva is more pleased than with the man who sees Him only in the temples. He who wants to serve the father must serve the children first. He who wants to serve Shiva must serve His children and must serve all creatures in the world first."[16]

## 13. POWER OF REASONING

We are to take care of ourselves—that much we can do—and give up attending to others; for a time. Let us perfect the means; the end will take care of itself. For the world can be good and pure, only if our lives are good and pure. It is an effect, and we are the means. Therefore, let us purify ourselves. Let us make ourselves perfect. Besides we should always remember that we have no separate identity.

Man, therefore, according to Vedanta philosophy, is the greatest being that is in the universe, and this world of work the best place in it, because only herein is the greatest and the best chance for him to become perfect. Angels or gods, whatever you may call them, have all to become men, if they want to become perfect. This is the great center, the wonderful poise, and the wonderful opportunity—this human life.

Reason is the lamp to show us the right and wrong, and the instrument for accomplishment of our desires: by reliance on right reason, one crosses over easily the wide ocean of the world.

## 14. WILL POWER

Medical experts should follow that good will, power and patience are basic to personality development. Both provide fibre and tone to it. Will is the motive power, driving force and patience is the period over which this force works to develop character.

All human endeavors achievements require minimum necessary time to mature and fulfil. Impatience only wastes vital energy, tires, confuses, sickens and impairs our will power. Our personality does not register on others if we are impatient with them who can benefit or be friend you without your giving him time.[17]

## CONCLUSION

Dr. S.S. Gupta has rightly said that our Rishis were social scientists par excellence and their social science included all the disciplines. Dr. Gupta suggests the following to improve human excellence:[18]

(i) The individual is the central point of the society and also the nation. So there should not be any scope of a conflict between interests of individuals, the society and the nation. There should be complete homogeneity and uniformity among the three. In the western thought this uniformity and homogeneity is missing. In socialist literature conflict is an essential ingredient.

(ii) That life is one whole. It should not be divided into watertight independent segments like social, political, economic, etc. By doing so, an invitation is given to tensions and split of life which will become competitive instead of complementary.

(iii) That the perfect coherence between individuals, between different segments of life and between individuals and these segments is possible when the guiding principles for fundamentals of all are same and not different. Today we find different guiding principles of all these segments of life leading to competition and conflicts among them. This is causing growing tensions in individuals and their split personalities.

(iv) That the guiding principles of the entire life, which can promote simultaneously, the happiness of individuals, the whole society and the world, should be natural, scientific and achievable. The Rishis-*cum*-Social Scientist of India gradually developed them and called them human-values or social values such as truth, simplicity, self-control, purity, non-stealing, non-anger. The number of these basic principles was not static. It went on changing as per the needs of time and new researches.

(v) That the sum total of these guiding principles will be called Dharma, which is distinct from the rituals of religion. It is unfortunate that today people, specially the politicians and even so-called scholars do not understand the meaning of Dharma and confuse it with religion. The ancient Rishis-*cum*-Social Scientists gave multi- dimensional meaning to Dharma. One important meaning was that every thing has a nature, i.e. Dharma. For example, fire has a Dharma (Nature) to burn and air has a Dharma to blow. Similarly, the Dharma of the people of the world should be these basic Human-values. So, by Dharma, they meant a code of conduct. Certainly, this is not Religion. Medical Experts must follow their Dharma, i.e. Service to ailing humanity.

To a person
Who is thoughtless, and
Negligent of Duties,
His enormous wealth
And Property
Will be of no value .

—*The Thirukkural*

## Notes and References


1. Walter R. Sharp, Field Administration in the United Nations System, London, 1961, p. 19.
2. Prof. Ramarajan Mukherji, Sanskrit and Human Excellence, in Souvenir, ed. Prof. Vachaspati Upadhyaya, World Sanskrit Conference, 5-9 April 2001, New Delhi, Stolri Lal Bahadur Shastri Rashtriya Sanskrit Vidyapeeth, pp. 14-16.
3. Complete Works of Swami Vivekananda, Vol. 111, p. 237.
4. *Ibid.*, Vol. II, p. 3.
5. *Ibid.*, p. 225.
6. Swami Vijaynanda, Gita on Karma Yoga, in *Yoga: Its Various Aspects*, Sri Ramakrishna Math, Madras; pp. 24-25.
7. *Ibid.*, pp. 25-26.
8. Isha Upanisad, 1.1.
9. Chondogya Upanisad, 3.4.1.
10. V. Jaganadham, Jawaharlal Nehru and Public Administration, *IJPA*, New Delhi, 1975.
11. Verinder Grover, Swami Vivekananda, A Biography of his Vision and Ideas, Deep & Deep, New Delhi, 1998, p. 114.
12. S. Radhakrishnan, The Bhagavad Gita, Harper Collins, New Delhi, 1996, p. 146.
13. *Ibid.*, p. 147.
14. Swami Jagadatmananda, Learn to Live, Vol. I, Chennai, Shri Ramakrishna Math, pp. 106-7
15. Complete Works of Swami Vivekananda, 1965 (ed.), Vol. 11, p. 78.
16. Ram Parshad Gupta, Food for Thought, New Delhi, 1996, pp. 18-23.
17. The Complete Works of Swami Vivekananda, Vol. IV, p. 324.
18. S.S. Gupta, *op. cit.*, pp. 159-60.

19

CHAPTER

# Modernizing Health Administration

## A. NEED AND NATURE OF MANAGEMENT IMPROVEMENT

People in advanced countries get their health services as much for granted as the essential utility services like water, electricity, public transport, etc. Despite the magic bullets of the modern medicine, the health services in the developing countries are far from satisfactory. The people living in the developing world, and especially 75 per cent of them living in rural areas, have little or no access to modern medical and health care resulting in high rates of morbidity and mortality from diseases which are preventable. If we want to reach the objective of providing decent quality health care to all by the first quarter of 21st century. We will have to introduce innovations in technical and administrative fields. It has been recognized by health experts in all the countries that the difficulties in meeting the health needs of the community are largely dependent upon the capabilities to design and manage the health care delivery system. The management of health care system can help in the greater achievement of goals through the optimum utilization of resources available—Men, Money and Material.

To quote Dr. Chi-Yuen Wu of UNDP:

> "To create administrative capabilities, commensurate with requirements, developing countries must be able among other things to use modern management techniques more, effectively than in the case of the industrially advanced countries."

Joginder Singh in his article, "Reducing Government Flab-Time to Drain the Swamp" in *Tribune* (March 16, 2000) rightly observes that it is amazing that the government is always emphasising on its employees to function with full coordination and assist the citizens with the quickest possible response. Notwithstanding all the Instructions/orders of the government, the position on the ground remains anything but people-oriented. The responsiveness of the administration to the people who matter is individual-oriented. There is hardly any response where the common good matters, unless powerful interests back it.

The need of the hour for our country, burdened with poverty, illiteracy, backwardness and rampant corruption, is effective and dynamic governance. Good governance and effective management can provide the panacea for all the ills and stumbling blocks in the system. Transformation of the country is possible only when the necessary changes are brought about. We need a revolution of a different kind led by the right-thinking and right-acting leaders, who should not only prepare but also implement a blueprint for future development in a fixed time schedule.

Unfortunately, present management systems are not functioning well as these are managed by untrained personnel. This is the common management challenge faced by those in charge of the health services. To quote a recently published book:[1]

> "In the field of health, we rarely have consciously trained executives. We have expected a vast army of professional care givers to fill individual human needs, mainly on a *laissez faire* basis, mostly without planning without coordination, without sufficient for (those) who either do not look for care, cannot afford it or cannot get to it."
> "With little or no formal training. Administrators . . . have arisen from our midst willy-nilly, too few through natural ability, too many by virtue of their staying-power on particular job, lack of available competition, or the administrator's uncritical need for power and control...."
> "In health administration, there are few theoreticians, few training centres. Few books, and an almost absolute dearth of strict scientific investigations."

Thus, there is a great need to improve the functioni of health care management with the help of modern management techniques. A modern management system is one which is designed to make the existing health care delivery process effective and efficient modern management methods and techniques are in reality, only techniques for improving this process by making it more accurate and reliable, by making the process respond faster, or by giving the health-manager the ability and capability to manage better.

Health administration in a country is a part of the total administration, and thus influences and is influenced by this general administrative culture. Let us have a look at the general administrative apparatus prevailing in developing countries. In India, for instance, the administrative machinery has not been adequate to handle the tasks of economic and social development. The administrative inadequacies in a national government has a retarding influence on economic and social development. This lack of efficiency in administration equally holds good for the health organisations as well. The widespread feeling of inefficiency of the administrative machinery was rightly sensed and expressed by Mrs. Gandhi in a broadcast to the nation shortly after assuming the high office of the Prime Minister. She said:

> "In economic development as in other fields of national activity, there is a disconcerting gap between intention and action. To bridge this gap, we should boldly adopt whatever far-reaching changes in administration may be found necessary. We must introduce new organisational patterns and modern tools and techniques of management and administration. We shall instil into the government machinery, greater efficiency and sense of urgency and make it more responsive to the needs of the people."[2]

In the health sector, it was emphasized that "better management of health services is essential if higher standards of health care are to be achieved . . . that progress. . . . today is to a higher extent dependent on education and development of the management, than it is on medical research and increase of material resources."[3]

The development of public administration remains an essential prerequisite for successful economic development of the country. Therefore, far-reaching improvements in public administration are required if the objectives of planned socio-economic development are to be realised.

Before we analyse the meaning, nature, scope and application of management techniques for administrative improvements and reforms let us be clear about the concept of administrative improvement first.

Administrative improvement means the act or the process of improving the administration. As stated in a United Nations Report: "Management improvement comprised the planning, implementation and evaluation of various measures conducive to the increase of organisational effectiveness and efficiency."[4]

Administrative reform is still widely regarded as a special type of improvement activity, even when it is often closely connected with other activities. The concept of the "administrative reform", as it is applied in practice, also has its weakness. In a report by the Secretariat of the United Nations Programme in Public Administration for the period from 1950 to 1966, it is stated that: "Efforts at administrative reform too often stop with the preparation of reports or promulgation of law."[5]

In a number of countries the word 'reform' has also a close relationship to political concepts and attitudes, which makes it less suited for general use than the broader concept of 'improvement' or 'effectiveness'.

Public administration in any country cannot remain static over a period of time. There are always scientific, economic, political, social, cultural and other changes taking place in a country. Health organisations like other organisations, must adjust themselves to these changes in order to be effective and responsive to the needs of the people. Peter Drucker, an expert in the field of management has said: "Social awareness is organisational self-interest. The needs of the society, if left unfilled, turn into social diseases. No institution whether business or hospital or University or Government agency is likely to survive in a diseased society."

The design of an administrative system is a basic aid to the achievement of its primary objectives; if the design is unsound, the achievement of objectives is likely to fall short of expectations. Therefore, there is a great need to improve the structure and functioning of the administrative organisations.

Most of the economic and social progress in the developing countries is halted because the administrative apparatus in these countries is not upto the mark. Therefore, there is an urgent need of administrative improvement in these countries. H. Paul Appleby has rightly remarked that the full success of the plan, therefore, turns rather exclusively on administrative reform to make the government as an organism equal to its identified goals.

The administrative capability of a Government and the manner in which the development programmes are likely to be carried out are intimately related. On the other hand, administrative inadequacies in a national Government have a retarding influence on economic and social development. These deficiencies prevent the vast flood of money, talent and material from achieving their objectives. As early as 1950, the Secretary General of the United Nations pointed out that, "Any systematic effort towards economic development must be preceded by or coupled with efforts to make more effective the functioning of Government machinery."[6]

During the last few decades, phenomenal changes are taking place at a fast rate in the field of science and technology as well as administration also, which today, has to shoulder multifarious task designed to fulfil the rising aspirations of the people. In the words of Prof. Waldo, Public Administration is, "a part of the cultural complex, and it not only is acted upon, it acts." It is a great creative force. There is an urgent need to re-orient (improve) the system of public administration to cope with changes in technology and social behaviour and maximise opportunities for raising productivity, and thus the standard of living of the people.

According to Sir Isaiah Berlin, "It is certainly a reasonable hypothesis that one of the principal causes of confusion, misery and fear is blind adherence to outworn notions, pathological suspicion of any form of critical examination, frantic efforts to prevent any degree of rational analysis of what we believe, we live by and for."

Thus, public administration including health administration must be recreated, renewed and revitalised to produce the predesigned changes and output in the modernization of societies. This necessitates a different trend and magnitude of administrative culture and capability.

## SCOPE OF MANAGEMENT IMPROVEMENT

If the need for change and effectiveness is to be fulfiled, management improvement must be considered to be an organisation-wide continuous activity. This important function must embrace the total needs based on the objectives and goals of the public administration and the resources available. The improvement efforts must be regarded as a whole involving a spectrum of different types and levels of activity. There is, in principle, no reason why 'administrative reform' and 'organisation and methods' should be set-up as separate and isolated activities. These and other new activities should rather be merged and coordinated into a total, carefully planned and organized 'management improvement programme', involving the whole organisation. The needs require centrally planned improvement programme, and for coordination purposes decentralized programmes in different ministries and institutions. Each agency or institution of importance should be responsible for its own programme, planned in cooperation with the central authorities.

As the implementation of significant changes in organisational structure and behaviour is complex and time-consuming task and is closely related to the long-term development planning of the country, improvement programme must be planned on long-term (from ten to fifteen years), medium-term (from four to five years) and short-term, (yearly) basis.

## STRATEGIES AND POLICIES IN ADMINISTRATIVE IMPROVEMENT

As stated in a UN publication[7] the following strategies and policies are necessary to bring about administrative improvement:

(a) Improvement work must be a systematically planned organized activity with specific work programmes, a continuous activity, and it should be based on long-term planning and development.
(b) Classification of objectives and goals is necessary to be able to measure or evaluate the effectiveness and manage the improvement work.
(c) Improvement work must be recognised as a responsibility of the management; and in planning and organising improvement projects, participation and involvement of management in the organisations affected by possible changes are of great importance.
(d) Special resources must be allocated to the improvement projects including the support of professional staff of high quality with special qualifications in the management fields.
(e) Improvement work must be based on the concept or the organisation as a socio-technical system where human and social factors are of primary importance.
(f) Training and development of the members of organisations—

both management and staff, usually constitute one of the most important parts of improvement work.

(g) Improvement projects should from the beginning be oriented towards implementation and change, step by step, and not only towards writing reports and giving recommendations. Such projects should include specific implementation plans.

(h) As a rule, there is need for both centralised and decentralized (though coordinated) improvement programmes. It is advisable first to build up a strong, central activity.

(i) An improvement work programme should be formalised as an obligation for the public administration institutions and tied with long-term development plans, and budgeting and accounting control procedures.

(j) The improvement project organisation should be flexible. A task force, under a responsible project leader and a Steering Committee is often a usual type of organisation.

(k) In larger projects, pilot studies of the implementation of new organisational structures in a limited part of the administration are often necessary and useful to demonstrate effects and results.

(l) Improvement projects must be planned in terms of activities, time and resources. The setting of deadlines or time-limits in the work programmes has frequently proved most helpful in the effort to obtain a high level activity and results.

After explaining the concept of administrative improvements, let us discuss the need, type and utility of management techniques as an instrument of administrative improvements and reforms.

## B. NEED FOR MANAGEMENT TECHNIQUES

In a developing country, such as ours, there is a great haste to achieve maximum growth and progress in the shortest time possible. It is felt that the scope of experimentation is a costly and slow process.

As such, we need to learn from the experience of others and use their results to help achieve our goals. A word of caution at this point is in order. Nothing succeeds like success. So too is the case of the glamorous instances of technology and management techniques and their tall claims of progress and development. Such a philosophy has done more harm than good. A few years before, modern management techniques were thought to be a panacea for all problems. Some problems did get solved while a host of others took birth as a result; many of the over popular techniques have found their graveyards whilst a lot of organisations which should have gone to the graveyards for not putting into use the 'over popular' techniques, have passed the test of time and resistance. In this context, Ernest Dale and L.C. Michelon observes that:

"Today's manager lives in a world of rapid change, and yet the rate of change is likely to increase in the years ahead. Unless, he can keep up with this change, he is likely to find himself obsolete—perhaps unpromotable or even unemployable."[8]

Thus, there is a great need to enhance the administrative capability of health administrators so that they can use these techniques profitably. Administrative capability is an important means of converting or processing programme inputs into outputs such as goods and services.

It has been mentioned by Gabriel that, "What makes the leadership variable so crucial in implementation process, is its dynamic, not passive quality, i.e. its capability to act and react on these critical inputs. It is this manipulative and transferring quality of leadership that could significantly determine the administrative capability of implementing organisation."[9] Administrative capability is "the capacity to obtain intended results through organisations."[10]

Katz says, "Administrative capability for development involves the ability to mobilize, allocate and combine the actions that are technically needed to achieve development objectives."[11]

Organisations are not simply structures but action-oriented system and the success and failure of the organisations are to be measured in terms of this action system. Action system is a structured device in which resources are mobilized and transformed by use of certain skill and technology to produce pre-designed output all taking place by the influence of administrative capability within an environmental context.

Health administrators should facilitate the accomplishment of desired objectives with the least friction and the most satisfaction to those for whom the task is done and those engaged in the enterprise, as has been shown in the Chart 19.1.

CHART 19.1

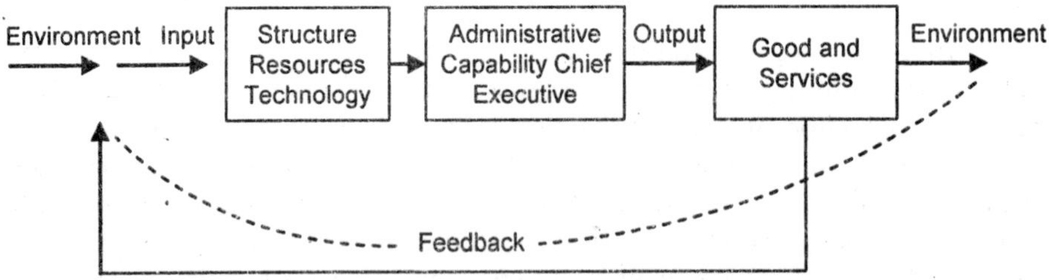


Thus, there is a need to understand and portray the management techniques in all its various facets. Management techniques are of added significance for the health sector as this sector deals with preventive, promotive, curative and rehabilitative aspects of health care activities and uses the services of Government, private and voluntary agencies. Most of the practitioners, academicians and political elite are not happy with the performance of this sector as the majority of people in the developing world do not have access even to rudimentary health care. After personal discussions with some of the health experts and top management of health personnel at Chandigarh, it was revealed that the present administration was in a bad state and needed radical reforms. It was confirmed by personal visits to some of the health institutions and their field establishments, as also by the health and medical personnel at District and Block levels. This is resulting in huge wastage of resources. There have been a large number of administrative problems which account for the unsatisfactory working of the health administration. These problems have already been examined in the earlier chapters. Some of the specific problems which need immediate solutions can be mentioned as:

(a) Absence of effective and time bound health policy to meet the needs of the people.
(b) Absence of coordination between the health and socio-economic sector; between Western and Indigenous system of medicine and among Government, Private and Voluntary administration.
(c) Lack of effective planning, monitoring, implementation and evaluation machinery.
(d) Lack of an effective manpower planning resulting in the concentration of health services in the urban sectors.
(e) Absence of people's participation in the health care delivery operations.
(f) Absence of decentralisation resulting in inefficiency of operations.
(g) Disproportionate investments for secondary and tertiary health care.
(h) Top heavy administrative set-up.
(i) Defective organisations and procedure—an obstacle in the way of efficient services.
(j) Lack of interest to improve administrative structure and procedure, i.e. absence of innovative leadership.

In reviewing the management of health services, the delegates who came to attend the 25th Regional Committee meeting of the South-East Asia Region of WHO, noted the following considerations and constraints."[12]

(a) lack of a clear development policy and clear objectives for health services in relation to socio-economic development;
(b) inadequate understanding of health problems and the problem of tackling it from the viewpoint of consumers and providers of health care;
(c) poor utilisation of existing resources and inadequate harnessing of potential resources, human and other for health;
(d) inadequate coordination and integration between different authorities and organisations providing health services in the same geographical areas;

(e) inadequate or no integration of preventive, curative and family planning services;
(f) the increasing cost of health services and their inequitable distribution, with the result that the basic health needs of all the people were not being met;
(g) the participation of communities in the promotion of their own health and in contributing to health services policy-making, financing and decision-making;
(h) the need to find ways of developing new types of health manpower, including local multi-purpose health workers, and of employing them on a wider scale;
(i) the need to develop an organisation in the countries of the region for improved delivery of health services within the existing constraints—both financial and manpower—for the masses in rural areas, which alone constitutes about 75 per cent of the population; and
(j) meagre allocation of fund (3 to 5 per cent) for health in the overall socio-economic development plans in most countries of the Region.

## C. NATURE AND CLASSIFICATION OF MANAGEMENT TECHNIQUES

### Nature

In order to understand the meaning of 'management techniques' we must be clear about the two concepts, namely, 'management' and 'techniques'. In simple words, management is the handling of tools and techniques to achieve a desired goal. In other words, management involves planning, organismg and controlling of human and other resources to achieve specified goals. A technique is a set of procedural steps which may be loosely or rigorously stated, which embody a multiple idea content and which are concerned with doing work to achieve an objective.

In other words, we can say that management technique is a set of procedural steps which may be loosely stated, embodying a multiple idea content and which are either concerned with decision-making in general or with decision relating to planning, organising or controlling of human and/or other resources with a view to achieving the specified objectives. Management techniques make positive efforts to analyse the situation in a systematic and scientific manner and provide a rational basis for decisions. Adoption of these techniques would encourage greater professionalism in administrative activities. If a new administrative culture is also developed side by side, it would be possible to make optimum use of available and potential resources. According to one of the ILO publications, management techniques are systematic procedures of investigating, planning, controlling and supervising which can be applied to management problems. Thus, modern management techniques in actuality, are the techniques for improving the management process by making it more accurate, by making the process respond faster, or by giving the manager greater control. From the above discussion, we can say that management techniques have the following features:

1. They are a set of procedural or formal steps. This is basic for any management technique. Procedural or formal steps lead to 'systematic' approach which has been the highlight of any scientific method, the root of all sound modern management theory. They take us from the known facts to the unknown parts of the problem.
2. They have a multiple-idea content. They do not have a single idea, but a number of them though related ones.
3. They help in decision-making in general or with decision relating either to planning, organising or controlling or to any combination of these three processes of planning, organising and controlling of human and/or other resources with a view to achieving certain specified objectives.
4. They give the idea of efficiency which, according to Clay, can further be broken into five components:
   (a) economy of efforts in terms of money and other resources;
   (b) speed;
   (c) quality;
   (d) stability; and
   (e) aesthetic or rhythmical approach.
5. They are consistent in their results.[13]

## FUNCTIONAL CLASSIFICATION OF MANAGEMENT TECHNIQUES

Management techniques can be classified in different ways. For example, they can be grouped according to the outlet and the department in which they are applied as, for example, preventive techniques, promotive techniques and curative techniques. This does not, however, cover all techniques. For example, where would we place the techniques of brain-storming or critical examination? An alternative can be classification according to parent discipline. But it is more an historical approach than a current use, because many of the techniques are developed in one field but later on used in a number of fields. Clay gives a classification which is based on the objective of the technique, i.e. what does the technique hope to achieve?[14]

### I. Detection

(To find out or discover something e.g., what is happening or what is wrong?): We can include such technique here as input-output Analysis. Attitude Survey, Production Study, Activity Sampling, Critical Examination, Break-even Analysis.

**2. Evaluation**

(To measure or estimate the value of an item): We can include such techniques here as Job Evaluation, Work Measurement, Work Estimation, Performance Appraisal, Cost-Benefit Analysis.

**3. Improvement**

(To improve performance): We can include such techniques here as Management by Objectives, Method Study, Value Analysis, etc.

**4. Optimization**

(To optimise performance): We can include such techniques here as Linear Programming, Ergonomics, Operations Research, etc.

**5. Specification**

(To specify a desired value or situation or action): Here we can include such technique as Layout Planning for Offices and Plants layout, designing, etc.

**6. Control**

Here we can include such techniques as Cost Control, Credit Control, Labour Control, Inventory Control, Production Control, Budget Control, etc.

**7. Communication**

(To communicate information): Here we can include such techniques as Visual Aids, Suggestion Schemes, Report Writing, Communication Theory, Information Theory, Management Information, etc.

**8. Demonstration**

(To demonstrate something): Here we can include such technique as Programmed Learning, Job Instruction, Management Development and Training, etc.

This achievement criteria tells us that these techniques can help us in discovering or finding something in evaluating the performance, in improving the performance, in optimizing the performance, in specifying a desired value or a situation, in controlling a variable, in communication or in demonstration.

The management techniques can also be classified in terms of various resources employed in an organisation, viz., human material, machinery and equipment, money and time. As such, some of the techniques which can be applied to bring about increased managerial capability, efficiency, effectiveness and productivity can be categorized as shown on next page..

## D. APPLICATIONS

Before we proceed to discuss the systematic applicability of management techniques according to the level of activities of management,

| Sl. No. | Source | Management Techniques |
|---|---|---|
| 1. | Human Resources | 1. Organisational analysis<br>2. Job evaluation<br>3. Training<br>4. Incentive schemes<br>5. Suggestion Schemes<br>6. Method Study<br>7. Work Measurement |
| 2. | Material | 1. Inventory Control<br>2. Value Analysis<br>3. Material Handling<br>4. Standardisation |
| 3. | Machinery and Equipment | 1. Method Study<br>2. Value Analysis |
| 4. | Space and Building | 1. Layout planning<br>2. Method Study |
| 5. | Money | 1. Cost Benefit Analysis<br>2. Budgetary control<br>3. Performance Budgeting<br>4. Management Accounting |
| 6. | Time | 1. Method study<br>2. Work Measurement<br>3. Network Analysis |

let us discuss in brief the meaning and utility of some of the important techniques.

**O&M**

It is generally used to describe the activities of groups of people in Government or other public bodies or in private institutions who are asked to advise health administrators or managers on the question of Organisation and Method so as to increase the efficiency of work for which they are responsible, either by providing a better service, or a cheaper one or both.

**Personnel Administration: Participative Management and Organisational Development (OD)**

The health of an organisation is measured in terms of its capability to adjust with internal and external environmental challenges. We find now-a-days that in big health organisations like hospitals, there is a lot of friction amongst the experts and other staff generating an atmosphere of frustration and low morale, resulting in the overall inefficiency. We can introduce the technique of OD in such large hospitals to maintain the healthy atmosphere of work. A comprehensive definition of OD has been given by Backhard. According to him:

> "Organisational Development is an effort: (1) Planned; (2) Organisation-wide; (3) Managed from the top to; (4) Increase organisation effectiveness and health through; (5) Planned Interventions in the organisations, Process using behavioural science knowledge."[15]

OD depends upon the purely internal initiative of the employees of an organisation. The present emphasis in health administration is only on structural changes but structural changes without personnel dedication and capabilities would be of no avail. It is high time that we introduce OD in all our big health institutions to ward-off the bureaucratic attitudes which result in low output and stagnation. We have also the other technique to achieve this objective, e.g. Management by Objectives, 'Participative Management'. We must try to integrate all these techniques for optimizing the efficiency of personnel in an organisation.

The most important task of Personnel Department must be to give abundant evidence of its belief that personnel in an organisation are key to development. This requires proper motivation of the employees. Motivation is of utmost importance as it constitutes the base for the management functions of planning and organising. It has been noticed that the performance of the personnel either as individuals or members of a group is less as compared to their capabilities in terms of skills, abilities and capacities. Finer, for example, states that demonstrated performance generally never exceeds more than fifty per cent of the individual's ability to perform.[16] Most individuals tend to balance their efforts around an assessment of relative costs (time and energy) and benefits:[17] A climate of creativity must be developed and maintained by management. Maier and Hayes say that the optimal climate for creativity, in whatever human conditions is optimal for individual freedom and self-expression in social setting.[18]

It is the duty of the officers of such units to make the employees feel that their work and their association with a given organisation represent a vehicle which will accelerate the achievement of personal goals as well as the achievement of goals of the organisation. This would require the active participation of the employees in the decision-making process of the organisation.[19]

> "Participation is . . . an individual's mental and emotional involvement in a group situation that encourages him to contribute to group goals and to share responsibility for them."[20]

## E. MANAGEMENT INFORMATION SYSTEM

The significance of information for administration can be compared to what Napoleon said about the army: "an army marches on its stomach," and administration marches on information. As the universe is saturated with information health administration must select pertinent information for their programmes otherwise it is difficult to make any rational policy or decision. This technique is tailored to provide such information to the decision-makers which is most relevant, accurate, Complete, concise, timely, economic, reliable and efficient. A good information system provides data for monitoring and evaluating the programmes and gives the requisite feedback to the administrators and planners at all levels.[21]

The development of a suitable technique for a health information system would improve the capacity of health administrators to make appropriate policy-decisions. The information system may not serve the purpose if the health administrators are not committed to use the information constructively. The health administrators should use the available information sensibly and logically rather than construct complex information system which may not be used. We can show with the help of the diagram the functions of information for policy formulation

CHART 19.2

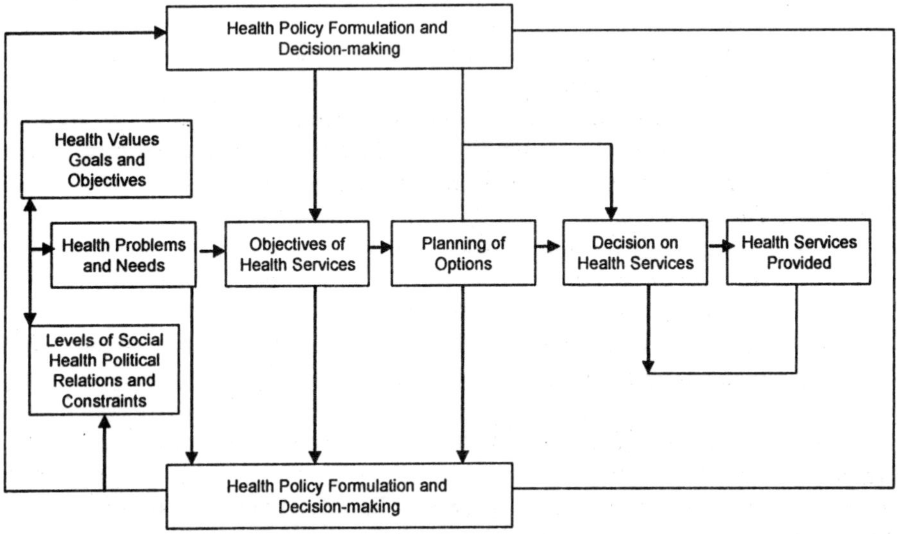


## F. ABC ANALYSIS

It is a technique which would enable a busy executive to chase those activities ardently which would quicken the wheels of administrative machinery. By arranging his work into an order of priorities, he can decide on which items to concentrate first. Which other to deal later, and yet which other to delegate to his assistants.

When done more systematically and in quantitative terms, this system of building up priorities of work is called the ABC analysis. ABC Analysis can be of great use in dealing with materials management in hospitals. Forty to sixty per cent of the total expenditure of an organisation is generally spent on materials. The other from of ABC Analysis is VED, i.e. arranging the activities in the orders of Vital, essential and Desirable which are essential to classify medicines.

## G. NET WORK ANALYSIS (PERT/CPM)

Both the Critical Path Method (CPM) and Programme Evaluation and Review Technique (PERT) emphasize efficient performance and temporal dimensions of a project. In the simplest form of PERT, a project is viewed as a total system and consists of setting up of schedule of dates for various stages and exercise of management control, mainly through project status reports, on its progress. The CPM is basically a technique to reduce the time required to implement a project. By breaking the project into activities that must be undertaken for its Implementation and by determining their time sequence, it is possible to isolate the most critical activities in the project and to compute the critical path schedule for their implementation. Network planning provides the basis for both CPM and PERT.

Moder and Philips enlist the following key advantages of using PERT:[22]

1. It encourages logical discipline in planning, scheduling and control of projects.
2. It encourages more long-range and detailed project planning.
3. It provides a standard method of documenting and communicating Project Plans, Schedules and Time and Cost Performance.
4. It identifies the most critical elements in the Plan, thus focusing management attention on the 10-20 per cent of the project that is most constraining on the schedule.
5. It illustrates the effects of technical and procedural changes on overall schedules.[23]

The application of PERT/CPM can be profitably utilised in the Programme and Projects of Health, e.g., Construction of Hospitals. Eradication of Communicable Diseases, Family Planning Programmes, Administration of Environmental Programmes, etc. Care should be taken that the cost of the PERT/CPM should not take away large resources of the Project.

## H. COST-BENEFIT ANALYSIS

This technique is designed to consider the social costs and benefits attributable to the project. The benefits are expressed in monetary terms to determine whether a given programme is economically sound, and to select the best out of several progrrammes. Its advantage lies not in making decision-making simpler, but in its possibilities for systematic examination of each part of a problem in hand, for putting diverse decision on a part and following logical sequence.[24]

Cost-Benefit Analysis is an aid to systematic thought and helps the planners to decide as to what should be done on the relative merits of different programmes. How far, for example, should resources be devoted to health education or maternal and child health services or immunization against particular disease? Any given budget for health may be distributed between programmes by including, first, those with the highest ratio of benefits to cost, then those with the next larger and so on, until the budget is fully allocated. The limitation of this method in the field of health administration is that it is difficult to express the benefits in monetary terms. We must encounter this limitation by making our tools of research methodology perfect.

## I. COST-EFFECTIVE ANALYSIS

Cost effectiveness methods are those that search for the least costly way of achieving a defined result. Cost effectiveness analysis are easier to make as the aim is clear. It helps the health administrator in managing health resources at the local level. The problem is to find the way of achieving the objective at lowest cost, e.g., to find effective ways of treating patients without sending them to hospital. Linear programming can help in this direction.

## J. SYSTEMS APPROACH

A systems is an integrated assembly of interacting elements, designed to carry out cooperatively a pre-determined function.[25] There are five major elements in a system approach—selecting objectives, designing alternatives, building models, weighing cost against effectiveness and the application of suitable criterion. It can be represented with the help of a Chart 19.3.

The application of systems analysis is useful in health management in that it provides for:[26]

1. consideration of all variables, over and above the biological and technical, that affect health intervention programmes
2. a planning approach that relates input to output;
3. an emphasis on quantification;
4. rigour in analytical methods;
5. orientation towards health problems rather than towards categories of service;
6. communication with key governmental decision-making centres that utilised comparable methods;

CHART 19.3

**Elements of Systems Analysis**

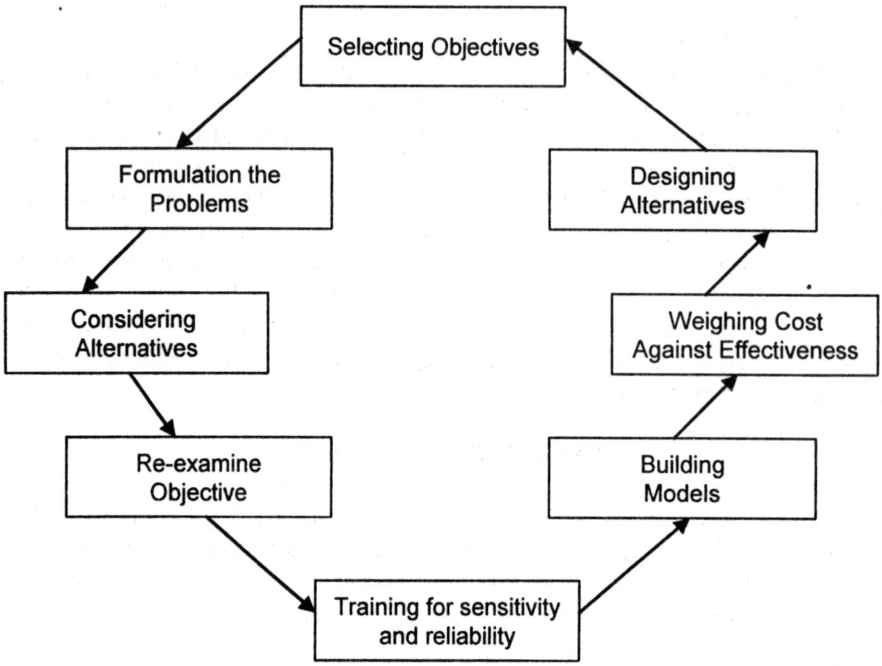


7. early attention to planning and priority setting;
8. improved interdisciplinary collaboration; and
9. the use of wide range of analytical models and methods of considerable power.

Application of Management Techniques for Administrative Improvement and Administrative Reforms (Chart 19.2)

Having discussed the importance and utility of some of the important Management Techniques, we shall explain the application of the management techniques at different levels of management and to situations covering time horizons with the help of a chart.

The chart reveals that one technique or the other is applied in one form or the other at all the three levels of management. Because the lowest level has to perform operational functions. Management techniques like World Study, Network Analysis, Capacity Utilisation Studies are adopted. At the middle level, where the policy is executed, some more important techniques like Manpower Planning. Cost Benefit Analysis Statistics and Forecasting, etc. are applied to effect improvements. The top management uses more strategic techniques like Technological Forecasting, Performance Budgeting, Operational Research Studies, etc.

## K. UTILITY AND LIMITATIONS

### Utility

Let us explain the use of these techniques in improving the health services with some examples:

1. In a case study. a 750-bedded hospital (Medical Institute) was facing acute shortage of nursing personnel. The study of the utilisation of nursing personnel in this hospital revealed that 33 per cent time of the nurses was being spent on non-nursing duties. Besides, there was 25 per cent turnover of the nurses. There was a great delay in appointing the new incumbents. The study suggested that if the nurses are not given non-nursing duties a saving of rupees three lakhs can take place. This was studied with the help of the techniques of organisational analysis.
2. A study was conducted by the author of a University Health Centre where there was a problem of pilferage of drugs. The Chief Medical Officer of the Centre was finding it very difficult to plug this loop-hole as he himself was busy in examining the patients for all the duty time. It was suggested that the whole stock of the medicine may be classified on the basis on the cost with the help of the technique of ABC analysis. It was suggested to the Chief Medical Officer to keep 'A' category of drugs under lock and key to be issued only under his signature. He could check for other drugs once a month concentrating only on A and B categories. This helped the Centre to save about Rs. 25,000 annually.
3. A study was carried out by C.R. Prasad on the Application of Quantitative methods in Hospital Management. He studied the problems of patients who were wasting a lot of their time to get the prescriptions (to pay the cash and to receive the medicine). The patients had to stand in line for about 45 minutes. Prasad applied Sampling techniques and used Simulation Procedures. He was able to suggest a model by which the average time of waiting could be reduced to 10 minutes from 45 minutes.[27]

The examples of the use of other techniques would be taken up in the relevant chapters.

Thus, we find that there is an ever-increasing array of methods and techniques available to assist the management for the acceleration of socio-economic development, with stated policies, objectives and priorities. Further, the impact of interdependence of the management techniques solely depend upon the development of improved management. But it is generally acknowledged that the availability and application of modern management skills do not meet the needs that are felt to exist.

Shortage and difficulties for the grater development and application of management skills are always encountered. Some of them are as under:

1. Shortage of experts in management techniques, and especially of those with knowledge and experience of the special problems of the health sector;
2. Difficulty in recruiting staff to specialise in health management and managerial technologies because of working conditions or lack of career prospects for personnel other than physicians;
3. Shortage of general management capability, together with lack of appreciation of 'systems thinking' and orientation to modern management on the part of doctors and health administrators;
4. Insufficient ability to identify situations in which the available consultants and other sources of expertise could best be used;
5. Lack of a form of organisation that can fully utilize the available management skills;
6. Shortage of staff of various kinds (not just those with specific management skills);
7. Shortage of teachers in management for medical schools, etc. and
8. Insufficient development of management methods for dealing with such difficulties, characteristic of health services as: defining objectives, public participation, coordination, motivation and supervision:

From the above, it is inferred that there is a room for improvement to make simultaneous progress on several fronts by:

(a) spreading the determination to overcome the difficulties mentioned and establishing confidence in using techniques;
(b) general management training and experience for health professionals;
(c) production of management specialists of various kinds, especially those with a broad experience in addition to their specialist skill;
(d) organisational changes necessary to utilise management skills and provide appropriate career and working conditions for their practitioners; and
(e) research and development to adapt management techniques to the health needs.[28]

No doubt, the theory of management techniques in the context of administrative improvement and administrative reforms can be learned in a classroom, from a text-book or through correspondence, but, these cannot replace the practical experience, only through which one acquires the skill of the technique.

## L. CRITICAL APPRAISAL OF MANAGEMENT TECHNIQUES

Although the needs for modern management technology differ from country to country and from situation to situation, it is not to be expected that these differences will always be accurately interpreted, or that the most appropriate techniques will automatically be invoked. In fact, techniques like most other things, are susceptible to the influences of fashion. Their value depends on the circumstances in which they are applied. In other words, the use of management techniques, just as the exploitation of any other resources, have to be subject to continuous feedback and review. There have been many instances when in a hurry to borrow from West. We blindly adopt the management techniques/technology in the 'as-it-is' form without even taking into consideration their limitations. John Argenti in one of his papers observes that "after all, many of the sophisticated techniques have not been employed by a great number of organisations in U.K. we should not blindly employ the technique. We should be sure of its potentialities and also skilled in its use.[29] This means that suitable technology has to be devised to provide for decent health care to the people much more economically than the affluent and advanced countries. Thus, there is a need to evolve appropriate management techniques and technology to suit our environment.

Modernizing Health Administration requires outstanding leadership. Eminent Industrialist, Mr. Rahul Bajaj, Chairman and Managing Director, Bajaj Auto Limited and President, CII, delivered the Convocation Address at the 49th Annual Convocation of the SNDT Women's University, Mumbai. He said, "To realize our goals and aspirations, we need outstanding leadership in every field and at every level. Leadership means that there is no substitute for excellence. No tolerance of mediocrity and no compromise with integrity. Leadership is not just charisma, not public relations, not showmanship. Leadership is performance, consistent behaviour and trust-worthiness."

We are in a hurry; we wish to achieve much; we cannot afford the luxury of wasting our resources for experimentation. What is, therefore, needed is a proper identification of opportunities, setting out of priority areas and accordingly, continually devising technology and techniques appropriate to our set-up, our value system and technologies that are compatible. The call is, therefore, to stress on the 'know-why' rather than just on the 'know-how' of techniques and technology. This can materialize only when we bear in mind the following motto:

THE RIGHT TECHNIQUE/TECHNOLOGY
AT THE RIGHT PLACE
AT THE RIGHT TIME
AT THE RIGHT COST
BY THE RIGHT METHODS/MEANS
BY THE RIGHT PERSONNEL

## NOTES AND REFERENCES

1. Milton Greenabltt, Myron Sharaf R. and Evelyn Stone M., Dynamics of Institutional Change, Pittsburgh, University of Pittsburgh Press, 1971, pp. 239-40
2. All India Radio Broadcast, June 26, 1966, Selected Speeches of Mrs. Indira Gandhi, January 1966, to 1969, Publication Division, March 1971.
3. WHO, Public Health Paper, 55, p. 68.
4. UN: "Inter-regional Seminar on Administration of Management Improvement Services" Vol. I, Copenhagen, Denmark, Oct. 1970, p. 24.
5. UN: United Nations Programmes in Public Administration (E/4296-ST/TAO/ M/38), pp. 11-12.
6. UN: Official Record of the Economic and Social Council (E 1708) Agenda Item No. 10, p. 3.
7. UN: Inter-regional of the Seminar on Administration of Management Improvement Services.
8. Earnest Dale and L.C. Michelon, "Modern Management Techniques", Penguin Books, 1974, p. 9.
9. Legiasis V. Gbriel.
10. Saul, M. Katz, "A Methodological note on appraising administrative capability for development".
11. *Ibid.*, pp. 99-100.
12. World Health Organisation, Regional Office of South-East Asia, New Delhi, (SEA/RC/26, pp. 31-32.
13. ILO: "Introduction to Work Study", Geneva, 1969, p. 26.
14. M.J. Clay, General Theory of Management Technques, Part I, in Work Study and Mangaement Services, London.
15. R. Bechhard: Organisation Development: Strategies and Models, Addison-Wesley, 1969, p. 9.
16. H. Finer, Theory and Practice of Modern Government, p. 106.
17. Eli Ginzberg: "Perspectives on Work Motivation", *Personnel*, Vol. 31, No. (July), 1959, pp. 48-49.
18. Norman Mair, R.F. and Hayes John, J. Creative Management, p. 36.
19. Davis Keith: "The Case for Participative Management", *Business Horizon*, Vol. 6, No. 3 (1963), p. 141.
20. Walters, Albert, F., "Management and Motivation Releasing Human Potential", Personnel, Vol. 39, No. 2, pp. 8-16.
21. For details refer: Information Systems for Modern Management by Murdicks Robert G. and Ross, Joel E., Prentice Hall of India (P) Ltd., Delhi, 1977.
22. For details see PERT & CPM, Principles and Applications by Srinath, L.S. Affiliated East West Press, Delhi, 1975.
23. J. Joseph, Moder and Cecil, Phillips, R., "Project Management with CPM and PERT", New York, Reinhold, 1964, pp. 5-6.
24. For details use Cost-benefit Analysis in Administration by Trevor Newton, George Allen & Unwin, Lond, 1972, and Weisbrod, B.A., "Concept of Costs and Benefits", in Chanse, S.B. (e.d), Problems in Public Expenditure Analysis Washington, D.C., Brookings, 1968, pp. 257-58.
25. Gilson, E. Ralph, "The Recognition of Systems Engineering, in Flagle, p. 58.
26. WHO Technical Report Series 596, "Application of System Analysis and Health Management", 1976, pp. 7-8.
27. Prasad, C.R., Applications of Quantitative Methods in Hospital Management in Management in Governmnet, Vol. IV, No. 3, Oct.-Dec. 1972, pp. 238-48.
28. WHO: Public Health Paper, 55, pp. 70-71.
29. John Argenti, "Whatever Happened to Management Techniques", in *Management Today*, April 1976.

## BOOKS BY THE SAME AUTHOR

1. International Administration: WHO South East-Asia Regional Office (New Delhi, 1977), Sterling Publishers
2. Principles, Problems and Prospects of Co-operative Administration (New Delhi, 1979), Sterling Publishers (Co-Author Dr. B.B. Goel)
3. Administration of Personnel in Co-operative (New Delhi, 1979), Sterling Publishers (Co-Author Dr. B.B. Goel)
4. Health Care Administration: Ecology, Principles and Modern Trends (New Delhi, 1980), Sterling Publishers
5. Health Care Administration: Policy-making and Planning (New Delhi, 1980), Sterling Publishers
6. Health Care Administration: Levels and Aspects (New Delhi, 1980), Sterling Publishers
7. International Civil Service: Principles, Problems and Prospects (New Delhi, 1984), Sterling Publishers
8. Public Health Administration (New Delhi, 1984), Sterling Publishers
9. Public Personnel Administration (New Delhi, 1984), Reprint 1987, Sterling Publishers
10. International Civil Services—Principles, Problems and Prospectives (New Delhi, 1984), Sterling Publishers.
11. Social Welfare Administration: Theory and Practice (Vols. I and II) (New Delhi, 1988), Deep & Deep Publications Pvt. Ltd.
12. Hospital Administration and Management (ed.) Co-Author Dr. R. Kumar in 3 volumes (New Delhi, 1989), Deep & Deep Publications Pvt. Ltd.
13. Policy and Administration: Family Planning & Beyond (New Delhi, 1990), Deep & Deep Publications Pvt. Ltd.
14. Modern Management Techniques (Revised and Reprinted) (New Delhi, 1990), Deep & Deep Publications Pvt. Ltd.
15. Development Planning and Administration (ed.) S. Bhatnagar (Co-editor) (New Delhi, 1992), Deep & Deep Publications Pvt. Ltd.
16. Financial Administration and Management (New Delhi, 1993), Sterling Publishers
17. Advanced Public Administration (New Delhi, 1993), Sterling Publishers

18. Personnel Administration and Management
(New Delhi, 1994), Deep & Deep Publications Pvt. Ltd.
19. Educational Policy and Administration
(New Delhi, 1994), Deep & Deep Publications Pvt. Ltd.
20. Slum Improvement Through Participatory Urban Based Community Structures
(New Delhi, 1999), Deep & Deep Publications Pvt. Ltd.
21. Distance Education in 21st Century
(New Delhi, 2000), Deep & Deep Publications Pvt. Ltd.
22. Health Care System and Management: Organization and Structure
(New Delhi, 2000), Deep & Deep Publications Pvt. Ltd.
23. Health Care System and Management: Policies and Programmes
(New Delhi, 2000), Deep & Deep Publications Pvt. Ltd.
24. Health Care System and Management: Management and Administration
(New Delhi, 2000), Deep & Deep Publications Pvt. Ltd.
25. Heath Care System and Management: Primary Health Care Management
(New Delhi, 2000), Deep & Deep Publications Pvt. Ltd.
26. Management Techniques: Principles and Practices
(New Delhi, 2001), Deep & Deep Publications Pvt. Ltd.
27. Encyclopaedia of Disaster Management in 3 Volumes
(New Delhi, 2001), Deep & Deep Publications Pvt. Ltd.
28. Management of Hospitals: Hospital Core Services
(New Delhi, 2002), Deep & Deep Publications Pvt. Ltd.
29. Management of Hospitals: Hospital Supportive Services
(New Delhi, 2002), Deep & Deep Publications Pvt. Ltd.
30. Management of Hospitals: Hospital Preventive and Promotive Services
(New Delhi, 2002), Deep & Deep Publications Pvt. Ltd.
31. Management of Hospitals: Hospital Managerial Services
(New Delhi, 2002), Deep & Deep Publications Pvt. Ltd.
32. Public Personal Administration
(New Delhi, 2002), Deep & Deep Publications Pvt. Ltd.
33. Public Financial Administration
(New Delhi, 2002), Deep & Deep Publications Pvt. Ltd.
34. Urban Development and Management
(New Delhi, 2002), Deep & Deep Publications Pvt. Ltd.
35. Public Administration: Theory and Practices
(New Delhi, 2003), Deep & Deep Publications Pvt. Ltd.
36. Advanced Public Administration (Revised and Enlarged Edition)

(New Delhi, 2003), Deep & Deep Publications Pvt. Ltd.

37. Panchayati Raj in India
(New Delhi, 2003), Deep & Deep Publications Pvt. Ltd.
38. Encyclopedia of Higher Education in 21st Century: Organisation and Structure
(New Delhi, 2004), Deep & Deep Publications Pvt. Ltd.
39. Encyclopaedia of Higher Education in 21st Century: Quality and Excellence
(New Delhi, 2004), Deep & Deep Publications Pvt. Ltd.
40. Encyclopedia of Higher Education in 21st Century, Extension Education Services
(New Delhi, 2004), Deep & Deep Publications Pvt. Ltd.
41. Stress Management and Education: An Indian Perspective
(New Delhi, 2004), Deep & Deep Publications Pvt. Ltd.
42. Human Values and Education:
(New Delhi, 2004), Deep & Deep Publications Pvt. Ltd.
43. Public Health Policy and Administration
(New Delhi, 2004), Deep & Deep Publications Pvt. Ltd.
44. Administration and Management of NGO's: Text and Case Studies
(New Delhi, 2004), Deep & Deep Publications Pvt. Ltd.
45. Nursing Services: Management and Administration
(New Delhi, 2005), Deep & Deep Publications Pvt. Ltd.
46. Population Policy and Family Welfare Administration
(New Delhi, 2005), Deep & Deep Publications Pvt. Ltd.
47. Human Resource Development in 21st Century
(New Delhi, 2005), Deep & Deep Publications Pvt. Ltd.
48. Encyclopaedia of Disaster Management (3 Volumes)
(New Delhi, 2006) Deep & Deep Publications Pvt. Ltd.
49. School Health Education
(New Delhi, 2007), Deep & Deep Publications Pvt. Ltd.
50. Health Education: Theory and Practices
(New Delhi, 2007), Deep & Deep Publications Pvt. Ltd.
51. Good Governance: An Integral Views
(New Delhi, 2007), Deep & Deep Publications Pvt. Ltd.
52. Right to Information and Good Governance
(New Delhi, 2007), Deep & Deep Publications Pvt. Ltd.
53. Disaster Management: Text and Case Studies
(New Delhi, 2007), Deep & Deep Publications Pvt. Ltd.
54. Hospital Administration: Theory and Practices
(New Delhi, 2007), Deep & Deep Publications Pvt. Ltd.
55. Environmental Health Values and Education,
(New Delhi, 2008), Deep & Deep Publications Pvt. Ltd.

56. Administrative and Management Thinkers: Revelvance in New Millennium
(New Delhi, 2008), Deep & Deep Publications Pvt. Ltd.
57. Principles and Practices of Human Values
(New Delhi, 2008), Deep & Deep Publications Pvt. Ltd.
58. Distance Education: Principles, Potentialities and Perspectives
(New Delhi, 2008), Deep & Deep Publications Pvt. Ltd.
59. Educational Administration and Management: An Integral View
(New Delhi, 2008), Deep & Deep Publications Pvt. Ltd.
60. Women Health Education
(New Delhi, 2008), Deep & Deep Publications Pvt. Ltd.
61. Health Care System and Hospital Administration
Vol. 1 (Organizational Structure)
(New Delhi, 2008), Deep & Deep Publications Pvt. Ltd.
62. Health Care System and Hospital Administration
Vol. 2 (Resources: Human, Finance and Material)
(New Delhi, 2008), Deep & Deep Publications Pvt. Ltd.
63. Health Care System and Hospital Administration
Vol. 3 ( Policy-making and Programmes)
(New Delhi, 2008), Deep & Deep Publications Pvt. Ltd.
64. Health Care System and Hospital Administration
Vol. 4 (Emerging and Thrust Areas)
(New Delhi, 2008), Deep & Deep Publications Pvt. Ltd.
65. Health Care System and Hospital Administration
Vol. 5 (Primary/Rural Health Care)
(New Delhi, 2008), Deep & Deep Publications Pvt. Ltd.
66. Health Care System and Hospital Administration
Vol. 6 (Secondary and Tertiary Health Care)
(New Delhi, 2008), Deep & Deep Publications Pvt. Ltd.
67. Health Care System and Hospital Administration
Vol. 7 (Management Techniques and Good Governance)
(New Delhi, 2008), Deep & Deep Publications Pvt. Ltd.
68. Education of Lifestyle and Lifetime Diseases
(Deep & Deep Publications Pvt. Ltd.)
69. Health Education Administration—From International Level to Village Level
(Deep & Deep Publications Pvt. Ltd.)
70. Education for Healthy Urban Cities
(Deep & Deep Publications Pvt. Ltd.)
71. Rural Health Education
(Deep & Deep Publications Pvt. Ltd.)

# Bibliography


Acton Society Trust, Hospitals and the State: Hospital Organisation and Administration under the National Health Service Series, London: Action Society Trust, 1956, 54p.

Acton Society Trust, Hospitals and the State: Hospital Organisation and Administration under the National Health Service, London: The Trust, 1959, iii, 80p.

Andhra Pradesh, Health and Local Administration Department Panchayats Executive Officers Regulations relating to Recruitment, etc., Hyderabad: The Author, 1956, l6p.

Bannington, B.G., English Public Health Administration, 2nd ed., London: P.S. King, 1929, 325p.

Berkov, Robert, The World Health Organisation: A Study in Decentralized International Administration, Geneva Droz, 1957, 173p.

Better Health by Community Projects Administration, Planning Commission, New Delhi: Community Projects, Planning Commission, n.d., 32p.

Blum, Henrik L., Public Administration: A Public Health Viewpoint, N.Y.: Macmillan, 1963, 532p.

Hugh Flanagan and Peter Spurgeon, Public Sector Managerial Effectiveness: Theory and Practice in the National Health Service, Buckingham: Open Univ. Press, 1996, 128p.

Freeman, Ruth B., Administration of Public Health Services and Edward M. Holmes, Philadelphia: Saunders, 1960, 507p.

Goddard, H.A., Principles of Administration Applied to Nursing Service by H.A. Goddard, Geneva: World Health Organisation, 1958, 106p.

Goel, Rajneesh, Community Health Care, New Delhi: Deep & Deep Publications Pvt. Ltd., 2004, 403p.

Goel, S.L., Health and Care Administration: Policy-making and Planning, Delhi: Sterling, 1980, 288p.

Goel, S.L, Health Care Administration: Ecology, Principles and Modern Trends, Delhi: Sterling, 1980, 233p.

Goel, S.L., Health Care Administration: Levels and Aspects, Delhi: Sterling, 1980, 245p.

Goel, S.L., Health Care System and Management, New Delhi: Deep & Deep Publications Pvt. Ltd., 2004, 4 Vols.

Goel, S.L., International Administration: WHO South-East Asia Regional Office, Delhi: Sterling, 1977, 344p.

Goel, S.L., Population Policy and Family Welfare: Reproductive and Child Health Administration, New Delhi: Deep & Deep Publications Pvt. Ltd., 2005, 526p.

Goel, S.L., Public Health Administration, Delhi: Sterling, 1984, 472p.

Goel, S.L, Public Health Policy and Administration, New Delhi: Deep & Deep Publications Pvt. Ltd., 2005, 651p.

Graduate Study in Public Administration: A Guide to Graduate Programs by Office of Education, Department of Health, Education and Welfare, Washington: United States Government Printing Office, 1961, 158+p.

Greenfield, Margert, State-Local Service for Mental Health, Bureau of Public Administration, Berkeley: The Bureau, 1955, 93p.

Guangde, Sun, Health Care Administration in China, Westport: Greenport, 1993, pp. 53-62.

Handbook on Human Services Administration, edited by Jack Rabin and Marcia B. Steinhauer, New York: Marcel Dekker, 1988, 604p.

Health Policy Research in South Asia: Building Capacity for Reform, edited by Abdo S. Yazbeck and David H. Peters, Washington, D.C.: World Bank, 2003, 428p.

Heaver, Richard, Managing Primary Health Care: Implications of the Health Transition, Washington, D.C.: World Bank, 1995, 41p.

Health Status of the Underprivileged, New Delhi: Centre for Urban Studies, Indian Institute of Public Administration, 1991, 225p.

Indian Institute of Public Administration, Centre for Urban Studies, Urban Health System, edited by P.K. Umashankar and Girish K. Misra, New Delhi: Reliance and IIPA, 1993, 259p.

Institute for Training in Municipal Administration, Administration of Community Health Services, Chicago: ICMA, 1961, 560p.

Johnston, Timothy, Investing in Health: Development Effectiveness in the Health, Nutrition, and Population Sector, Washington, D.C.: World Bank, 1999, 69p.

Khandewale, Shreekant V., Health Administration and the Weaker Sections in an Indian Metropolis, Delhi: Devika, 1996, 231p.

Klinoubol, Kriengkrai, Public Health Development and Administration: A Study of Developing Economy, Delhi: Deep & Deep Publications Pvt. Ltd., 1989. 436p.

Local Self-Government Administration in States of India, 1956, New Delhi: Ministry of Health, 1956, 149p.

Local Self-government Administration in States of India, 1962, Ministry of Health, Delhi: The Manager of Publications, 1962, 161+p.

Legislature Committee on Local Administration by Health, Education and Local Administration Department, Madras, Madras: Health, Education and Local Administration Department, 1958, 5 Parts.

Morden, Margaret Gorsuch, Cooperative Health Administration in Metropolitan, Los Angeles: The Bureau, 1949, 52p.

Panchayat Manual, Madras: Health, Education and Local Administration Department, 1956, 368+p.

Papers in Public Administration, No. 6, Ann Arbor: The Bureau, 1950, 85p.

Public Services M.B.A. Induction Module: India-U.K. context (August-September, 1999: Indian Institute of Public Administration, New Delhi), Gender-related Issues (course material), New Delhi: Indian Institute of Public Administration, 1999, vp.

Report of the Regional Training Seminar on Social Security Administration, New Delhi: Regional Office for Asia and Oceania, 1979, 75p.

Rowbottom, R., Hospital Organisation: A Progress Report on the Brunel Health Services Project, London: Heinemann, 1973, 314p.

Survey of Research in Public Administration, 1980-90, edited by V.A. Pai Panandiker, Delhi: Konark, 1997, 631p.

Tebow, Hilda P., Staff-Development as an Integral Part of Administration, Washington, D.C.: Department of Health, Education and Welfare, 1959, 33+p.

The Indo-US Symposium on Community Mental Health at National Institute of Mental Health and Neuro Sciences, Bangalore: National Institute of Mental Health and Neuro Sciences, 1992, 520p.

Weaver, Jerry L., Conflict and Control in Health Care Administration, Beverly Hills: n.p., 1975, 197p.

Welfare Administration and Social Welfare Around the World, by Department of Health, Education and Welfare, United States, Washington: Government Printing Office, 1963, 9p.

Wishwakarma, R.K., Health Status of the Underprivileged, New Delhi: Centre for Urban Studies, Indian Institute of Public Administration, 1993, 283p.

# Index